Rodchok

NEUROLOGIC CLINICS

VOLUME 6 / NUMBER 4
NOVEMBER 1988

EVOKED POTENTIALS

Robin Gilmore, MD, *Guest Editor*

W. B. SAUNDERS COMPANY
Harcourt Brace Jovanovich, Inc.

Philadelphia London Toronto
Montreal Sydney Tokyo

W. B. SAUNDERS COMPANY
Harcourt Brace Jovanovich, Inc.

The Curtis Center
Independence Square West
Philadelphia, PA 19106–3399

Neurologic Clinics is covered in *Excerpta Medica*

NEUROLOGIC CLINICS
November 1988   Volume 6, Number 4   ISSN 0733–8619

The following information is published in accordance with the requirements of the United States Postal Code.

Neurologic Clinics is published quarterly by W. B. Saunders Company, The Curtis Center, Independence Square West, Philadelphia, Pennsylvania 19106–3399. Second class postage paid at Philadelphia, PA 19106, and additional mailing offices. POSTMASTER: Send address changes to W. B. Saunders Company, The Curtis Center, Independence Square West, Philadelphia, PA 19106–3399. The subscription price is $66.00 per year for individuals, $72.00 per year for foreign individuals, and $75.00 for institutions. There is a postage charge of $5.00 for subscriptions billed to U.S. addresses and shipped outside the U.S.

The editor of this publication is Brenda D. Frank, W. B. Saunders Company, The Curtis Center, Independence Square West, Philadelphia, Pennsylvania 19106–3399.

Printed by the Maple-Vail Book Manufacturing Group, York, Pennsylvania.

Contributors

MICHAEL J. AMINOFF, M.D., F.R.C.P., Professor of Neurology, Department of Neurology, University of California School of Medicine, San Francisco, California

JOSEPH C. AREZZO, Ph.D., Associate Professor of Neuroscience and Neurology, Albert Einstein College of Medicine, Bronx, New York

DARWIN R. BOOR, M.D., Assistant Professor of Neurology, Emory University School of Medicine, Atlanta, Georgia

GASTONE G. CELESIA, M.D., Chairman and Professor of Neurology, Loyola University of Chicago, Stritch School of Medicine, Maywood; Hines Veterans Administration Hospital, Hines, Illinois

KEITH H. CHIAPPA, M.D., Associate Professor of Neurology, Harvard Medical School; Director, EEG and Evoked Potentials Laboratory, Massachusetts General Hospital, Boston, Massachusetts

ANDRÉE DURIEUX-SMITH, Ph.D., Associate Professor of Otolaryngology, University of Ottawa; Director of Audiology, Children's Hospital of Eastern Ontario, Canada

ANDREW EISEN, M.D., F.R.C.P.(C.), Professor, Division of Neurology, Department of Medicine, University of British Columbia; Director, Neuromuscular Disease Unit, Department of Diagnostic Neurophysiology, Vancouver General Hospital, Vancouver, British Columbia, Canada

RONALD G. EMERSON, M.D., Assistant Professor of Neurology and Assistant Professor of Pediatrics, Neurological Institute, Columbia Presbyterian Medical Center, New York, New York

CHARLES M. EPSTEIN, M.D., Associate Professor of Neurology, Emory University School of Medicine, Atlanta, Georgia

C. WILLIAM ERWIN, M.D., Assistant Professor of Medicine (Neurology) and Professor of Psychiatry, Duke University Medical Center, Durham, North Carolina

ROBIN GILMORE, M.D., Director, Clinical Neurophysiology Program, and Associate Professor, Department of Neurology, University of Kentucky Medical Center, Lexington, Kentucky

ALAN D. LEGATT, M.D., Ph.D., Assistant Professor of Neurology and Neuroscience and Director of Intraoperative Neurophysiology, Montefiore Medical Center and the Albert Einstein College of Medicine, Bronx, New York

KEVIN NELSON, M.D., Assistant Professor of Neurology, and Director, Electromyography Laboratory, University of Kentucky, Lexington, Kentucky

MARC R. NUWER, M.D., Ph.D., Associate Professor, Neurology, UCLA Department of Neurology, Reed Neurological Center, Los Angeles, California

TERENCE W. PICTON, M.D., Ph.D., F.R.C.P.(C.), Professor of Medicine, University of Ottawa; Attending Physician, Ottawa General Hospital; and Consultant Physician, Children's Hospital of Eastern Ontario, Canada

RODNEY A. RADKE, M.D., Assistant Professor of Medicine (Neurology), Division of Neurology, Duke University Medical Center, Durham, North Carolina

PAOLO M. ROSSINI, M.D., Associate Professor of Clinical Neurophysiology, Department of Public Health, The University of Rome "Tor Vergata," Rome, Italy

HERBERT G. VAUGHAN, JR., M.D., Professor of Neuroscience, Neurology, and Pediatrics, and Director, Rose F. Kennedy Center for Research in Mental Retardation and Human Development, Albert Einstein College of Medicine, Bronx, New York

THORU YAMADA, M.D., Professor of Neurology, Division of Clinical Electrophysiology, Department of Neurology, College of Medicine, University of Iowa Hospitals, Iowa City, Iowa

Contents

Preface xi

> Robin Gilmore

Principles of Signal Analysis and Averaging................................ 649

> Charles M. Epstein and Darwin R. Boor

> Averaging is the primary method for detecting small evoked
> potentials in the midst of surrounding electrical noise. Not
> all types of noise can be removed by averaging, however.
> The condition of the patient, electrodes, amplifiers, and
> filters are equally important for successful recording.

Anatomy and Physiology of Visual Evoked Potentials and
Electroretinograms... 657

> Gastone G. Celesia

> ERGs are electrical potentials originating in the retina and
> recorded directly from the corneal surface of the eyes.
> Flash ERGs are elicited by high intensity flashes either on
> scotopic or photopic conditions. The origin of the A and B
> waves of ERG are a combination of photoreceptor poten-
> tials, K+ mediated current flow and DC potentials within
> Müller cells, whereas the C waves are altered K+ fluxes
> induced by light in the pigment epithelia. Oscillatory
> potentials are probably related to feedback circuits of the
> inner layer of the retina. Electroretinograms evoked by
> pattern are mostly originated in ganglion cells. The use of
> various visual stimuli allow the selective activation of
> different retinal structures. Flashes selectively activate
> retina luminance and color detectors, whereas small pattern
> stimuli preferentially activate contrast and edge detectors.
>   Visual evoked potentials recorded from the scalp prob-
> ably originate from multiple cortical visual areas. P-100
> response of the visual evoked potential to pattern stimula-

tion is a cortically originated wave either produced exclusively by area 17 or 18 or by a multiplicity of cortical neuronal pools. Visual evoked potentials have important application for the diagnosis of optic nerve disease, assessment in conjunction with pattern ERG of the prognosis of recovery of visual function, and the evaluation of visual physiology and physiopathology.

Anatomic and Physiologic Bases of Brain Stem Auditory Evoked Potentials 681

Alan D. Legatt, Joseph C. Arezzo, and Herbert G. Vaughan, Jr.

The human short-latency or "brain stem" auditory evoked potentials consist of a series of phasic waves derived from action potentials within a short-latency, low-jitter subset of the subcortical auditory pathways; a superimposed slower component is derived from synaptic potentials. Most waves are composites of contributions from multiple generators. Their probable anatomic sources are identified based on data from near-field intracranial recordings, lesion studies, and far-field mapping studies.

Anatomic and Physiologic Bases of Median Nerve Somatosensory Evoked Potentials 705

Thoru Yamada

Diagnostic utilization of somatosensory evoked potentials has made much progress in recent years. Introduction of far-field or stationary field potentials has opened a new dimension but also added further complexity in understanding the physioanatomic mechanisms of nerve impulse propagation. Exploring further the anatomic, physiologic, and psychological substrates of somatosensory evoked potentials would enhance diagnostic utilities of the test.

Anatomic and Physiologic Bases of Posterior Tibial Nerve Somatosensory Evoked Potentials 735

Ronald G. Emerson

Somatosensory evoked potentials following posterior tibial nerve stimulation reflect the activation of both white and gray matter structures in the large-fiber afferent sensory system. This article briefly reviews the mechanisms of generation of body surface recordable evoked potentials and then discusses specific generators of spinal, subcortical, and cortical short-latency responses to posterior tibial nerve stimulation.

Anatomic and Physiologic Bases of Motor Evoked Potentials 751

Paolo M. Rossini

The anatomophysiologic mechanisms underlying noninvasive stimulation of brain, spinal cord, and roots via electric and magnetic impulses are surveyed. Different types of technical approaches as well as the methods for measurements of the conduction times of central motor tracts are fully described. Safety aspects are also reviewed. This new neurophysiologic technique, since its recent introduction, has explosively expanded both in its research and clinical applications.

Brain Stem Auditory Evoked Potentials in the Evaluation of the Central Nervous System 771

Charles M. Epstein

Brain stem auditory evoked potentials (BAEPs) are sensitive to anatomic disturbances of the brain stem auditory pathways, especially those caused by disruption of myelin. They are influenced by temperature but are virtually unaffected by level of consciousness, drugs, and metabolic disequilibrium. These properties make BAEPs useful in evaluating many posterior fossa disorders.

Auditory Evoked Potentials in the Assessment of Hearing 791

Terence W. Picton and Andrée Durieux-Smith

The auditory evoked potentials are the best available technique for identifying infants with a hearing impairment before the age of 6 months. They are also very important in the evaluation of patients with suspected retrocochlear hearing loss. New developments may soon allow the determination of hearing thresholds at different frequencies and a more accurate assessment of patients with central auditory dysfunction.

Somatosensory Evoked Potentials in the Evaluation of the Central Nervous System 809

Michael J. Aminoff

Somatosensory evoked potentials (SEPs) are easily elicited in the clinical neurophysiology laboratory. They have been used to detect lesions in central somatosensory pathways, to serve as a prognostic guide in patients who are either comatose or who have had a hemispheric stroke, and to monitor cord function to prevent or minimize neurologic problems. They have also been used to define the extent of neuropathologic involvement in patients with a wide variety of neurologic disorders, but in this context they provide information that is often of more academic relevance than clinical importance. These various applications of SEPs are reviewed in this article.

Somatosensory Evoked Potentials for the Evaluation of the Peripheral Nervous System.. 825

Andrew Eisen

Use of the somatosensory evoked potential (SEP) in the evaluation of the peripheral nervous system is described. When using SEPs to evaluate peripheral nervous system disease, it is assumed that the central nervous system is intact. SEPs can be used to measure conduction through nerves that, by nature of their anatomic site, are difficult to assess. By reason of central amplification they can indicate return of nerve continuity following trauma before peripheral sensory action potentials are recordable. For the same reason, it is possible to use them to measure peripheral sensory conduction velocity when conventional methods cannot be applied. They are helpful in the localization of plexopathies. Considerable effort has been devoted to their use in radiculopathies, but, for the most part, their role here is limited.

Somatosensory Evoked Potentials in Infants and Children.................. 839

Robin Gilmore

Somatosensory evoked potentials (SEPs) are a useful, reliable means of assessing function of the somatosensory system. Factors of complex maturational changes of the CNS, such as synaptogenesis and myelination, as well as body growth, complicate interpretation of SEPs. Understanding of these factors enhances clinical interpretation in infants and children.

Evoked Potentials for Diagnosis of Multiple Sclerosis 861

Keith H. Chiappa

The author discusses visual evoked potentials, brain stem auditory evoked potentials, somatosensory evoked potentials, motor evoked potentials, and MRI for the diagnosis of MS. Most patients with MS will eventually have an MRI scan. However, certain specific questions regarding function and anatomic regions are better studied with evoked potentials, especially those of optic nerve, brain stem, and spinal cord.

Use of Somatosensory Evoked Potentials for Intraoperative Monitoring of Cerebral and Spinal Cord Function..................................... 881

Marc R. Nuwer

Somatosensory evoked potentials can be used in the operating room to monitor the function of the spinal cord or the cerebral hemispheres. Several techniques are available, including recordings taken from epidural spinal electrodes, from the scalp, or from the exposed cortex. These provide sensitive monitoring methods that can identify impairment from inadvertent or excessive compression, ischemia, hypoxia, or distraction. Quick identification of such problems can lead to prompt correction of the cause, preventing postoperative neurologic deficits.

Intraoperative Monitoring of Auditory and Brain Stem Function 899
Rodney A. Radke and C. William Erwin

Extensive clinical experience has demonstrated that intraoperative brain stem auditory evoked potentials (BAEPs) are a reliable method of monitoring auditory and brain stem function during posterior fossa surgery. An intraoperative BAEP change identifies possible neurophysiologic compromise and allows adjustment of the surgical approach in an attempt to avoid permanent neurologic injury. The use of BAEPs intraoperatively has been associated with a significant decline in postoperative auditory morbidity. Supplementation of this technique with direct eighth nerve recordings and/or upper extremity somatosensory evoked potentials offers further improvement in identifying possible surgical threat to auditory or brain stem function.

Use of Peripheral Nerve Action Potentials for
Intraoperative Monitoring 917
Kevin R. Nelson

Intraoperative peripheral nerve action potential recording (INAP) detects regenerating axons crossing the site of physical injury earlier than clinical or EMG/NCS examination and prior to developing severe changes in distal tissues. With an INAP present, neurolysis is usually performed. If an INAP is absent, resection of the neuroma is undertaken followed by end-to-end suture or grafting. Peripheral nerve tumor resection can be aided by INAP identification of intact nerve fasicles.

Index 935

Subscription Information .... **Inside back cover**

FORTHCOMING ISSUES

February 1989
> NEUROGENETIC DISEASES
> William Johnson, MD, *Guest Editor*

May 1989
> PAIN
> Russell Portenoy, MD, *Guest Editor*

August 1989
> NEUROLOGIC MANIFESTATIONS OF SYSTEMIC DISEASE
> Jack E. Riggs, MD, *Guest Editor*

PREVIOUS ISSUES

February 1988
> ENDOCRINOLOGY OF NEUROPSYCHIATRIC DISORDERS
> Walter A. Brown, MD, *Guest Editor*

May 1988
> NEUROLOGIC COMPLICATIONS OF TRANSPLANTS
> Roy Patchell, MD, *Guest Editor*

August 1988
> MUSCLE DISEASE
> Jack E. Riggs, MD, *Guest Editor*

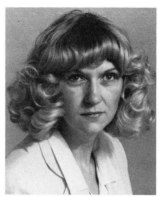

ROBIN GILMORE, MD
Guest Editor

Preface

Evoked potentials (EPs) as a specialty of clinical neurophysiology has evolved with contributions from basic scientists and clinicians of many disciplines. These contributors include neurophysiologists, neuroanatomists, audiologists, physiatrists, psychiatrists, pediatricians, pediatric neurologists, neurosurgeons, and, finally, but not least, neurologists. Although Caton is generally credited with describing EPs recorded from animals in the 1870s, it was Dawson who first developed the strategy of recording EPs using the photographic overtrace technique in the 1940s. Dawson and others developed the electronic averaging instruments for signal analysis that are so essential to high quality recording. Since the 1970s, EPs have been increasingly used in many clinical settings.

EPs are important diagnostic tools for clinicians caring for patients suspected of harboring central nervous system (CNS) disease or dysfunction. Although several techniques have been developed for imaging the *structure* of the CNS over the last quarter century, there have been fewer with which to study *function* of the CNS. EPs have allowed us to study directly *function* of primary sensory and now, motor systems in humans. We are able to evaluate auditory function, visual function, somatosensory, and, most recently, motor functions for diagnostic and prognostic purposes.

Visual evoked potentials and electroretinograms are a means by which one may extend physical examination of the visual system. Visual EPs are a sensitive method of judging anterochiasmatic pathways in a variety of clinical settings including suspected multiple sclerosis (MS), compressive lesions (such as tumor), spinocerebellar degenerations, B12 deficiency, and functional visual loss, among many others.

There is much interest in the comparison of magnetic resonance imaging (MRI) of the optic nerve and visual EPs in the evaluation of patients with suspected MS. Earlier this year, Miller and colleagues[1] reported on their experience using the advanced technology of short inversion time inversion recovery (STIR) to image the optic nerve. They found that visual EPs in the symptomatic eye were 100 per cent sensitive, whereas STIR-MRI detected lesions in only 84 per cent. In the asymptomatic eye, visual EPs were again more sensitive than MRI. Thus, they concluded that visual EP remained the preferred investigation for demonstrating abnormalities in optic neuritis.

Brain stem auditory EPs (BAEPs) are very useful in evaluating patients for possible brain-stem dysfunction, whether related to acoustic neuromas, brain-stem gliomas, or nonstructural lesions of the brain stem such as Leigh's disease. BAEPs are invaluable in evaluating infants, young children, and uncooperative children or adults for hearing loss. After being identified in early infancy, infants can be provided with amplification in order to facilitate speech and language development.

Somatosensory EPs (SEPs) provide a means by which to study the function of peripheral nerve, spinal cord, and brain. Establishing the diagnosis of many disorders can be aided by SEPs. Peripheral nervous system and CNS are readily assessed. Prognosis in coma associated with different conditions, including hypoxia and trauma, may be suggested by SEPs. Evaluating the sensory system of infants and children is a particular challenge to the clinician. SEPs provide a means to study the nervous system of infants and children noninvasively.

Monitoring the nervous system intraoperatively allows the physician to continuously assess portions of the nervous system at risk for compromised function. Monitoring sensory systems of the spinal cord and cerebrum and the brain stem are in widespread use as "guardians" of neural function. Monitoring motor systems of the CNS and peripheral nervous system are becoming more important as the techniques are developed and disseminated.

Finally, the study of evoked potentials offers clinicians the means to measure sensory and motor dysfunctions they can see, those they cannot see, and those at which they can only guess.

ROBIN GILMORE, MD

Guest Editor

REFERENCE

1. Miller DH, Newton MR, van der Poel JC, et al: Magnetic resonance imaging of the optic nerve in optic neuritis. Neurology 38:175–179, 1988

Department of Neurology/MS 129
University of Kentucky Medical Center
800 Rose Street
Lexington, Kentucky 40536-0084

Principles of Signal Analysis and Averaging

Charles M. Epstein, MD* and Darwin R. Boor, MD†

An evoked potential (EP) is a change in the electrical activity of the nervous system in response to an external stimulus. EPs may be produced in any neural structure—sensory or motor, central or peripheral—by any perceivable input. In contemporary clinical neurology, however, "evoked potentials" refer most commonly to studies that record averaged potentials from the central nervous system.

EPs recorded at the scalp or spine are tiny signals. They vary in size from the range of conventional EEG (50 μV) to 100 times smaller. EPs must be separated from other sources of electrical activity, which constitute unwanted noise and may be many orders of magnitude larger. Various types of noise and their size in relation to EPs are shown on a logarithmic scale in Figure 1. Methods for extracting an EP despite these and other kinds of interference are best understood in relation to the sources of noise and the different components of an evoked response system. The major sections are the input system and amplifiers; a digital microprocessor, which performs averaging, counting, and display functions; and an analog-to-digital (A/D) converter, which serves as the interface between the other two. Optimum recording and interpretation of evoked potentials are dependent on an understanding of each section and its relationship with the others.

INPUT SYSTEM AND AMPLIFIERS

The input system consists simply of the electrodes, a jack box, and a set of switches that direct the proper electrodes on the head to the amplifiers for each designated channel. Electrode selection may be manual or under

*Associate Professor of Neurology
†Assistant Professor of Neurology

From Emory University School of Medicine, Atlanta, Georgia

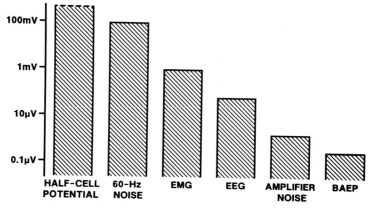

Figure 1. Relative amplitude of the BAEP in comparison to other sources of electrical noise arising from the head, the electrical environment, and the recording system. Note the logarithmic scale.

software control. This relatively simple section of the recording system is also the source of one of the largest unwanted signals. At the point where each electrode contacts the body, a significant voltage develops in the form of a half-cell potential created by the interface between dissimilar conductors (that is, the electrode, the scalp, and the electrolyte solution that connects them).[2] In most EP studies the half-cell potentials remain relatively constant and are adequately blocked by the use of AC coupling. If the electrode connections are not electrically and mechanically stable, then rapid voltage swings may occur at the scalp-electrode interface that will be passed on to the sensitive EP amplifiers, overwhelming the individual evoked potentials and frequently corrupting the averaged potentials.[1]

An equally important source of interference is the 60-cycle AC power in modern buildings. The scalp potentials induced by the associated electromagnetic fields may reach 100 mV, or 100,000 times larger than short-latency EPs. Even worse, these relatively huge potentials lie squarely in the frequency range of interest for most EPs. To remove them, we take advantage of the fact that the 60-cycle field is about the same intensity on different parts of a human body, and we use a special device called a differential amplifier to subtract out the common 60-cycle signal. The typical differential amplifier incorporates two active leads and a "ground" reference. It senses the potential difference between each active lead and the "ground" electrode, and then precisely subtracts one from the other removing any common signals—especially 60 Hz noise and EKG artifact. The portion of the signal that is different at the two active electrodes is the "differential mode" signal, the portion they have in common is the "common mode" signal, and the ability to amplify the former while attenuating the latter is known as common mode rejection, which is frequently expressed as a ratio (CMRR).

The three-wire differential input system has several implications for clinical neurophysiology.[1] *Both* active electrodes record physiologic signals equally, even when one is called a "reference."[2] A poor (that is, high impedance or mechanically unstable) connection in any of the three leads will cause problems, of which increased 60-cycle noise is only the most obvious.[3] Naive personnel may mistakenly believe that the "ground" electrode should be connected to earth ground, as represented by lightning rods and water pipes. Attaching patients to earth ground is potentially dangerous because it encourages leakage currents to pass through the patient on the way by. Commercial EP machines generally have protection devices in the jack box to prevent this, and the protection should not be circumvented when there is any possibility of the patient's contacting another AC-powered electrical device.

Once the common-mode contaminants have been removed, the amplifier magnifies the remaining signals according to the desired gain and filter settings. The spontaneous EEG and EKG are present all over the scalp, and vigorous EOG or EMG artifacts can easily be 100 to 1000 times larger than the smallest EPs. The amplitudes of these signals tend to vary with scalp location, and significant differential mode signals frequently develop between recording sites. All these unwanted signals can often be reduced by judicious use of the low-frequency (LF) and high-frequency (HF) filters. These filters are usually built from combinations of resistors and capacitors. The amount of noise that can be eliminated by such analog filters is limited, because the frequency ranges of EPs and other neurophysiologic signals overlap extensively. Furthermore, analog filters can induce phase shifts—changing the apparent latency and shape of EP waves even when there seems to be little effect on amplitude. As a general guideline, to avoid phase shifts, both the low- and high-frequency filters should be separated from the major frequencies in the signal by a factor of 10. Thus the ratio of HF to LF should be 100 or more, which results in passbands such as 1 to 100 Hz or 30 to 3000 Hz. When the filters are set tighter than this, as is the case with many BAEP recordings, EP features become especially sensitive to additional small changes in the filter settings.

Finally, even high-quality amplifiers generate random noise that may be larger than BAEPs or SSEPs. Thus the residual noise from all these sources is usually large enough to obscure the EP produced by a single sensory stimulus. To define the EP better, the amplified signal is digitized and passed on to a small computer, where further noise reduction is most commonly carried out by averaging.

ANALOG-TO-DIGITAL CONVERTER

Before the amplified electrical signal can be processed further, it must be converted to a digital form suitable for computer manipulation. The incoming signal is sampled at regular intervals generally ranging from 1 μsec to 1 msec. An analog-to-digital (A/D) converter assigns every sample an integer value according to the magnitude of the signal at that instant. Each value is then assigned to a specific location in the computer memory, known as an address or bin. When the data are displayed graphically with each address corresponding to a point on the horizontal axis of the display, a tracing resembling the original analog signal appears. Most averagers have at least 1000 addresses, so that the many separate points merge to give the appearance of a continuous line.

The precision of the sampling operation depends on the sampling rate and on the resolution of the A/D converter. The maximum A/D precision is expressed in "bits," which are the decimal places of a binary number. An 8-bit A/D converter can define up to 2^8 (256) different signal values, numbered from 0 to 255; a 12-bit A/D converter can assign 4096 values, numbered from 0 to 4095. The full-scale range of an A/D converter describes the highest and lowest input voltages it can accurately handle (Fig. 2). The resolution describes the smallest change in voltage that can be distinguished. If the incoming signal is too small, then the A/D converter will not record the small changes in signal amplitude due to the EPs (Fig. 2B). If the incoming signal is too large, then the A/D converter will truncate the signal to the maximum or minimum value it can assign (Fig. 2C). In either case, the computer will receive a distorted image of the analog signal. Thus the amplitude of the signal must always be matched to the input range of the A/D converter. In most EP systems the full-scale range is called the sensitivity, and is calibrated in terms of the original input amplitude rather than the amplified signal that is actually fed to the A/D converter.

Because excessively large signals are the most distorted and also the most likely to contain artifact, all modern EP systems contain an "artifact rejection" option that automatically discards faulty data sets when the range of the A/D converter is exceeded.

AVERAGER

In averaging, the onset of each sensory stimulus triggers the computer to acquire a brief segment of brain activity over a fixed time period, generally ranging from 10 to 1000 msec. Each segment appears on the display screen as a single sweep. The top line of Figure 3 shows one such sample, recorded over 256 msec following a visual stimulus. The EP is hidden obscurely in the background. However, consecutive samples of brain activity collected during a train of stimuli can be added on top of one another. The EPs, which occur a fixed time after the stimulus, tend to summate and grow larger. The background activity, which is random in regard to the stimulus, tends to average out. If the resulting sum is normalized (divided by the number of responses it contains), the amplitude of the averaged evoked response remains fixed and the noise appears decreased. Thus the EP becomes progressively better defined as more

---

Figure 2. A hypothetical 4-bit A/D converter, allowing 16 digital values over the full-scale range from $-V$ to $+V$ numbered 0 to 15. The signal is a sine wave, broken up into discrete points separated by the sampling interval. A, The signal amplitude is appropriate to the input range, and takes on values from 4 to 12 on the central scale. B, The signal is too small compared to the input range, and varies only between the digital values of 7 and 8. C, The signal is too large, so that the tops and bottoms of the sine wave are chopped off above 15 and below 0; if this data were sent to the computer, it would be badly distorted.

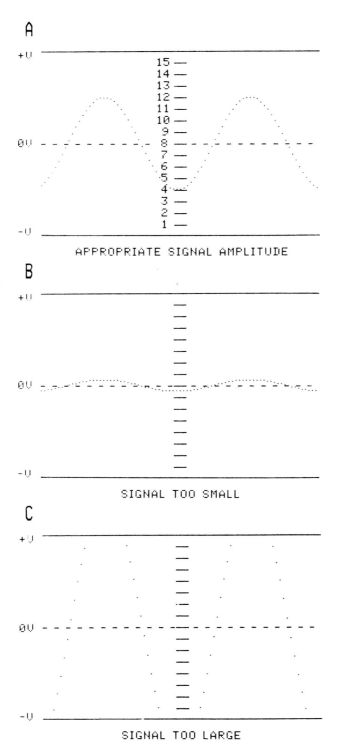

Figure 2. *See legend on opposite page*

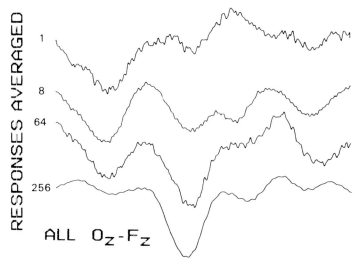

Figure 3. Increasingly better resolution of a VEP with increasing numbers of responses in the average.

responses are averaged (Fig. 3, bottom). When there is only one stimulus per sweep, and the data sample is longer than the duration of the EP, the result is called a "transient" EP. Transient EPs are the type most commonly used in clinical studies.

After a few hundred or few thousand stimuli, averaging of transient EPs allows measurement of salient characteristics like amplitude, shape, and latency from onset of the stimulus. Assuming that the EP is the signal we wish to detect, and the background EEG, artifact, and so on are considered random noise, then theoretically averaging may improve the signal-to-noise ratio by a factor equal to the square root of the number of responses in the average. Summing the response to 100 stimuli can therefore decrease the background noise 10 times; 2500 samples can decrease it 50 times.

The validity of signal averaging depends on the accuracy of two underlying assumptions, which should be familiar to researchers and clinicians alike.

1. The evoked response to every stimulus in a train has the same latency and configuration. This assumption holds well for BAEPs and SSEP components out to N19, is adequate with some reservations for midlatency components such as VEPs (which may be affected by the level of wakefulness or attention), and is at best questionable for long-latency "cognitive" EPs such as P300.

2. The background noise is random with respect to the stimulus. A common type of nonrandom noise occurs when the EP stimulus rate is a whole number that divides evenly into the 60 cps frequency of AC power lines. The small amount of 60 cps noise that escapes differential subtraction will then be augmented by averaging, just like the EP signal, and may be large enough to overwhelm it. To avoid this, the stimulus rate should be offset slightly from a whole number (for example, 5.1 or 10.3) to keep 60-Hz contaminants from synchronizing in successive sweeps.

Other types of noise time-locked to the average include electrostatic artifacts from a somatosensory stimulator or electromagnetic earphones, inadvertent auditory EPs related to sounds generated by some types of visual stimulators, and short-latency EMG bursts ("microreflexes") that can follow strong auditory and visual stimuli. In long-latency EPs used to test cognition, there may be effects due to anticipation of a regularly occurring stimulus. Careful technique, and not further averaging, is the only way to eliminate these problems.

In the presence of continuous muscle contraction artifact, relaxing or sedating the subject will generally be more effective than increasing the number of trials or sweeps. Muscle contraction artifact often comes in bursts during speech, swallowing, or body movement. An alert technician will get the best results by stopping the averager whenever such activity occurs.

SPECIAL METHODS FOR ANALYZING EPs

In addition to conventional averaging, many other techniques have been used in attempts to improve the quality, accuracy, or speed of evoked potential estimates. The general goals are to reduce noise or to avoid some of the assumptions on which averaging is based. Although most such methods are highly mathematical, and it is not possible to review them here in great detail, the fundamental concepts are usually straightforward.[3]

Digital Filtering

Unlike conventional analog filters, digital filters implemented on a computer can be designed to avoid phase shifts. The waveform distortions introduced by analog filters can thus be avoided; alternatively, the effective passband of the recording can be reduced, thus enhancing the signal/noise ratio and reducing the number of responses necessary to obtain a stable averaged result.

Fourier Transformation

Many types of analysis are based on shifting evoked potentials into the "frequency domain" via Fourier transform. If the EP is well defined and free of noise, its separate frequency components can then be measured precisely. If considerable noise is present, various types of frequency-domain filtering can be used to sort out which frequencies contain the most signal and which the most noise. In subsequent studies the noisier components can be discarded and a relatively noise-free signal reconstituted.

Pattern Recognition and Signal Extraction

Correlation techniques and other forms of pattern recognition such as "time warping" can adjust the latency of each data segment to obtain a better overall fit in the final average. A special model, or template, of the EP waveform can be used to detect EPs without assuming that they always come at the same time after the stimulus. With relatively large EPs, such as P300, it is possible to detect the response in a single trial according to how well it matches the template. Obviously, the validity of such techniques depends on the accuracy of the template chosen for analysis and the techniques used to form it. So-called autoregressive and "moving-average" techniques adjust the template to each subject, and the template can be recalculated after each stimulus.

Although on a research basis such methods have some advantages over conventional averaged evoked potentials, their implementation requires considerable expertise in signal analysis, considerable computation, and a separate set of assumptions about the nature of the underlying signal. These drawbacks have thus far impeded their adoption for routine clinical use.

REFERENCES

1. American Electroencephalographic Society: Guidelines for clinical evoked potential studies. J Clin Neurophysiol 1:3–53, 1984
2. Geddes LA, Baker LE: Principles of Applied Biomedical Instrumentation. 2nd ed. New York, Wiley, 1975
3. Gevins AS: Analysis of the electromagnetic signals of the human brain: Milestones, obstacles, and goals. IEEE Trans Biomed Eng 31:833–846, 1984

Department of Neurology
Emory University School of Medicine
Atlanta, Georgia 30322

0733–8619/88 $0.00 + .20

Anatomy and Physiology of Visual Evoked Potentials and Electroretinograms

Gastone G. Celesia, MD*

Electroretinograms (ERGs) and visual evoked potentials (VEPs) have been successfully employed to study the physiology and physiopathology of the visual system.

Holmgren[88] in 1865 first demonstrated the possibility of recording ERGs from the eye. The cellular sources of the ERG are reasonably well known and are related to the type of stimulus employed to evoke them.[9–11, 16, 19, 20, 30, 31, 66, 74, 77, 147] ERGs evoked by bright flashes have a different source than ERGs evoked by patterned stimuli.

Visual evoked potentials were first recorded from the scalp in the early 1950s.[50, 56] The sources of VEPs are complex and somewhat controversial.[17, 36, 47, 80, 94, 95, 123, 126, 143, 170] The utilization of these techniques permits the evaluation of the functional integrity of the visual pathways from the retina to the visual cortex in humans.[38]

ELECTRORETINOGRAPHY

Anatomy and Physiology of the Retina

ERGs are electrical potentials originated in the retina and recorded directly from the corneal surface of the eye.[9, 31, 35, 66, 74] The anatomy and physiology of the eye are briefly summarized as they relate to these electrical potentials. For further information the reader is referred to recent textbooks on the subject.[60, 132]

The eye is both an optical and a neuronal device. The light entering the eye must pass through transparent media—the cornea, the aqueous

---

*Chairman and Professor of Neurology, Loyola University of Chicago, Stritch School of Medicine, Maywood; Hines Veterans Administration Hospital, Hines, Illinois

This work was supported in part by the Veterans Administration.

humor, the lens, and the vitreous humor—to reach the retina. Prerequisite for normal retinal function is an intact optic system. Thus, for example, a cataract or a vitreous hemorrhage may prevent a checkerboard pattern stimulus from reaching the retina and be transformed into electrical signals to be transmitted to the visual cortex and perceived by the subject. The condition of the eye optics must be considered in recording and interpreting ERGs or/and VEPs.[40, 51]

The retina represents a miniature brain with both receptors and processing neurons in close proximity to one another. The characteristics of the retinal neuronal circuitry are very complex. The retina can be considered a useful model of the central nervous system.[60–62] Dowling aptly defined the retina as "an approachable part of the brain."[60]

The amount of light entering the lens and reaching the retinal surface is controlled by the iris, a diaphragm that can be contracted or dilated by the ciliary muscles. The opening of the iris diaphragm, the pupil, determines the amount of light reaching the photoreceptors.[76]

The retina contains five layers[62, 139]: the outer nuclear layer, the outer plexiform layer, the inner nuclear layer, the inner plexiform layer, and the ganglion cell layer. The outer surface of the retina is covered by the pigment epithelium. The pigment epithelium is close to the outer segments of the photoreceptors. The outer nuclear layer contains the cell bodies of the photoreceptors. The outer plexiform layer contains the synapses among photoreceptors and horizontal and bipolar neurons. The inner nuclear layer contains the cell bodies of horizontal bipolar amacrine neurons and the cell body of the glial cells of Müller. The inner plexiform layer contains the synaptic interconnections among bipolar, amacrine, and ganglion cells. The ganglion cell layer contains the cell bodies of the ganglion cells as well as some amacrine cells.[30, 61, 62, 89, 139, 147]

There are two types of photoreceptors: cones and rods.[54, 60, 62, 132, 147] The function of the two photoreceptors is different: cones mediate color vision at high intensity of light, and rods are utilized in nocturnal dim vision. The photoreceptors are the first-order neurons and act as transducers converting optic images into electrical neuronal signals by a process called phototransduction. The outer segment of the photoreceptors is constituted of double-membrane disks or saccules that contain visual pigments. The light sensitivity of the visual pigments is due to the "retinal," a vitamin A aldehyde bound to "opsin," the visual pigment protein. Rodopsin is the visual pigment for the rods. The human retina contains three subtypes of cones, each sensitive to a particular wavelength: blue, green, or red light. Each of the three types of cones has a specific visual pigment with peak sensitivity to a particular wavelength in the spectrum of visible light.[60, 61, 88, 121] The three types of cones are named for their response to the peak sensitivity of the visual spectrum: long-wavelength–sensitive (LWS) cones (or blue cones), middle-wavelength–sensitive (MWS) cones (or green cones), and short-wavelength–sensitive (SWS) cones (or yellow cones). Less is known of the chemical characteristics of the three cone pigments. The photoreceptors produce selective responses to light of varying wavelength and intensities. These responses are transmitted to the second-order neurons synaptically by both conversion and divergence.

Second-order neurons, the bipolar cells, segregate "on" and "off" channels, develop surrounding inhibition, and participate in the development of encoding of color specificity and interaction of rod and cone signals.[157] Rich lateral connections are provided by horizontal and amacrine cells.

The functional specialization of the various regions of the retina is reflected by the differences in local concentration of cells. At the center of the eye's visual axis is the fovea. Within the center of the fovea is a region containing exclusively cones: the foveola. The human retina contains about 100 million rods and 6 million cones.[138] In the foveola the concentration of cones is 150,000/mm^2; the concentration then drops abruptly to about 4000–5000 cones/mm^2 outside the fovea. Rods are absent in the foveola and increase in concentration at the periphery of the retina. The rod density peaks at 20 degrees from the fovea, then falls gradually, reaching 30,000–40,000 at the extreme periphery of the retina.

The distribution of ganglion cells in the retina shows the highest concentration around the fovea.[136, 169] Ganglion cells are absent in the fovea in an area equal to the diameter of the capillary-free zone. There is a high correlation among the cell distribution of cones, ganglion cells, and visual acuity. Frisen and Frisen[69] have shown that the diminution of visual acuity as we move away from the fovea is not so much related to the variation of cone density but to that of ganglion cells that receive information from the cones. At the periphery of the retina many photoreceptors converge toward one ganglion cell, whereas at the foveola the ratio of cones to ganglion cells approaches 1:1.[129] This ratio optimizes high visual discrimination. Conversely, the ability of the rods to detect light in a very dim surround is related to the high ratio of convergence of rods to a single ganglion cell.

The axons of the ganglion cells travel into the optic nerve to the lateral geniculate body. Ganglion cells transmit information to the lateral geniculate body via action potentials. Each ganglion cell responds to light stimulation only in a certain retinal area called the "receptive field." If stimulation of the center of the receptive field induces on-discharges, stimulation of the periphery of the field results in off-discharges.[106] This center-surround opponent arrangement represents the initial coding step of the central visual system. Three major subgroups of physiologic responses have been described in cat and primate ganglion cells.[59, 63, 93, 164] Ganglion cells that gives transient bursts of spikes (action potentials) to the stimulus placed in their receptive fields are called Y cells. Y cells have fast conduction velocity, have a center-surround opponent mechanism, fire preferentially to movement of edges, and probably provide analysis of movement and initiation of visual fixation reflexes. Other smaller cells give a sustained firing to visual stimuli and have a small receptive field. These cells are called X cells; they are slow conducting, have a color spectral opponency mechanism, and provide fine spatial discrimination. A third class of ganglion cells, W cells, show no center-surround mechanism, are very slow conducting, and are either excited or inhibited by contrast. The complexity of the ganglion cells has been demonstrated in the cat retina, where 23 morphologically different types of ganglion cells have been described.[102]

Visual information is processed into separate, although interrelated,

Table 1. *Relationship between F-ERG and Retinal Cells*

WAVE	CELL TYPE	PHYSIOLOGIC EVENT
ERP	Photoreceptors	Molecular transition of visual pigment molecules in photoreceptors
a-wave	Photoreceptors	Photoreceptor light response
b-wave	Müller cells	K^+-mediated current flow and DC potential
c-wave	Pigment epithelium	Altered K^+ fluxes induced by light
Oscillatory potentials	Bipolar cells (?) or inner layer of retina	Feedback circuits of inner layer of the retina

retinal circuits or modules where particular features such as color, contrast, and luminance are extracted. The information is processed by parallel channels of ganglion cells.[73, 114, 117, 123, 150–152, 155, 174] W, X, and Y ganglion cells represent at least three major parallel retinal pathways.[155] Neurotransmitters and neuromodulators have been found in the retina. Acetylcholine, dopamine, GABA, taurine, serotonin, glutamate, various amino acids, and several peptides have been demonstrated in the vertebrate retina.[130–132, 142] The study of retinal transmitters and modulators is one of the most rapidly developing areas of research in neuroscience. Retinal neuropharmacology studies can frequently be extrapolated to the central nervous system, as the retina represents a model for the brain.[130–132]

In the diagnostic armamentarium of the clinician two types of ERGs are useful: flash and pattern ERGs. The nature of the two ERGs is different and will be discussed separately.

Flash Electroretinography

Flash-evoked ERG (F-ERG) consists of a series of negative-positive deflections labeled a-wave, b-wave, and c-wave. The use of very intense or bright flashes evokes a positive potential that precedes the a-wave; such potential is named the early receptor potential (ERP). Small wavelets superimposed on the b-waves have been named oscillatory potentials. The source of the various potentials has been identified by intracellular recordings and selective pharmacologic intervention on the retina.[9, 30, 31, 60–62, 70, 71, 134, 147, 173]

Understanding the cellular origin of the various waves and how these potentials are generated is important for the logical application of F-ERG to the study of retinal function. F-ERG represents the algebraic summation of four basic components: (1) the photoreceptor potential, (2) a DC potential, (3) the b-wave, and (4) the c-wave. The negative a-wave results from the rising phase of the photoreceptor potential; the large positive b-wave originates in the retinal glial cells (Müller cells) and is related to K^+-mediated current flow in these cells.[134] The DC potential is of uncertain origin and adds algebraically with the other basic ERG components to influence the amplitude of the a- and b-waves. The onset of the DC potential participates in the onset of the b-wave to the abrupt termination of the a-wave. The c-wave is generated in the pigment epithelium (Table 1).

The morphology and parameters of ERGs vary in relation to dark (scotopic) or light (photopic) adaptation of the retina and the intensity and wavelength of the stimulus.[11, 19, 20, 48, 49, 77] It is therefore possible by using

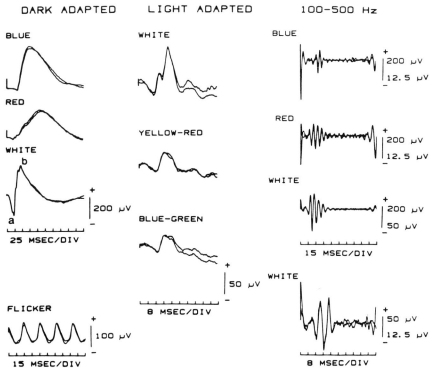

Figure 1. Flash ERG in a normal 32-year-old man. Each response represents the average of five ERGs; two averages are superimposed to demonstrate reproducibility. The left column represents ERG to dim suprathreshold and scotopically matched blue and red flashes to white flashes and to 32-Hz flicker in the absence of background light. The center column represents ERG to white and photopically matched yellow-red and blue-green flashes in the presence of background light. The right column represents the oscillatory potentials obtained with digital filters (100–500 Hz). Note the different amplitude and time calibration for the three columns.

sequential stimuli, varying from blue to white in the dark-adapted state and from white to blue-green in the light-adapted state, to separate the contribution of the rod and cone system to the ERG. The seven quantitative tests using Ganzfeld full-field stimulation, proposed by Berson and Gouras[19, 20, 74, 75] and by Chatrian and co-workers,[48, 49] optimize the evaluation of retinal function in clinical settings. The ERG to a dim blue flash in the dark-adapted state is exclusively a rod-mediated response (see Fig. 1), whereas the ERG to flicker is exclusively a cone-mediated response.[19, 20, 48, 49, 73–75] Rods can follow stimuli repeating only at a frequency below 20 flashes/sec.[11] Therefore, responses obtained by stimulation frequencies of 30 Hz are generated by the cone system. The ERG to dim red flash in the dark-adapted state contains early oscillations that are generated in the cone system, followed by a b-wave generated by the rods. Background light greater than 8 foot-Lamberts is sufficient to eliminate the rod response. The ERG to white flashes in the dark-adapted state consists of an a-wave generated both by rods and cones and a b-wave generated mostly by rods. ERGs obtained in the light-adapted state by white, yellow-red, and blue-green flashes are generated exclusively by cones.

The shortcoming of this protocol for clinical F-ERG recordings is that unless efforts are made to reduplicate stimulus and recording conditions, the normative data and the F-ERG pathologic interpretations are laboratory specific and cannot be easily applied from one laboratory to another.[124, 176] Furthermore, amplitude and latency measurements do not allow interpretation of retinal pathophysiology.[124] These difficulties have been bypassed by the measurements of the amplitude intensity response functions and the application of the Naka-Rushton equation.[133] F-ERG b-wave amplitude increases as a function of log stimulus luminance and can be expressed by

$$R = \frac{R_{max}I^2}{I^n + K^n}$$

where R is the ERG amplitude in uV, R_{max} is the maximum b-wave amplitude in uV, I is the stimulus luminance of the flash in cd/m^2, K is the half-saturation constant in cd/m^2, and n is the slope of the function. It has been demonstrated that the three parameters R_{max}, K, and n can be used clinically and interpreted in relation to retinal pathophysiology.[124, 176] Changes in R_{max} relate either to response compression owing to retinal "gain" loss or to regional losses of retinal function; changes in K relate either to changes in retinal sensitivity or to changes in preretinal light absorption; and changes in n may be due to heterogeneous losses of retinal sensitivity (Fig. 2). The validity of this method has now been shown in many retinal disorders in different laboratories.

Superimposed on the ascending slope of the F-ERG are a series of four to six wavelets, the *oscillatory potentials* (OPs). Frequency analysis of the OPs reveals they have a frequency in the region of 100–160 Hz. Their frequency varies depending on the state of dark adaptation. In the fully dark-adapted state they have a frequency of 150–160 Hz, whereas in the lighter state of the dark-adaptation curve they have a frequency of 120–130 Hz.[3, 100, 171, 173] OPs can then be easily recorded by selective filtering, with a low bandpass of 100 Hz and a high bandpass of 500 Hz (see Fig. 1). OPs have a different source of origin than the a-, b-, and c-waves of the F-ERG. Occlusion of the central retinal artery in the monkey results in the disappearance of the OPs.[31] This dependence of OPs on retinal circulation suggests they originate in the inner layer of the retina. The persistence of OP in patients with optic atrophy further suggests they are not related to ganglion cells.[172] Heynen and colleagues,[85] studying the current source and the sink profiles of the OP in the macaque retina, suggest that they are generated in the bipolar cells. However, these authors could not rule out that OPs could be originating in the interplexiform neuronal cells.

Neurotransmitters such as GABA and dopamine selectively depress the OPs, whereas acetylcholine and carbacholine have no effect on them. These findings suggest that the OPs are related to inhibitory feedback synaptic circuits within the retina.[31, 161] Although the true origin of these potentials remains controversial, they are certainly related to the normal functioning of the inner layer of the retina. OPs can therefore be utilized for diagnostic purposes.[28, 161]

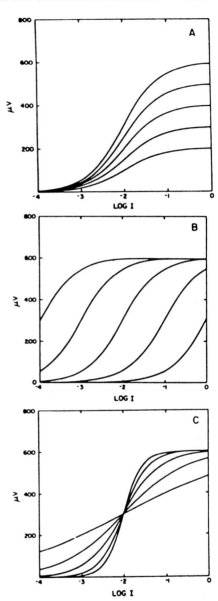

Figure 2. A, Schematic ERG intensity-response functions generated by the Naka-Rashton equation employing different values of R_{max}. B, Schematic ERG intensity-response functions generated by the equation employing different values of K. C, Schematic ERG intensity-response functions generated by the equation employing different values of n. (From Wu L, Massof RW, Starr SJ: Computer-assisted analysis of clinical electroretinographic intensity response functions. Doc Ophthalmol Proc Series 37:231, 1983; with permission.)

Pattern Electroretinography

Pattern ERG (P-ERG) is evoked by pattern-reversal stimuli, where the pattern alternates while the mean luminance is kept constant. P-ERG evaluates primarily the function of the retina serving the central visual field and mostly the macular region.[12, 14, 44, 45, 57, 58, 87, 97, 105, 118–120, 153, 154]

In 1981 Maffei and Fiorentini[120] studied steady-state P-ERG in cats and demonstrated that the P-ERG disappeared after section of the optic nerve. They correlated the abolition of the P-ERG with retrograde degeneration of the ganglion cells. These and other studies[58, 66, 118, 119, 125] suggest that the P-ERG originates in ganglion cells. On the other hand, detailed physiologic study of P-ERG in humans showed that P-ERG may reflect nonlinearity of local luminance components and therefore may represent preganglionic activity.[8, 105, 145, 154, 160]

The issue of the source of P-ERG is central to the value of P-ERG as a marker of ganglion cell activity and therefore as a possible indicator for prognosis of visual recovery following a lesion in the optic nerve.[45, 97] Tobimatsu and co-workers[165] looked at the source of P-ERG evoked by pattern reversal checks of high luminance and various spatial frequencies. The same stimulation and recording parameters used in humans were employed.

Spatial frequency functions were studied both for transient and steady-state responses. The amplitude of the major positive wave ($b_{(p)}$-wave) and the succeeding negative wave ($c_{(p)}$-wave) of the transient P-ERG showed a bimodal distribution with a peak amplitude around 0.60–0.75 and 0.30 cycle/degree (Fig. 3). Steady-state P-ERG showed a similar bimodal distribution. Section of the optic nerve was carried out in four cats. There were no changes in the flash ERG before and after surgery, indicating that no significant damage had occurred to the outer retina and that both rod and cone systems were functioning normally. However, both transient and steady-state P-ERGs to stimulation with checks smaller than 0.30 cycle/degree were absent, whereas P-ERG to stimuli larger than 0.30 cycle/degree persisted. Retrograde degeneration of ganglion cells was demonstrated histologically in all cats.

One of the most controversial issues in P-ERG is whether it represents a luminance[105, 135, 145] or a contrast[148, 168] response. Low spatial frequency amplitude attenuation (so-called "spatial frequency tuning") of the P-ERG cannot be explained without lateral inhibition of retinal cells. Lateral inhibition occurs in cells with center-surround receptive field organization.[64] Therefore, the source of the signal showing lateral inhibition is located in bipolar, or ganglion, cells. The data of Tobimatsu and colleagues[165] indicate that the spatial frequency functions for transient $b_{(p)}$- and $c_{(p)}$-waves and for the steady-state P-ERG in the cat have a preferred frequency at about 0.6–0.75 cycle/degree with a low frequency attenuation at about 0.5 cycle/degree, but with a second amplitude increase at frequencies lower than 0.5. This bimodal behavior indicates that at spatial frequencies above 0.5 cycle/degree (or smaller than 1.4 degrees of arc), the tuning is due to a "contrast response" originating in cells with center-surround organization. At spatial frequencies below 0.5 cycle/degree (or 1.4 degrees of arc), the "luminance response" becomes predominant and the P-ERG at these low frequencies represents a response from cells sensitive to mean luminance changes. These suggestions are confirmed by the results of the section of the optic nerve. Retrograde degeneration of the ganglion cells is associated with disappearance of P-ERG evoked by stimuli above 0.3 cycle/degree (or 2.4 degrees of arc), whereas stimuli of lower spatial frequencies evoked a P-ERG. It is reasonable to conclude that P-ERG to alternating checks is a

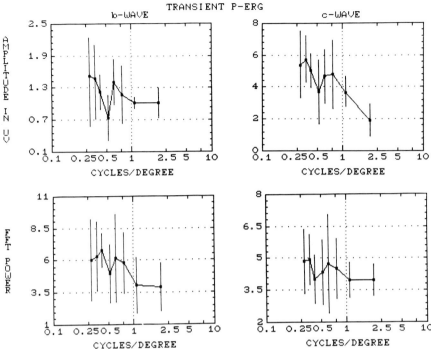

Figure 3. Spatial frequency functions of P-ERG in cats. The left column represents the amplitude of the $b_{(p)}$-wave, the right column the amplitude of the $c_{(p)}$-wave. The two upper graphs represent the peak-to-peak amplitude, whereas the lower two graphs represent the power of the spectrum for the same waves. Note that the function is similar for the two methods of measurement. There is a bimodal distribution for both waves with a peak at 0.6 cycle/degree and a trough at 0.5 cycle/degree. The curve is the mean of four cats, and the bars represent the SD.

mixture of contrast and luminance responses. P-ERG to small checks (above 0.5 cycle/degree or smaller than 1.4 degrees) is generated in the ganglion cells, whereas P-ERG to larger checks is generated in preganglionic retinal cells. The specific cells of origin for this latter response are unclear at this time.

These data suggest that in clinical practice the size of the stimulating pattern is a crucial parameter. The size of the pattern that will be primarily a ganglion cell response may be different in humans than cats. Indeed, the contrast sensitivity of the cat is displaced to lower spatial frequencies by a factor of 10 compared with humans.[33]

If P-ERG reflects postreceptor retinal activity and possibly ganglion cell activity, it can be used as a marker to determine retinocortical transient time, provided visual evoked scalp potentials are simultaneously recorded with the P-ERGs. Retinocortical transient time (RCT) then reflects activity outside the retina in the visual pathways.[44, 45, 97] RCT is defined as the difference in milliseconds between the latency of VEP waves and ERG. Two retinocortical times have been calculated: RCT($b - N70$) = latency of $N70$ minus latency of b-wave, and RCT($b - P100$) = latency of $P100$ minus latency of b-wave.

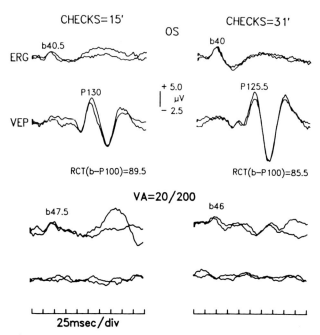

Figure 4. The upper half of the illustration shows the P-ERG and VEPs on a patient with definite multiple sclerosis (MS) and small central scotoma in the left eye (OS). Note the normal P-ERGs but the prolonged VEPs and RCT. These findings suggest demyelination of the optic nerve. The lower half of the figure shows the findings in a patient with definite MS and severely impaired vision in the left eye (visual acuity 20/200 and large central scotoma). Note the small P-ERGs and the absent VEPs indicating block of transmission in the optic nerve and early axonopathy.

Celesia and Kaufman[44] studied patients with macular lesions and described abnormal transient P-ERGs in 89 per cent of cases with checks of 15 degrees and in 67 per cent of patients with checks of 31 degrees. In early cases of senile macular degeneration P-ERG was present but delayed.[44, 97, 158] Similar absent or greatly depressed P-ERGs were described by Sherman[154] and Trau and colleagues[167] in macular diseases.

Abnormalities of P-ERG are not limited to maculopathies. They are also present in optic nerve lesions whenever there is an associated retrograde degeneration of ganglion cells.[23, 44, 57, 65, 119, 140]

In summary, delayed P-ERG occurs only in macular diseases; absent or markedly depressed P-ERGs are present in either maculopathies or severe optic nerve diseases associated with axonal involvement and retrograde degeneration of the ganglion cells (Fig. 4).

Conclusions

The data reviewed support the principle of "selective activation": different structures of the retina can be preferentially activated by varying the type of visual stimulation.[38] Flashes selectively activate retinal luminance and color detectors, and small-pattern stimuli preferentially activate contrast and edge detectors. Furthermore, different cellular structures and different retinal functions are tested by the different stimuli.

Pragmatically retinal function can be studied by two conventional methods: F-ERGs and P-ERGs.

F-ERG can be used to determine the presence, nature, and extent of retinal dysfunction and determine whether retinal dysfunction involves rods, cones, or both systems. The amplitude-latency functions of F-ERG allow the interpretation of pathology in relation to retinal function. Oscillatory potentials assess the functional integrity of the inner layers of the retina.

P-ERG can be used to assess macular and ganglion cell function. Maculopathies and optic nerve diseases may selectively alter P-ERGs.

VISUAL EVOKED POTENTIALS

Visual evoked potentials are extensively used in clinical practice since the initial demonstration by Halliday's group that the latency of pattern VEPs is affected by demyelination in cases of optic neuropathy even when visual symptoms are absent. It is presumed that these potentials are near-field potentials from the visual cortices.[36, 47, 63, 94, 95] It is therefore important to briefly review the anatomy and physiology of the central visual system.

Anatomy and Physiology

The optic nerve is about 50 mm long from the eye to the chiasma and comprises nerve fibers originating in the ganglion cells. Nerve fibers from ganglion cells in the macula form the papillomacular bundle, which occupies the entire temporal side of the optic disk. The human retina projects to both ipsi- and contralateral sides of the cortex. Crossing of the fibers from the nasal retina occurs in the chiasma. Crossed and uncrossed fibers begin to separate at the termination of the optic nerve. Macular fibers also are subdivided into crossed and uncrossed fibers; the macular fibers from the nasal portion of the macula cross in the chiasma into the contralateral optic tract, whereas the macular temporal fibers travel into the ipsilateral optic tract.[132, 136, 173]

Different types of retinal ganglion cells project in parallel but separately to the geniculate body and the cortex. In animals it has been demonstrated that X ganglion cells project almost exclusively to the A and A1 layers of the lateral geniculate body (LGB), whereas Y cells terminate in A, A1, and C layers of the LGB and also in the superior colliculi.[149] In the cat X cells deal with fine detail and pattern detection; Y cells are important for change and movement.[93, 108, 109, 174]

Information from the contralateral hemifield travels in the optic tract and, after synaptic transfer to lateral geniculate body neurons, continues into the striate area 17 via the geniculocalcarine tract. In humans information to the two other visual areas, 18 and 19, are via area 17. No direct geniculocortical projection to the parastriate (area 18) or peristriate (area 19) cortex has yet been demonstrated. Recently, however, some evidence has been presented suggesting the possibility of a true parallel representation of retinal inputs transmitted to the cortex through the thalamus via the superior colliculi and/or the pretectum.[53, 155]

At least nine visuotopically organized areas have been demonstrated in monkeys.[4] Some of these areas are located in the parietal and temporal lobe.[4, 78, 177, 178] This cortical organization of multiple visual areas with multiple reduplication of the retinotopic representation of the visual fields appears to be a general phenomenon in the phylogenetic scale. Marr[123] suggested that the representation of multiple cortical area is similar to the modular design used in computers, where any large computation is broken into a collection of smaller modules as independent as possible of one another. Then replication of cortical sensory representation may provide the structure on which new information capabilities are developed. Zeki[177] suggested that different aspects of a visual stimulus are represented in different extrastriate visual areas. He suggested that area V4 may represent color, whereas area STS may represent movement. Extrastriate neurons respond preferentially to moving stimuli of a certain range of velocities. This may represent a motion perception.[53] Although there is no comparable study of the detailed mapping of primate visual cortex, it is expected that a similar if not more complex system exists in humans.[36, 47, 67, 68, 146]

Over half the visual cortex of primates is devoted primarily to visual function[78]; most likely a comparable amount of human cortex is similarly involved in visual processing. This may explain why VEPs of relatively large amplitude can be recorded from various regions of the scalp from the vertex to the occipital protuberance. It has been demonstrated with positron emission tomography (PET) and regional cerebral blood flow[36, 47, 67, 68] that visual stimulation not only activates areas 17, 18, and 19, but also an area in the lateral temporal region comparable to the middle temporal visual area of primates. Multiple and discrete extrastriate responses were demonstrated with PET by Fox and colleagues.[67, 68] It is then reasonable to assume that the distribution of surface-recorded potentials to flashes or pattern reflects the complex interaction of electrical field potentials within at least four cortical areas, rather than the sole volume transmission of striate dipoles.

Visual neurons respond selectively to a visual pattern of progressively greater complexities as ascending levels in the hierarchy of the cortex.[16, 90-92, 174] Individual neurons can be selectively sensitive to the orientation and direction of movement and the width, length, velocity, and contrast of the stimulus. Each neuron must be considered as a multichannel coding device that responds to specific information represented in the stimulus.[38, 73, 86] There is anatomic and electrophysiologic evidence that the primate visual cortex is subdivided into distinct anatomic regions that process different types of visual information and has a separate connectivity with prestriate cortex.[86, 114-116, 166] The new techniques of ^{14}C-deoxyglucose autoradiography and cytochrome oxidase staining have demonstrated the existence of dots, stripes, and columns representing complex units of cortical organization in the visual system.[86, 114-116]

How neurons process visual information is still uncertain. Among the various theories the most active debate is between the advocates of "feature detectors" and proponents of "spatial frequency filters." According to some physiologists cortical cells are feature detectors or extractors, therefore responding optimally to special features of the stimulus such as edges or bars.[90–92, 114–116, 123, 174] According to other physiologists neurons are spatial frequency filters reducing visual information to Fourier components.[2, 33, 34, 107, 166] The debate may be groundless because the two hypotheses are complementary and not exclusive.[55, 107, 117] To understand the computation basis of vision, John and Schwartz[96] have suggested that a third paradigm is necessary—"spatial mapping." The spatial or anatomic rearrangement of visual data is important in visual analysis.[149] These authors point out that the visual system is organized mostly along spatial lines; the retinotopic and orientation column organization of the visual cortex is spatially and not frequency referenced.[149]

In spite of this controversy, it is generally agreed that the visual system is a multichannel device that processes information via parallel channels[6, 73, 114, 115, 143, 151] and that each channel constitutes a set of sequential processes.[38] Form, color, and spatial information are processed along independent and parallel pathways in the brain.[115] However, parallel processing should not be considered incompatible with serial processing. Michael[127] has shown that although luminance-contrast information and color-contrast information are processed along separate parallel channels at the cortical level, color cell population processes color in a serial manner.[127]

Visual Evoked Potentials

Visual evoked potentials (VEPs) result from the transient change of brain activity following an intermittent stimulus. VEPs are critically dependent on many parameters: stimulus brightness or luminance, contrast level, type of photic stimulus (patterned or unpatterned), type and size of patterned stimuli, total field size, and method and rate of presentation.[5, 7]

Although VEPs can be elicited by a variety of visual stimuli, including flashes, LEDs, gratings, vernier offset, windmill-dartboard patterns, and so on,[24–26, 32, 103, 112, 113, 162] the most frequently used stimuli are checkerboard pattern reversal. Checkerboard pattern-reversal stimuli are preferred because they evoke reproducible and relatively large potentials. Checks have sharply defined borders, and neurons are selectively sensitive to borders. There is evidence that vision occurs by the movement of borders of contrast across a retinal mosaic by the continuous micronystagmus of the normal eye.[73] Kelly[99] eliminated these micronystagmoid movements by stabilization of the image on the retina, and demonstrated that all vision was lost. Borders are further enhanced in the human visual system by the Mach band phenomenon.[141] This phenomenon is explained by lateral and reciprocal inhibitory interaction occurring at the retinal level.[60]

Check sizes and contrast are important variables in the use of patterned stimuli. Checks or gratings of less than 30 degrees of arc predominantly stimulate contrast and spatial frequency detectors, whereas patterns at low spatial frequency (with checks larger than 40 degrees) inevitably stimulate luminance channels.[118] Checks equal to or smaller than 15 degrees of arc not only stimulate contrast and spatial frequency channels, but preferentially stimulate the fovea.[39, 84, 126, 144] The retina outside the fovea detects objects, leaving to the fovea the task of identifying them following eye movement fixation.[175] In peripheral vision the premium is on object detection, whereas in central vision pattern discrimination and color detection are most important.[150, 175]

The choice of the field size and check size may have to be changed according to the region of the visual pathways one wishes to study. To detect small demyelinating lesions that affect optic nerve fibers originating in ganglion cells subserving the fovea (the papillomacular bundle), checks equal to or smaller than 30 degrees with a small total field should be used. On the other hand, to stimulate areas outside the fovea to detect chiasmal or retrochiasmal lesions, large fields with check size greater than 1 degree may be preferable.[38]

Halliday and co-workers[83] in 1972 demonstrated the usefulness of VEPs to checkerboard pattern reversal in the diagnosis of optic neuritis. Since that time delayed or absent VEPs to pattern-reversal stimulation have been employed effectively to detect optic nerve pathology. Abnormal pattern VEPs have been reported in many disorders affecting the optic nerve, including retrobulbar neuritis, papillitis, ischemic optic neuropathy, toxic optic neuropathy, optic nerve compression, and optic atrophy.[13, 25, 37, 42, 43, 72, 80–83, 101]

VEPs are quite useful in helping to establish the diagnosis of multiple sclerosis (MS). The presence of delayed or absent VEPs in the absence of retinal pathology suggests the presence of an optic nerve lesion. The demonstration of such a lesion in a subject with evidence of central nervous system disorders may establish the presence of multiple lesions, the hallmark for the diagnosis of MS. VEPs were delayed or absent in 72 per cent of patients suffering with MS.[42, 45] More important is the great sensitivity of VEPs in detecting subclinical optic nerve lesions when other clinical signs of visual impairment are lacking. Fifty-four to 70 per cent of MS patients without visual dysfunction and normal neuro-ophthalmologic examination had delayed VEPs.[13, 18, 23, 25, 27, 42, 45, 82, 83] Although the advent of magnetic resonance imaging (MRI) has made possible the demonstration of cortical and brain-stem white matter demyelination, its impact on the demonstration of optic nerve deficits has been less effective.[128, 137] VEPs were abnormal in all cases of optic neuritis studied by Miller and co-workers,[128] whereas MRI was abnormal in only 84 per cent of cases. Similarly, Ormerod and colleagues[137] concluded that VEPs were more sensitive than MRI in detecting lesions of the optic nerve.

In assessing optic nerve function the use of more than one stimulus parameter allows the testing of more than one of the "parallel information processing channels" and therefore improves detection of abnormalities.[38] Pathologic processes can differentially affect these channels. Patients with suspected MS have been found to have delayed VEPs only when the pattern was presented in a specific orientation or with a specific spatial frequency.[32, 52] A pattern presented in a different orientation or specific frequency often evoked normal potentials in the same patient.

VEPs can detect compression of the chiasma.[72, 81] Patients with CT evidence of suprasellar extension and normal visual fields had abnormal VEPs.[72] Absent or prolonged T-VEPs to full-field pattern stimulation indicate direct compression of the optic nerve or optic nerve compromise by vascular impairment. Detection of chiasmatic lesions in the absence of optic nerve involvement requires the use of hemifield stimulation. Absence or prominent amplitude depression of responses to stimulation of both temporal or both nasal hemifields is unequivocal evidence of chiasmatic impairment.

VEPs must be interpreted with caution. Refractive errors and retinal diseases may affect both the latency and amplitude of the responses. Delayed or absent P100 have been reported in retinal diseases, particularly in maculopathies.[44]

The simultaneous recording of P-ERGs and VEPs in patients with MS (see Fig. 4) reveals three types of abnormalities: (1) normal P-ERGs, delayed VEPs, and prolonged retinocortical time (RCT); (2) normal P-ERGs, absent VEPs; and (3) absent P-ERGs and absent VEPs.[44, 97] Normal P-ERGs with prolonged VEPs and RCT indicate demyelination of the optic nerve, whereas normal P-ERGs with absent VEPs indicate total block of the optic nerve fibers stimulated by the specific pattern. Impaired P-ERGs with absent or delayed VEPs suggest a severe axonal involvement with retrograde degeneration of ganglion cells. Kaufman and colleagues[98] have suggested that in cases of recent optic neuritis an abnormal P-ERG (absent or greatly reduced P-ERG) indicates poor prognosis for visual recovery, whereas the preservation of P-ERGs is usually associated with visual function recovery. These authors further demonstrated that progressive loss of P-ERG amplitude correlated with the development of optic nerve atrophy.

The value of VEPs in the diagnosis of retrochiasmatic lesions is still highly controversial. Part of the difficulty is related to the complexities of the topographic distribution of VEPs and their variations in normal subjects.[46] Amplitude asymmetry to full-field pattern reversal has proven unreliable as a diagnostic indicator.[46, 110] Hemifield stimulation with checks greater than 50 degrees of arc is recommended by the American EEG Society guidelines for clinical potential studies[5] to study retrochiasmatic function.

Full-field stimulation produces symmetrical amplitude distribution of VEPs over both occipital regions in about 63 per cent of subjects and mild asymmetrical responses in the remaining 37 per cent of subjects.[42, 110] Hemifield stimulation evokes asymmetrical amplitude responses in 64 per cent of cases with higher amplitude potentials ipsilateral to the stimulated hemifield. Symmetrical responses to hemifield pattern stimulation over both lateral occipital regions are recorded in about 36 per cent of normal subjects. Contralateral occipital lateralization, that is, larger-amplitude VEPs over occipital regions contralateral to the hemifield stimulated, was never observed in normal subjects.[17, 21, 22, 46, 80] The greater amplitude of P100 over the scalp ipsilateral to the stimulated hemifield (paradoxical lateralization of P100) has been explained by the mesial location of the generators in the hemisphere contralateral to the stimulated hemifield.[17, 21, 22] The location of the ipsilateral electrode is optimal for recording potentials from the posteromedial aspect of the contralateral occipital lobe (area 17). These explanations are based on the hypothesis that the major response P100 is generated in the striate cortex. Vaughan,[170] in analyzing the scalp topography of visual evoked potentials in monkeys, cautioned that as primary (area 17) and secondary (extrastriate areas) activity is temporally overlapping and generated in contiguous areas, it may be rather difficult to resolve their relative contributions from the scalp topography. Multichannel topographic scalp distribution and statistical analysis have been applied to VEPs with mixed results.[111, 156] Although there is consensus that $P100$ is a cortical-originated wave, it is unclear if it is exclusively produced by area 17 or 18 or by a multiplicity of cortical neuronal pools. Ducati and colleagues[63] recorded directly from the human visual cortex with depth electrodes during surgical procedures for dyskinesias. They noted reversal of polarity of the $N75$–$P100$ VEP complex when the stereotactic electrode crossed the cortex, thus demonstrating the local origin of the two waves. They could not, however, establish whether the generator was located primarily in area 17 or in parastriate cortices.

VEPs to hemifield pattern-reversal stimulation detects 75 to 85 per cent of patients with known lesions of the visual pathways and homonymous field defects.[21, 22, 46, 79, 121]

It is generally acknowledged that the sensitivity of VEPs in diagnosing abnormalities of retrochiasmatic lesions is poor. The 15 to 25 per cent failure of hemifield VEPs is probably related to the topographic variability of the striate cortex in humans and to the large cortical representation of the macular region.[36, 38, 47, 143] The striate cortex does not always reach the occipital pole, and often the lateral exposed part of the striate cortex is asymmetrical, being larger in the left hemisphere.[29, 163] An even more important factor is the large representation of the macula in the striate cortex.[29, 47, 146, 163] Pattern-reversal hemifield stimulation activates the hemi-macula, and its magnified cortical representation results in normal topographic distribution of VEPs. Improvement of diagnostic yield in retrochiasmatic lesions will require the development of methodology to preferentially stimulate the periphery of the visual field.

Bilateral lesions of the occipital lobes, if sufficiently extensive, result in cortical blindness. Surprisingly, VEPs have been found to be present in most of the cases studied.[1, 24, 41, 47, 104, 159] Responses to flashes are often prolonged and simplified, and responses to pattern evoked by small gratings or checks are affected, whereas responses to larger-size patterns are preserved. There are two possible explanations for the preservation of VEPs in cortical blindness: (1) EPs originate in extrastriate areas (areas 18 and 19) via retino-tectal-cortical pathways[159] or (2) EPs are generated by small islands of striate cortex that have survived the pathologic process, causing the occipital lobe destruction.[36, 47] In favor of the latter hypothesis is the demonstration of functioning islands of striate cortex in a cortical-blind patient by positron emission tomography. In this case glucose metabolism and regional cerebral blood flow showed a functioning area of cortex in the anterior aspect of the left striate area.[47] These areas most likely represent peripheral retinal fields, and are insufficient for conscious visual perception or capable only of rudimentary visual perception.

Conclusions

Visual evoked potentials are ancillary methods to study the function of the visual system. They have three important applications: (1) diagnosis of optic nerve diseases, (2) assessment in conjunction with P-ERGs of the prognosis for the recovery of visual function, and (3) evaluation of visual physiology and physiopathology.

REFERENCES

1. Abraham FA, Melamed E, Levy S: Prognostic value of visual evoked potentials in occipital blindness following basilar artery occlusion. Appl Neurophysiol 32:126, 1975
2. Albrecht DG, De Valois RL, Thorell LG: Visual cortical neurons: Are bars or gratings the optimal stimuli? Science 207:88, 1980
3. Algvere P, Westbeck P: Human ERG in response to double flashes of light during the course of dark adaptation: A Fourier analysis of the oscillatory potentials. Vision Res 12:195, 1972
4. Allman JM, Baker JF, Newsome WT, et al: Visual topography and function. Cortical visual areas in the owl monkey. In Woolsey CN (ed): Cortical Sensory Organization, Vol. 12: Multiple Visual Areas. Clifton, New Jersey, Humana Press, 1981, pp 171–185
5. American Electroencephalographic Society: Guidelines for Clinical Evoked Potential Studies. J Clin Neurophysiol 1:3, 1984
6. Arden GB: The importance of measuring contrast sensitivity in cases of visual disturbance. Br J Ophthalmol 62:198, 1978
7. Arden GB, Bodis-Wollner I, Halliday AM, et al: Methodology of patterned visual stimulation. In Desmedt JE (ed): Visual Evoked Potentials in Man: New Developments. New York, Oxford University Press, 1977, pp 3–15
8. Arden GB, Vaegan, Hogg CR: Clinical and experimental evidence that the pattern electroretinogram (PERG) is generated in more proximal retinal layers than the focal electroretinogram (FERG). Ann NY Acad Sci 388:580, 1982
9. Armington JC: The Electroretinogram. New York, Academic Press, 1974, p 478
10. Armington JC: The electroretinogram, the visual evoked potential, and the area-luminance relation. Vision Res 8:263, 1968
11. Armington JC, Biersdorf WR: Long-term adaptation of the human electroretinogram. J Comp Physiol Psychol 51:1, 1958
12. Armington JC, Brigell M: Effects of stimulus location and pattern upon the visually evoked cortical potential and the electroretinogram. Int J Neurosci 14:169, 1981
13. Asselman P, Chadwick DW, Marsden CD: Visual evoked responses in the diagnosis and management of patients suspected of multiple sclerosis. Brain 98:261, 1975
14. Baker CL, Hess RF: Linear and nonlinear components of human electroretinogram. J Neurophysiol 51:952, 1984
15. Barlow HB: Why have multiple cortical areas? Vision Res 26:81, 1986
16. Barlow HB: Summation and inhibition in the frog's retina. J Physiol (London) 119:60, 1953
17. Barrett G, Blumhardt LD, Halliday AM, et al: A paradox in the lateralization of the visual evoked response. Nature 261:253, 1976
18. Becker WJ, Richards IM: Serial pattern shift visual evoked potentials in multiple sclerosis. Can J Neurol Sci 11:53, 1984
19. Berson EL, Gouras P, Gunkel RD: Rod responses in retinitis pigmentosa, dominantly inherited. Arch Ophthalmol 80:58, 1968
20. Berson EL, Gouras P, Hoff M: Temporal aspects of the electroretinogram. Arch Ophthalmol 81:207, 1969
21. Blumhardt LD, Barrett G, Halliday AM: The asymmetrical visual evoked potential to pattern reversal in one half-field and its significance for the analysis of visual field defects. Br J Ophthalmol 61:456, 1977
22. Blumhardt LD, Barrett G, Kriss A, et al: The pattern evoked potential in lesions of the posterior visual pathways. Ann NY Acad Sci 388:264, 1982
23. Bobak P, Bodis-Wollner I, Harnois C, et al: Pattern electroretinograms and visual evoked potentials in glaucoma and multiple sclerosis. Am J Ophthalmol 96:72, 1983
24. Bodis-Wollner I, Atkin A, Raab E, et al: Visual association cortex and vision in man: Patterned evoked potentials in a blind boy. Science 198:629, 1977
25. Bodis-Wollner I, Hendley CD, Mylin LH, et al: Visual evoked potentials and the visuogram in multiple sclerosis. Ann Neurol 5:40, 1979
26. Bodis-Wollner I, Onofrj M: System diseases and visual evoked potential diagnosis in neurology: Changes due to synaptic malfunction. Ann NY Acad Sci 388:327, 1982
27. Bottcher J, Trojaborg W: Follow up of patients with suspected multiple sclerosis: A clinical and electrophysiological study. J Neurol Neurosurg Psychiatry 45:809, 1982

28. Bresnick GH, Korth K, Groo A, et al: Electroretinographic oscillatory potentials predict progression of diabetic retinopathy. Preliminary report. Arch Ophthalmol 102:1307, 1984

29. Brindley GS: Sensory effects of electrical stimulation of the visual and paravisual cortex in man. *In* Joung R (ed): Handbook of Sensory Physiology. Berlin, Springer-Verlag, 1973, pp 583–594

30. Brown KT: Physiology of the retina. *In* Mountcastle VB (ed): Medical Physiology. St. Louis, Mosby, 1980, pp 504–543

31. Brown KT: The electroretinogram: Its components and their origin. Vision Res 8:633, 1968

32. Camisa J, Mylin LH, Bodis-Wollner I: The effect of stimulus orientation on the visual evoked potential in multiple sclerosis. Ann Neurol 10:532, 1981

33. Campbell FW, Maffei L, Piccolino M: The contrast sensitivity of the cat. J Physiol (London) 229:719, 1973

34. Campbell FW, Robson JC: Application of Fourier analysis to the visibility of gratings. J Physiol (London) 197:551, 1968

35. Celesia GG: Visual evoked potentials and electroretinograms. *In* Niedermeyer E, Lopes da Silva F (eds): Electroencephalography. Baltimore, Urban and Schwarzenberg, 1987, pp 665–684

36. Celesia GG: Neuronal generators of human visual evoked potentials: Correlation between visual evoked potentials and visualization of regions of cortical activation by positron emission tomography. *In* Morocutti C, Rizzo PA (eds): Evoked Potentials: Neurophysiological and Clinical Aspects. Amsterdam, Elsevier, 1985, pp 245–254

37. Celesia GG: Visual evoked responses. *In* Owen JH, Davis H (eds): Evoked Potential Testing: Clinical Applications. Orlando, Grune and Stratton, 1985, pp 1–54

38. Celesia GG: Evoked potential techniques in the evaluation of visual function. J Clin Neurophysiol 1:55, 1984

39. Celesia GG: Steady state and transient visual evoked potentials in clinical practice. Ann NY Acad Sci 388:290, 1982

40. Celesia GG: Visual evoked potentials in neurological disorders. Am J EEG Technol 18:47, 1978

41. Celesia GG, Archer CR, Kuroiwa Y, et al: Visual function of the extrageniculocalcarine system in man. Arch Neurol 37:704, 1980

42. Celesia GG, Cone S: Visual evoked potentials: A practical approach within the guidelines for clinical evoked potential studies. Am J EEG Technol 25:93, 1985

43. Celesia GG, Daly RF: VECA: A new electrophysiological test for the diagnosis of optic nerve lesions. Neurology (Minneapolis) 27:637, 1977

44. Celesia GG, Kaufman D: Pattern ERGs and visual evoked potentials in maculopathies and optic nerve diseases. Invest Ophthalmol Vis Sci 26:726, 1985

45. Celesia GG, Kaufman D, Cone S: Simultaneous recording of pattern electroretinography and visual evoked potentials in multiple sclerosis: A method to separate demyelination from axonal damage to the optic nerve. Arch Neurol 43:1247, 1986

46. Celesia GG, Meredith JT, Pluff K: Perimetry, visual evoked potentials and visual spectrum array in homonymous hemianopsia. Electroencephalogr Clin Neurophysiol 56:16, 1983

47. Celesia GG, Polcyn RE, Holden JE, et al: Visual evoked potentials and positron emission tomographic mapping of regional cerebral blood flow and cerebral metabolism: Can the neuronal potential generators be visualized? Electroencephalogr Clin Neurophysiol 54:243, 1982

48. Chatrian GE, Lettich E, Nelson PL, et al: Computer assisted quantitative electroretinography, I: A standardized method. Am J EEG Technol 20:57, 1980

49. Chatrian GE, Nelson PL, Lettich E, et al: Computer assisted electroretinography, II: Separation of rod and cone components of the electroretinogram in congenital achromatopsia and congenita nyctalopia. Am J EEG Technol 20:79, 1980

50. Ciganek L: Potentiels corticaux chez l'homme, évoqués par les stimuli photiques. Rev Neurol 99:194, 1958

51. Collins DW, Carroll WM, Black JL, et al: Effect of refractory error on the visual evoked response. Br Med J 1:231, 1979

52. Coupland SG, Kirkham TH: The orientation-specific visual evoked potential deficits in multiple sclerosis. J Neurol Sci 9:331, 1982

53. Creutzfeldt O: Multiple visual areas: Multiple sensory-motor links. *In* Rose D, Dobson VG (eds): Models of the Visual Cortex. Chichester, Wiley, 1985, pp 54–61

54. Curcio CA, Sloan KR, Packer O, et al: Distribution of cones in human and monkey retina: Individual variability and radial asymmetry. Science 236:235, 1987

55. Daugman JG: Representational issues and local filter models of two-dimensional spatial visual encoding. *In* Rose D, Dobson VG (eds): Models of the Visual Cortex. Chichester, Wiley, 1985, pp 96–107

56. Dawson GD: A summation technique for the detection of small evoked potentials. Electroencephalogr Clin Neurophysiol 1:65, 1954

57. Dawson WW, Maida TM, Rubin ML: Human pattern-evoked retinal responses are altered by optic atrophy. Invest Ophthalmol Vis Sci 22:796, 1982

58. Dawson WW, Startton RD: Tissue responses of the monkey retina: Tuning and dependence on inner layer integrity. Invest Ophthalmol Vis Sci 27:734, 1986

59. deMonasterio FM: Properties of concentrically organized cells of the macaque retina. J Neurophysiol 41:1394, 1978

60. Dowling JE: The Retina: An Approachable Part of the Brain. Cambridge, Belknap Press, 1987, p 282

61. Dowling JE: Information processing by local circuits: The vertebrate retina as a model system. *In* Schmitt FO, Worden FG (eds): The Neurosciences: Fourth Study Program. Cambridge, MIT Press, 1979, pp 163–181

62. Dowling JE: Organization of vertebrate retinas. Invest Ophthalmol 9:655, 1970

63. Ducati A, Fava E, Motti EDF: Neuronal generators of the visual evoked potentials: Intracerebral recording in awake humans. Electroencephalogr Clin Neurophysiol 71:89, 1988

64. Enroth-Cugell C, Robson JG: The contrast sensitivity of retinal ganglion cells of cats. J Physiol (London) 187:517, 1966

65. Fiorentini A, Maffei L, Pirchio M, et al: The ERG in response to alternating gratings in patients with diseases of the peripheral visual pathways. Invest Ophthalmol Vis Sci 21:490, 1981

66. Fishman GA: Basic principles of clinical electroretinography. Retina 5:123, 1985

67. Fox PT, Miezin FM, Allman JM, et al: Retinotopic organization of human visual cortex mapped with positron emission tomography. J Neurosci 7:913, 1987

68. Fox PT, Raichle ME: Stimulus rate dependence of regional cerebral blood flow in human striate cortex, demonstrated by positron emission tomography. J Neurophysiol 51:1109, 1984

69. Frisen L, Frisen M: A simple relationship between the probability distribution of acuity and the density of retinal output channels. Acta Ophthalmol 54:437, 1976

70. Gallego A, Gouras P: Neurocircuitry of the Retina: A Cajal Memorial. New York, Elsevier, 1985, p 274

71. Galloway NR: Early receptor potential in the human eye. Br J Ophthalmol 51:261, 1967

72. Gott PS, Weiss MH, Apuzzo M, et al: Checkerboard visual evoked response in evaluation and management of pituitary tumors. Neurosurgery 5:553, 1979

73. Gouras P: Parallel processing of color-contrast detectors in the visual cortex. *In* Rose D, Dobson WG (eds): Models of the Visual Cortex. Chichester, Wiley, 1985, pp 242–252

74. Gouras P: Electroretinography: Some basic principles. Invest Ophthalmol Vis Sci 9:557, 1970

75. Gouras P: Rod and cone independence in the electroretinogram of the dark adapted monkey's perifovea. J Physiol (London) 187:455, 1966

76. Graham CH, Bartlett NR, Brown JL, et al: Vision and Visual Perception. New York, Wiley, 1965, p 637

77. Granit R: Receptor and Sensory Perception. New Haven, Yale University Press, 1955, p 366

78. Gross CG, Bruce CJ, Desimone R, et al: Cortical visual areas of the temporal lobe: Three areas in the macaque. *In* Woolsey CN (ed): Cortical Sensory Organization, Vol 2. Multiple Visual Areas. Clifton, New Jersey, Humana Press, 1981, pp 187–216

79. Haimovic IC, Pedley TA: Hemifield pattern reversal visual evoked potentials. II. Lesions of the chiasm and posterior pathways. Electroencephalogr Clin Neurophysiol 54:121, 1982

80. Halliday AM: Clinical applications of evoked potentials. *In* Matthews WB, Glaser GH

(eds): Recent Advances in Clinical Neurology. Edinburgh, Churchill and Livingstone, 1978, pp 47–73

81. Halliday AM, Halliday E, Kriss A, et al: The pattern-evoked potential in compression of the anterior visual pathways. Brain 99:357, 1979

82. Halliday AM, McDonald WI, Mushin J: Visual evoked potentials in patients with demyelinating disease. In Desmedt JE (ed): Visual Evoked Potentials in Man: New Developments. Oxford, Clarendon Press, 1977, pp 438–449

83. Halliday AM, McDonald WI, Mushin J: Delayed pattern-evoked responses in optic neuritis in relation to visual acuity. Lancet 1:982, 1972

84. Harter MR, White CT: Evoked cortical responses to checkerboard patterns: Effects of check-size as a function of visual acuity. Electroencephalogr Clin Neurophysiol 28:48, 1970

85. Heynen H, Wachtmeister L, van Norren D: Origin of the oscillatory potentials in the primate retina. Vision Res 25:1365, 1985

86. Hendrickson AE: Dots, stripes and columns in monkey visual cortex. Trends Neurosci 8:406, 1985

87. Hess RF, Baker CL: Human pattern-evoked electroretinogram. J Neurophysiol 51:939, 1984

88. Holmgren F: En method att objektivera effectenaf ljusintryck pa retina. Upsala Lakare-forenings Forhandlingar 1:177, 1865–1866

89. Hubbell WL, Bownds MD: Visual transduction in vertebrate photoreceptors. Annu Rev Neurosci 2:17, 1979

90. Hubel DL, Wiesel TN: Uniformity of monkey striate cortex: A parallel relationship between field size, scatter and magnification factor. J Comp Neurol 158:295, 1974

91. Hubel DM, Wiesel TN: Receptive fields and functional architecture of monkey striate cortex. J Physiol (London) 195:215, 1968

92. Hubel DM, Wiesel TN: Receptive fields of single neurons in the cat's striate cortex. J Physiol (London) 148:574, 1959

93. Ikeda H, Wright MJ: Receptive field organization of "sustained" and "transient" retinal ganglion cells which subserve different functional roles. J Physiol (London) 222:769, 1972

94. Jeffreys DA, Axford JC: Source location of pattern-specific components of human visual evoked potentials: I: Component of striate cortical origin. Exp Brain Res 16:1, 1972

95. Jeffreys DA, Axford JC: Source location of pattern-specific components of human evoked potentials: II: Component of extrastriate cortical origin. Exp Brain Res 16:22, 1972

96. John ER, Schwartz EL: The neurophysiology of information processing and cognition. Annu Rev Psychol 29:1, 1978

97. Kaufman D, Celesia GG: Simultaneous recording of pattern electroretinogram and visual evoked responses in neuro-ophthalmologic disorders. Neurology (Minneapolis) 35:644, 1985

98. Kaufman D, Lorance R, Wray SH: Pattern electroretinogram: A prognostic indicator of optic nerve lesions. Neurology (Minneapolis) 35, Suppl 1:130, 1985

99. Kelly DH: Spatiotemporal variation of chromatic and achromatic contrast thresholds. J Opt Soc Am 73:742, 1983

100. King-Smith PE, Loffing DH, Jones R: Rod and cone ERGs and their oscillatory potentials. Invest Ophthalmol Vis Sci 27:270, 1986

101. Kirkham TH, Coupland SG: The pattern electroretinogram in optic nerve demyelination. Can J Neurol Sci 10:256, 1983

102. Kolb HR, Nelson R, Mariani A: Amacrine cells, bipolar cells and ganglion cells of the cat retina: A Golgi study. Vision Res 21:1081, 1981

103. Kooi KA, Marshall RE: Visual Evoked Potentials in Central Disorders of the Visual System. Hagerstown, Maryland, Harper and Row, 1979, p 169

104. Kooi KA, Sharbrough FW: Electrophysiological findings in cortical blindness. Report of a case. Electroencephalogr Clin Neurophysiol 20:260, 1966

105. Korth M: Pattern-evoked responses and luminance-evoked responses in the human electroretinogram. J Physiol (London) 337:451, 1983

106. Kuffler SW: Discharge patterns and functional organization of mammalian retina. J Neurophysiol 16:37, 1953

107. Kulikowski JJ, Bishop PO: Fourier analysis and spatial representation in the visual cortex. Experientia 37:160, 1981

108. Kulikowski JJ: Pattern and movement detection in man and rabbit: Separation and comparison of occipital potentials. Vision Res 18:183, 1978
109. Kulikowski JJ: Spatial resolution for the detection of pattern and movement (real and apparent). Vision Res 18:237, 1978
110. Kuroiwa Y, Celesia GG: Visual evoked potentials after hemifield pattern stimulation in the diagnosis of retrochiasmatic lesions. Arch Neurol 38:86, 1981
111. Lehmann D, Darcey TM, Skandries W: Intracerebral and scalp fields evoked by hemiretinal checkerboard reversal and modeling of their dipole generators. In Courjon J, Manguiere F, Revol M (eds): Clinical Applications of Evoked Potentials in Neurology. New York, Raven Press, 1982, pp 41–48
112. Lesser RP, Luders H, Klem G, et al: Visual potentials evoked by light-emitting diodes mounted in goggles. Cleveland Clin Q 52:223, 1985
113. Levi DM, Manny RE, Klein SA, et al: Electrophysiological correlates of hyperacuity in the human visual cortex. Nature 306:468, 1983
114. Livingstone MS: Art, illusion and the visual system. Sci Am 258:78, 1988
115. Livingstone MS, Hubel DH: Anatomy and physiology of a color system in the primate visual cortex. J Neurosci 4:309, 1984
116. Livingstone MS, Hubel DH: Thalamic input to cytochrome oxidase-rich regions in monkey visual cortex. Proc Natl Acad Sci USA 79:6098, 1982
117. MacKay D: Strife over visual cortical function. Nature 289:117, 1981
118. Maffei L: Electroretinographic and visual cortical potentials in response to alternating gratings. Ann NY Acad Sci 388:1, 1982
119. Maffei L, Fiorentini A: Generator sources of the pattern ERG in man and animals. In Maffei L, Fiorentini A (eds): Evoked Potentials. New York, Alan R. Liss, 1986, pp 101–116
120. Maffei L, Fiorentini A: Electroretinographic responses to alternating gratings before and after section of the optic nerve. Science 211:953, 1981
121. Maitland MJ, Aminoff C, Kennard C, et al: Evoked potentials in the evaluation of visual field defects due to chiasmal or retrochiasmal lesions. Neurology (Minneapolis) 32:968, 1982
122. Mansfield RJW: Primate photopigments and cone mechanisms. In Fein A, Levine JS (eds): The Visual System. New York, Alan R. Liss, 1985, pp 89–106
123. Marr D: Vision: A Computational Investigation into the Human Representation and Processing of Visual Information. San Francisco, Freeman, 1982, p 397
124. Massof RW, Wu L, Finkelstein D, et al: Properties of electroretinographic intensity-response functions in retinitis pigmentosa. Doc Ophthalmol 57:279, 1984
125. May JG, Ralston JV, Reed JL, et al: Loss in pattern-elicited electroretinograms in optic nerve dysfunction. Am J Ophthalmol 93:418, 1982
126. Meredith JT, Celesia GG: Pattern-reversal visual evoked potentials and retinal eccentricity. Electroencephalogr Clin Neurophysiol 53:243, 1982
127. Michael CR: Models of the Visual Cortex. Chichester, Wiley, 1985, p 301
128. Miller DH, Newton MR, van der Poel JC, et al: Magnetic resonance imaging of the optic nerve in optic neuritis. Neurology 38:175, 1988
129. Missotten L: Estimation of the ratio of cones to neurons in the fovea of the human retina. Invest Ophthalmol 13:1045, 1984
130. Morgan WW: Retinal Transmitters and Modulators: Models for the Brain, Vol I. Boca Raton, CRC Press, 1985, p 164
131. Morgan WW: Retinal Transmitters and Modulators: Models for the Brain, Vol II. Boca Raton, CRC Press, 1985, p 166
132. Moses RA, Hart WM: Adler's Physiology of the Eye: Clinical Application. St. Louis, Mosby, 1987, p 709
133. Naka KI, Rushton WAH: S-potentials from colour units in the retina of fish (Cyprinidae). J Physiol 185:587, 1966
134. Newman EA: Regulation of potassium levels by glial cells in the retina. Trends Neurosci 8:156, 1985
135. Ohzawa I, Freeman RD: Pattern evoked potentials from the cat's retina. J Neurophysiol 54:691, 1985
136. Oppel O: Untersuchungen über die verteilung und zahl der retinalen ganglienzellen beim menschen. Albrecht v. Graefe Arch Klin Exp Ophtalmol 172:1, 1967

137. Ormerod IEC, Miller DH, McDonald WI, et al: The role of NMR imaging in the assessment of multiple sclerosis and isolated neurological lesions. Brain 110:1579, 1987
138. Osterberg G: Topography of the layer of rods and cones in the human retina. Acta Ophthalmol 13(Suppl 6):1, 1935
139. Polyak S: The Retina. Chicago, University of Chicago Press, 1941, p 607
140. Porciatti V, von Berger GP: Pattern electroretinogram and visual evoked potential in optic nerve disease: Early diagnosis and prognosis. Doc Ophthalmol Proc Series 40:101, 1984
141. Ratliff F: Mach Bands: Quantitative Studies on Neural Networks in the Retina. San Francisco, Holden-Day, 1965, p 365
142. Redburn DA, Madtes P: GABA: Its role and development in retina. Prog Retinal Res 6:69, 1986
143. Regan D: Evoked Potentials in Psychology, Sensory Physiology and Clinical Medicine. London, Chapman and Hall, 1972, p 328
144. Regan D, Richards W: Independence of evoked potentials and apparent size. Vision Res 11:679, 1971
145. Reimslag FCC, Ringo JL, Spekreijse H, et al: The luminance origin of the pattern electroretinogram in man. J Physiol 363:191, 1985
146. Reivich M, Cobb W, Rosenquist A, et al: Abnormalities in local cerebral glucose metabolism in patients with visual field defects. J Cereb Blood Flow Metabol 1(suppl 1):S471, 1981
147. Rodieck RW: The Vertebrate Retina: Principle of Structure and Function. San Francisco, Freeman, 1973, p 1044
148. Schuurman RP, Berninger T: Luminance and contrast responses recorded in man and cat. Doc Ophthalmol 59:187, 1985
149. Schwartz EL: Local and global functional architecture in primate striate cortex: Outline of a spatial mapping doctrine for perception. In Rode D, Dobson WG (eds): Models of the Visual Cortex. Chichester, Wiley, 1985, pp 146–156
150. Shapley R: The importance of contrast for the activity of single neurons, the VEP and perception. Vision Res 26:45, 1986
151. Shapley R: Parallel pathways in the mammalian visual system. Ann NY Acad Sci 388:11, 1982
152. Shapley R, Perry VH: Cat and monkey retinal ganglion cells and their visual functional roles. Trends Neurosci 9:229, 1986
153. Sherman J: ERG and VEP as supplemental aids in the differential diagnosis of retinal versus optic nerve disease. In Cracco RQ, Bodis-Wollner I (eds): Evoked Potentials. New York, Alan R. Liss, 1986, pp 343–353
154. Sherman J: Simultaneous pattern-reversal electroretinograms and visual evoked potentials in diseases of the macula and optic nerve. Ann NY Acad Sci 388:214, 1982
155. Sherman SM: Parallel W-, X- and Y-cell pathways in the cat: A model for visual function. In Rose D, Dobson VG (eds): Models of the Visual Cortex. New York, Wiley, 1985, pp 75–84
156. Skandries W: Visual evoked potentials topography: Methods and results. In Duffy FH (ed): Topographic Mapping of Brain Electrical Activity. Boston, Butterworth, 1986, pp 7–28
157. Slaughter MM, Miller RF: The role of glutamate receptors in information processing in the distal retina. In Gallego A, Gouras P (eds): Neurocircuitry of the Retina: A Cajal Memorial. New York, Elsevier, 1985, pp 51–65
158. Sokol S: An electrodiagnostic index of macular degeneration: Use of a checkerboard pattern stimulus. Arch Ophthalmol 88:619, 1972
159. Spehlmann R, Gross RA, Ho SU, et al: Visual evoked potentials and postmortem findings in a case of cortical blindness. Ann Neurol 2:531, 1977
160. Spekreijse H, Apkarian P: The use of a system analysis approach to electrodiagnostic (ERG and VEP) assessment. Vision Res 26:195, 1986
161. Speros P, Price J: Oscillatory potentials: History, techniques and potential use in the evaluation of disturbances of retinal circulation. Surv Ophthalmol 25:237, 1981
162. Srebro R, Osetinsky MV: The localization of cortical activity evoked by Vermier offset. Vision Res 27:1387, 1987
163. Stensaas SS, Eddington DK, Dobelle WH: The topography and variability of the primary visual cortex in man. J Neurosurg 40:747, 1974

164. Stone J, Hoffman KP: Very slow conducting ganglion cells in the cat's retina: A major new functional type? Brain Res 43:610, 1972

165. Tobimatsu S, Celesia GG, Cone S: Pattern-ERG to alternating checks in cats: Evidence of retinal spatial frequency tuning, and effect of optic nerve section. Noninvasive assessment of the visual system. 1988 Technical Digest Series, Vol 3:90, 1988

166. Tootell RBH, Silverman MS, De Valois RL: Spatial frequency columns in primary visual cortex. Science 214:813, 1981

167. Trau R, Van Looy H, Meckaert I, et al: Une nouvelle méthode d'exploration clinique: l'ERG et VER simultanés au pattern. Bull Soc Belge Ophthalmol 198 II:111, 1982

168. Vaegan, Burke W: Pattern and focal electroretinogram separation by barbiturate anesthesia in decerebrate cat. Doc Ophthalmol Proc Series 40:49, 1984

169. Van Buren JM: The Retinal Ganglion Cell Layer. Springfield, Illinois, Charles C. Thomas, 1963

170. Vaughan HG: The neural origins of human event-related potentials. Ann NY Acad Sci 388:125, 1982

171. Wachtmeister L: Spatial characteristics of the oscillatory potentials of the electroretinogram. Acta Ophthalmol 64:681, 1986

172. Wachtmeister L, el Azazi M: The oscillatory potentials of the electroretinogram in patients with unilateral optic atrophy. Ophthalmologica 191:38, 1985

173. Weale RA: Focus on Vision. Cambridge, Harvard University Press, 1982, p 194

174. Wiesel TN, Gilbert CD: Visual cortex. Trends Neurosci 9:509, 1986

175. Williams DR: Seeing through the photoreceptor mosaic. Trends Neurosci 9:193, 1986

176. Wu L, Massof RW, Starr SJ: Computer assisted analysis of clinical electroretinographic intensity-response functions. Doc Ophthalmol Proc Series 37:231, 1983

177. Zeki SM: Uniformity and diversity of structure and function in rhesus monkey prestriate visual cortex. J Physiol 277:273, 1978

178. Zeki SM: Color coding in the superior temporal sulcus of rhesus monkey visual cortex. Proc R Soc (London) 197:195, 1977

Loyola University of Chicago
Stritch School of Medicine
Maywood, Illinois 60153

Evoked Potentials 0733–8619/88 $0.00 + .20

The Anatomic and Physiologic Bases of Brain Stem Auditory Evoked Potentials

Alan D. Legatt, MD, PhD,* Joseph C. Arezzo, PhD,†
and Herbert G. Vaughan, Jr., MD‡

The human short-latency or "brain stem" auditory evoked potentials (BAEPs) are a series of positive and negative waves recorded within the first 10 msec after the onset of a transient auditory stimulus. Although they have attained wide clinical usage, including applications in audiology,[76] neurology,[10, 23] and intraoperative monitoring,[24] there is still considerable controversy about the specific identities of the generators. The relative contributions of action potentials and synaptic potentials, and the effects of fiber tract geometry and tissue impedances on the surface waveforms, are also being questioned. To maximize the power of the BAEPs for localizing lesions affecting the auditory pathways, the generators of the various component waves must be identified. In this article we describe the currently available evidence for, and theories about, the BAEP generators.

We refer to these potentials as BAEPs because the term is widely used and understood, even though they are more accurately called short-latency auditory evoked potentials.[3] The roster of generators clearly includes the distal cochlear nerve (in this article, "distal" refers to the eighth nerve at the cochlea, and "proximal" to the nerve at the brain stem), which is not within the brain stem, and may also include the thalamocortical auditory

*Assistant Professor of Neurology and Neuroscience, and Director of Intraoperative Neurophysiology, Montefiore Medical Center and the Albert Einstein College of Medicine, Bronx, New York

†Associate Professor of Neuroscience and Neurology, Albert Einstein College of Medicine, Bronx, New York

‡Professor of Neuroscience, Neurology, and Pediatrics, and Director, Rose F. Kennedy Center for Research in Mental Retardation and Human Development, Albert Einstein College of Medicine, Bronx, New York

The authors were supported by grants GM-07288, HD-01799, MH-0623, and NS-25041 from the USPHS.

radiations. Other synonyms include the auditory brain-stem response, far-field electrocochleography, and brain-stem audiometry.

Surface-recorded human auditory evoked potential components with latencies of less than 10 msec were first described by Sohmer and Feinmesser[85] and attributed to either "repetitive firing of auditory nerve fibers" or "the discharge of neurons in brain stem auditory nuclei." They were further characterized by Jewett and co-workers,[47, 48] who clearly identified their far-field nature, ascribed several of the waves to central generators, and established the roman numeral nomenclature used in most laboratories. Reports of neurologic and audiometric applications followed soon thereafter.

Recording Techniques

Brief click stimuli produced by delivering 50 to 100 μsec duration square pulses to electromechanical transducers (headphones or ear insert transducers) are usually used to elicit BAEPs; filtered clicks or tone pips may also be employed. Because reversal of click polarity may alter the BAEP waveforms,[11, 73, 96] a single polarity is preferable. Typical filter settings for recordings in adults are 100 to 3000 Hz,[11, 96] but the low cutoff frequency can substantially alter the BAEP waveform and should be lowered in infants, whose BAEPs comprise lower frequencies.[77]

Human BAEPs are typically recorded between a scalp electrode at the vertex (Cz in the International 10–20 System) and another electrode at the mastoid or earlobe ipsilateral to a monaural stimulus. In this configuration up to seven vertex-positive peaks, labeled waves I through VII, are recorded. A slow negativity (SN), which is wider than the individual positivities, follows wave V and is useful in the identification of that component. Vertex positivity is usually displayed as an upward deflection,[3] though this is not universal.

Only waves I, III, and V are recorded reliably enough to be routinely used in clinical applications.[3] Waves IV and V are often fused in a complex of variable morphology,[12] sometimes obscuring component identification. The SN, whose wave shape and amplitude are influenced by the choice of filter settings, may also be useful for interpretation of BAEPs.[18, 27, 101]

Additional recording montages, most commonly including the contra-lateral mastoid or earlobe, are used to emphasize and help identify certain of the waves.[96] Other approaches currently under investigation include mapping of BAEP three-channel Lissajous' trajectories[34, 46, 84] and analysis of BAEP scalp topographies recorded from arrays of electrodes,[34, 44, 82] which may be coupled with mathematical modeling of the putative generators within a volume conductor.[34, 82]

METHODS OF SOURCE IDENTIFICATION

Evidence about the identities of the BAEP generators can be derived from several approaches: investigation of far-field topographies, intracranial recordings within or near the subcortical auditory pathways, and analysis of the effects of lesions, all of these either in human or animal subjects.

Each of these has advantages and disadvantages, and the optimal understanding of the generators comes from consideration and integration of all the available data.

Surface mappings help to dissect out the overlapping subcomponents of the BAEPs, but do not directly identify the generators. Scalp potential distributions predicted by generator hypotheses based on other data must, however, conform to the observed component topographies.

Intracranial recordings from sites within or near the generators provide the most direct evidence for BAEP sources. There are occasional opportunities for intracranial BAEP recordings in humans during neurosurgery. Although electrodes may be placed in the vicinity of the subcortical auditory pathways[16, 37, 39, 62–66, 102, 103] and within the ventricular system,[39] serial recordings cannot be made within the brain-stem fibers and nuclei in humans. More extensive depth recordings can be performed in animals, including measures of unit activity.[42, 55]

It is important to realize that some of the activity recorded within a brain-stem structure may not contribute to the far-field BAEP waveform owing to the geometrical arrangement of the active cellular elements. Their activation may produce a closed field that is not recorded beyond the immediate vicinity of the structure,[59] or an equivalent dipole oriented so as not to contribute to the vertex-to-ipsilateral ear waveform. Thus, temporal coincidence of a surface BAEP component and a large peak within a brain-stem nucleus does not by itself identify a generator. Moreover, components generated by propagating action potentials may show latency shifts as the recording electrode is moved along the axis of propagation in the near field, and the latency may match that of the far-field component only at the terminus of the pathway.[4, 55] Thus, structures studied with depth recordings should be conclusively identified as generators of BAEP components only if their contributions can be traced as they are volume-conducted to the far field.

Studies of BAEPs in patients with discrete lesions of the nervous system may help to identify the generators, though the anatomic correlation between the visualized lesion and the area of tissue dysfunction is not always clear. Complete identification of all generators is not possible from clinical data alone. However, comparison of a patient's BAEPs with those associated with known lesions may give a localization to a region of the neuraxis, for example, the rostral brain stem, which is adequate in some clinical applications.

Precisely positioned lesions and detailed intracranial recordings may be performed in experimental animals. There are, however, major differences in the anatomic relationships of the brain stem, brain, and head between humans and nonprimates; in some of the latter the head is not in the far field of the BAEPs owing to its small size.[78] Data from subhuman primates[53–55] are more directly applicable to the interpretation of human BAEPs. In all cases, however, drawing inferences about the human BAEP generators requires making assumptions about cross-species homologies, which must be carefully evaluated. Differences in the length of the pathways, especially the eighth nerve, are important.[65, 66]

ANATOMIC SOURCES OF BAEPS

Efforts to identify the generators using depth recordings and lesions in experimental animals began simultaneously with the initial reports of the BAEPs.[45, 58] Soon thereafter BAEPs were studied in human patients with brain damage.[86, 89, 90, 93, 97]

As Jewett and Williston first noted,[48] most human BAEP peaks are composites of contributions of multiple generators. This is supported by the bifid wave III seen in some normal BAEPs,[12, 96] containing two components that overlap in most subjects, and by the results of intraoperative recordings.[39] Detailed intracranial mapping studies have demonstrated multiple generators for many BAEP components in animals.[1, 55] Such complexity derives in part from the pattern of connections within the auditory pathways, with ascending fibers both synapsing in and bypassing various relay nuclei.[98–100] It is also due to the presence of two bursts of activity in the eighth nerve, the N1 and N2 action potentials (recorded by electrocochleography), which can drive the more rostral pathways.

Although most reports of generators based on clinical-pathologic correlations stated that their conclusions and summary figures were probably simplifications,[90, 93, 96, 97] many subsequent discussions and clinical papers have assumed a one-peak-to-one-generator correspondence. Inasmuch as the human intracranial and clinical data tend to identify only the major generator of each wave, it is important to realize that other generators may provide significant contributions that could be unmasked if the major contribution is lost. If these were construed as the contribution of the major generator, clinical interpretation of these BAEPs could be erroneous.

BAEPs are the summated activity of pools of neurons. The short duration of most BAEP peaks indicates that they derive from action potentials rather than postsynaptic potentials. Furthermore, their generators must comprise a subset of subcortical auditory neurons with the shortest latencies and a high degree of synaptic security that minimizes temporal dispersion, as shown by single-unit recordings in the cat.[42] Neurons with these characteristics are required for sound localization; there is an anatomically distinguishable neuronal subsystem for sound localization within the brain stem[25] that appears to correspond to the BAEP generators. In human patients, BAEP abnormalities are highly correlated with difficulty in correctly lateralizing click pairs with interaural time delays.[40, 106] In contrast, pure tone audiometry and speech discrimination may be normal in patients with grossly abnormal BAEPs.[40, 49, 70]

Wave I

Wave I has been clearly identified with the N1 component of the eighth nerve compound action potential (8NCAP) in many studies, including simultaneous recordings from surface electrodes and ear canal, tympanic membrane, or transtympanic electrodes.[14, 38, 48, 79, 85] Its origin in the distal portion of the eighth nerve is consistent with its surface topography, which shows a circumscribed negativity ipsilateral to the stimulated ear,[44] its presence in some patients who fulfill clinical and EEG criteria for brain death[33, 88, 89, 92, 95] (see Figs. 1 and 2), and its persistence after section of the

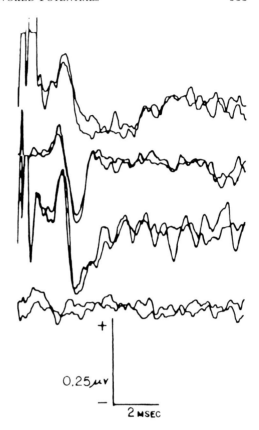

Figure 1. BAEPs from four patients fulfilling clinical and EEG criteria for brain death. Wave I is present in three cases, followed by an even larger wave IN in two. Positivity is plotted as an upward deflection in the waveform. (*Adapted from* Starr A: Auditory brain-stem responses in brain death. Brain 99:543–554, 1976; with permission.)

0.25 μv

2 MSEC

intracranial portion of the eighth nerve in some cases of surgery for acoustic neuroma[56, 80] (see Fig. 3). Wave I may be absent or abnormal preoperatively in some patients with eighth-nerve tumors[56, 81, 94, 95] or basilar artery thrombosis,[29] presumably owing to interference with the blood supply of the cochlea.[19, 21, 29] It is usually intact with lesions confined to the brain stem.[38, 90] A case of unilateral wave I absence with a brain-stem glioma infiltrating the cochlear nuclei has been reported,[89, 90] but that loss of wave I could have been due to vascular compromise or to coincidental ear disease.

Recordings from the intracranial eighth nerve[39, 87] contain an initial positivity corresponding to wave I and reflecting outward transmembrane current flow driven by the depolarization in the distal part of the nerve (see Fig. 4). This is followed by a negative peak (N1) whose latency varies with recording electrode position, reflecting the arrival of the propagating action potential at the site of the recording electrode.

Wave I may also receive a contribution from the cochlear summating potential, which precedes and overlaps with the N1 8NCAP in recordings from the human external auditory meatus[9] and contributes to the homologue of wave I in the monkey.[54, 55] The cochlear microphonic is usually obscured by the electrical stimulus artifact unless piezoelectric headphones are used.[43]

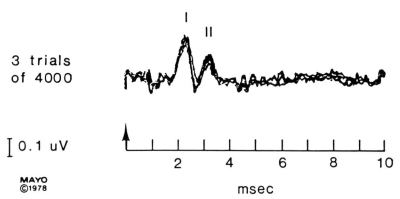

♀ : age 52

3 trials
of 4000

I 0.1 uV

MAYO
©1978

msec

Figure 2. BAEPs in a patient with complete brain death, including necrosis of the cochlear nuclei, verified at postmortem examination. Waves I and II are both present. Simultaneous electrocochleography suggested that the latter originated in the N2 component of the 8NCAP. Positivity plotted upward. (*From* Stockard JJ, Stockard JE, Sharbrough FW: Brainstem auditory evoked potentials in neurology: Methodology, interpretation, and clinical application. *In* Aminoff MJ (ed): Electrodiagnosis in Clinical Neurology. Ed 2. New York, Churchill Livingstone, pp. 467–503, 1986; with permission.)

Wave IN

Wave I is often followed by a prominent negative peak, IN, corresponding to positivity at the mastoid[44] and in the electrocochleogram.[14, 79, 85] A negativity at the same latency is recorded from the eighth nerve at the internal auditory meatus[39] (see Fig. 4), suggesting that the IN peak reflects the reversal of eighth-nerve transmembrane current flow with arrival of the N1 volley at the internal auditory meatus. This is confirmed in experimental animals where inactivation of the intracranial eighth nerve reduces or eliminates the second peak at each recording site but spares the initial

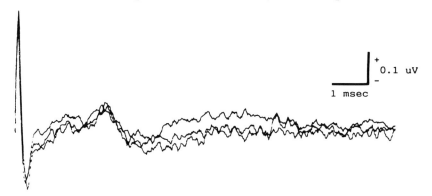

Figure 3. Intraoperative BAEP to left ear stimulation, recorded after sacrifice of the intracranial eighth nerve during resection of a left-sided acoustic neuroma. Wave I is still present. Vertex to left earlobe recording, bandpass 150 Hz to 3000 Hz, three averages of 2000 sweeps superimposed. Positivity plotted upward.

Figure 4. BAEPs recorded directly from the human eighth nerve at the internal auditory meatus (*top*) and at the cerebellopontine angle (*middle*) compared with the far-field scalp BAEPs (*bottom*). The onset and peak of P1 are coincident with those of the scalp-recorded wave I. Negativity plotted upward. (*From* Hashimoto I, Ishiyama Y, Yoshimoto T, et al: Brain stem auditory evoked potentials recorded directly from human brain stem and thalamus. Brain 104:841–859, 1981; with permission.)

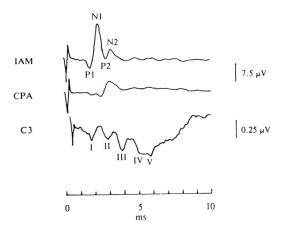

(wave I) peak.[57] A clear IN potential is visible in many of the published recordings from brain-dead patients who also exhibit a wave I[88, 89] and is sometimes even larger than wave I (see Fig. 1).

Wave II

The origin of wave II is controversial. Possible generators include the distal eighth nerve, the proximal eighth nerve, and the cochlear nucleus and/or its outflow.

Wave II has the same latency as the N2 component of the 8NCAP recorded from ear canal, tympanic membrane, and transtympanic middle ear electrodes.[31, 85] Recordings from the eighth nerve at the internal auditory meatus reveal two positive/negative biphasic components[39, 87] (see Fig. 4). The positivities, which coincide with waves I and II, at least in part reflect depolarization of the distal eighth nerve. When BAEP topography is analyzed with a volume conduction model, the source that gives rise to wave I, and thus represents the distal eighth nerve, also makes a large contribution to wave II.[82]

The contribution to wave II from the second volley (N2) in the distal eighth nerve is clearly a significant one. It accounts for the presence of wave II in patients with acoustic neuromas that eliminate all later waves[90, 95] (see Fig. 5), in a patient with a lower brain-stem lesion that compromised the proximal eighth nerve as far as the internal auditory meatus (wave IN was eliminated),[17] and in some brain-dead patients[33, 95] (see Fig. 2).

Intracranial recordings from the human eighth nerve are dominated by a large negativity that recordings at multiple sites along the nerve reveal to be the propagating 8NCAP[39, 65] (see Fig. 4). At the brain stem, the peak latency of this negativity approximates that of wave II, suggesting a contribution to that wave from the N1 volley in the proximal eighth nerve.

Wave II is the earliest component affected by pontomedullary cerebrovascular accidents involving the cochlear nucleus.[93] This has usually been taken to imply that a major generator of wave II is within the brain stem, probably the cochlear nucleus or its outflow. Wave II is also abnormal

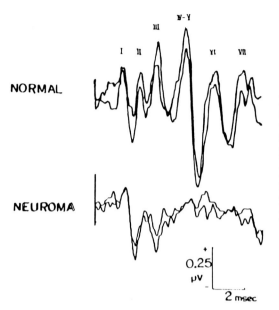

Figure 5. Presence of waves I, IN, II, and IIN but absence of all subsequent waves in a patient with an acoustic neuroma. Positivity plotted upward. (*Adapted from* Starr A, Hamilton AE: Correlation between confirmed sites of neurological lesions and abnormalities of far-field auditory brainstem responses. Electroencephalogr Clin Neurophysiol 41:595–608, 1976; with permission.)

in some patients with cerebellopontine angle tumors damaging the eighth nerve in whom wave I is unaffected.[93]

Hashimoto and colleagues[39] concluded from their intracranial recordings that wave II contains contributions from both the eighth nerve and the brain stem. They recorded a phasic positivity coincident with wave II over the dorsal pons (see Fig. 6), with gradients demonstrating its near-field nature. This peak can be traced continuously to the far field, although it undergoes a complex series of latency shifts at serial recording sites within the ventricular system.[39] In contrast, from their recordings from the intracranial eighth nerve and estimates of eighth-nerve conduction times, Møller and Jannetta[65, 66] felt that timing considerations rule out a contribution of postsynaptic cochlear nucleus activity to wave II.

A contribution to wave II from postsynaptic cochlear nucleus activity can be reconciled with the timing of the 8NCAP at the brain stem, because the BAEPs are derived from the fastest subsystem within the subcortical auditory pathway. Activity in the fastest eighth nerve fibers reaches its proximal end earlier than the peak latency of the 8NCAP, which reflects the summated activity of the entire eighth nerve. Indeed, the onset of the near-field wave II negativity over the proximal eighth nerve[39, 65] or medial to the cochlear nucleus[62] precedes its peak by 0.5 to 1.0 msec in published data not subjected to digital filtering (see Figs. 4 and 7). Digital filtering tends to narrow the peaks and may even convert the leading edge of the negativity into a positivity (see Fig. 7A and 7B). With a 0.6 msec synaptic delay for the fastest synapses within the cochlear nucleus,[55, 75] the earliest cochlear nucleus outflow will coincide with the peak of the total 8NCAP.

The estimates of eighth-nerve conduction times[66] were based on two studies[22, 51] reporting that over 75 per cent of cochlear division fibers are less than 5 μm in diameter. In contrast, a more recent study[72] found that

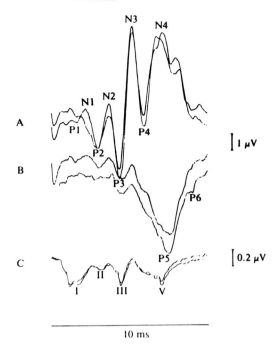

Figure 6. Human BAEPs recorded at operation from the midline dorsal pons at the level of the facial colliculi (A) and from the midline dorsal mesencephalon at the level of the inferior colliculi (B), compared with the far-field BAEP (C). Negativity plotted upward. Binaural stimulation. (*From* Hashimoto I, Ishiyama Y, Yoshimoto T, et al: Brain-stem auditory evoked potentials recorded directly from human brain stem and thalamus. Brain 104:841–859, 1981; with permission.)

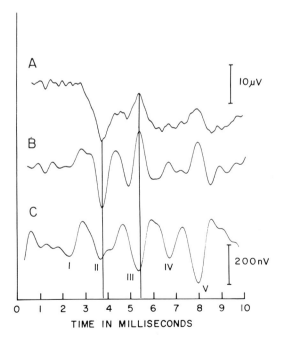

Figure 7. Human BAEPs recorded at operation from the medial side of the inferior cerebellar peduncle, presumably in close proximity to the cochlear nucleus, during surgery in a patient with a fourth ventricular tumor, before (A) and after (B) digital filtering, compared to far-field BAEPs (C). Negativity plotted upward. (*From* Møller AR, Jannetta PJ: Auditory evoked potentials recorded from the cochlear nucleus and its vicinity in man. J Neurosurg 59:1013–1018, 1983; with permission.)

almost half the fibers are larger than 5 μm. A large population of fibers between 3 and 5 μm in diameter[72] would give rise to an 8NCAP peak propagating at between 10 and 20 m/sec, as confirmed by intracranial recordings.[39, 65] But 25 per cent of the fibers are larger than 7 μm[72]; their activity could easily reach the eighth nerve terminals 0.5 to 0.6 msec earlier than the peak of the total 8NCAP.

The pathologic data are compatible with a purely peripheral origin for wave II, because the far-field peak generated by the distal eighth nerve may originate in the nerve terminals,[55] which are within the substance of the cochlear nucleus and will be damaged by any lesion affecting it. Conversely, postsynaptic cochlear nucleus activity may give rise to the large wave II recorded near the cochlear nucleus (see Fig. 7), which Møller and Jannetta[62] interpreted as arising from the eighth nerve. The existence of a postsynaptic, centrally generated contribution to wave II is demonstrated by intracranial recordings[39] and supported by clinical evidence.[41]

Furthermore, a purely peripheral origin of wave II implies that wave III must be generated by the cochlear nucleus outflow owing to timing considerations,[62] but the bilateral origin of wave III (see below) implies a generator at or above the level of the trapezoid body/superior olivary complex. Moreover, the length of the conduction pathway from cochlear nucleus to contralateral inferior colliculus in humans is approximately 46 mm.[68] The human lateral lemniscus contains "a relatively homogeneous population of lightly myelinated axons, 2–4 μm in diameter,"[67] diameters similar to those used in the estimates of eighth-nerve conduction times.[65] Assuming a similar conduction velocity of 10 to 20 m/sec, the conduction time from cochlear nucleus to the contralateral mesencephalon would be 2.3 to 4.6 msec. Because wave V is generated, at least in part, in the contralateral mesencephalon (see below), and the average normal III–V interpeak latency is 1.8 to 1.9 msec,[12, 28, 93, 96, 97] wave III cannot represent the earliest cochlear nucleus activity. This supports the presence of postsynaptic cochlear nucleus activity at the latency of wave II.

Wave IIN

As is wave I, BAEP wave II is sometimes followed by a negative peak, labeled IIN. It appears in part to reflect arrival of the N2 component of the 8NCAP at the internal auditory meatus, where a negativity of approximately the same latency may be recorded[39] (see Fig. 4). As with IN, IIN may be recorded from patients in whom acoustic neuromas have eliminated all centrally generated BAEP components[90] (see Fig. 5).

Wave III

Human lesion data localize the major generators of wave III to the caudal pontine tegmentum. Most patients with lesions in this region that involve the superior olivary complex have a normal wave II but abnormal wave III.[93, 97, 105] Wave III is present and usually normal in patients with lesions confined to the middle or upper pons or mesencephalon,[89, 90, 93, 97] though occasionally it is delayed (see Fig. 8). In most patients with asymmetrical lesions, wave III is more abnormal following stimulation of the ear ipsilateral to the major pathology,[5, 28] but occasionally it is more

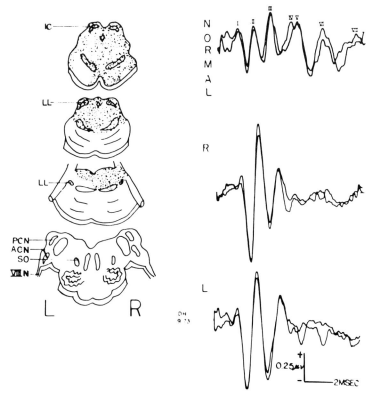

Figure 8. Presence of waves I through III, but loss of later waves, in a patient in whom a germinoma destroyed most of the mesencephalon and pons, including the right but not the left lateral lemniscus. The latencies of waves II and III were abnormally delayed, but those of wave I were normal. Positivity plotted upward. (*From* Starr A, Hamilton AE: Correlation between confirmed sites of neurological lesions and abnormalities of far-field auditory brainstem responses. Electroencephalogr Clin Neurophysiol 41:595–608, 1976; with permission.)

abnormal with contralateral stimulation.[93] This localizes a major generator of wave III to a level at or above the pontine tegmentum where the ascending auditory pathways decussate.

Human intracranial recordings demonstrate a large phasic positivity over the dorsal pons that coincides with wave III (see Fig. 6), but they do not precisely localize the generator.[39] The positivity is smaller over the dorsal mesencephalon, perhaps reflecting the termination of some axons in pontine structures, so that fewer reach the inferior colliculus. Latency shifts as a function of rostrocaudal position in human intracranial recordings[16, 39] support a contribution from activity ascending in the lateral lemniscus.

The human wave III is most likely a composite, as is suggested by its occasional bifid waveform[12] and its alteration by unilateral lesions of either side. It may therefore reflect activity originating in the superior olives and ascending in the lateral lemnisci bilaterally.

Møller and Jannetta[62] ascribed wave III to the cochlear nucleus, based on the presence of a large-amplitude peak of the same latency recorded in the vicinity of that structure, and they concluded that wave II is generated

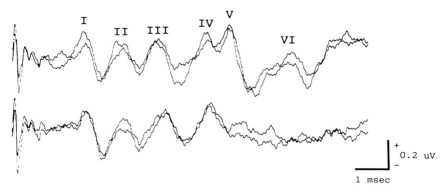

Figure 9. BAEPs recorded during surgery for a basilar artery aneurysm. The aneurysm ruptured immediately after the upper recordings were taken, and the basilar artery was transiently clipped in order to control the bleeding. The lower recordings, taken after the clip was removed, demonstrate a loss of wave V and VI, which persisted. Waves I through IV were unaffected. Left ear stimulation, vertex to left earlobe recording, bandpass 150 Hz to 3000 Hz, two averages of 2000 sweeps superimposed. Positivity plotted upward.

entirely within the eighth nerve (as previously mentioned). Again, however, activity of postsynaptic cochlear nucleus neurons at the latency of wave II is both compatible with the eighth-nerve data and supported by other experimental data, and the largest peak recorded near the cochlear nucleus corresponds to wave II (see Fig. 7). Thus, a contribution to wave III from third-order auditory neurons of the superior olivary complex is not ruled out by timing considerations. A contribution from second-order auditory neurons, driven by eighth-nerve fibers firing at the peak of the 8NCAP, is also possible.

Because waves I, IN, II, and IIN all originate, at least in part, in the eighth nerve, they may be recorded in patients with total brain-stem necrosis. The presence of wave III, however, is not compatible with brain death.

Wave IV

The major generators of wave IV are in close proximity to those of wave V, because they are usually either both affected or both unaffected by brain-stem lesions. They are not identical, however, because they may be differentially affected by multilevel demyelination.[93] Intraoperative BAEP monitoring has also demonstrated dissociation of the generators (see Fig. 9).

Absence of wave IV in a single patient with a brain-stem lesion does not identify its generator, because a separate wave IV cannot be identified in all normal subjects.[12] However, wave IV has been noted to be abnormal, along with wave V, in a series of patients with tumors or cerebrovascular accidents of the midpons or rostral pons.[90, 93, 97]

Intracranial recordings demonstrate a large phasic positivity over the dorsal pons that coincides with wave IV[39] (see Fig. 6). It is smaller over the dorsal mesencephalon, perhaps reflecting the termination of some lemniscal axons caudal to the inferior colliculus. In intraventricular recordings,[39] the latency of the wave IV peak systematically increases as the electrode is

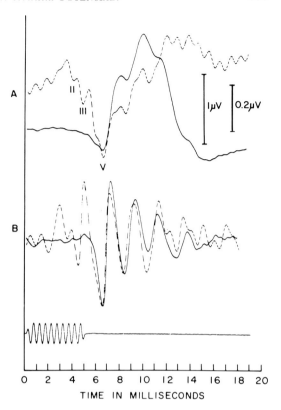

Figure 10. BAEPs recorded at operation from the human inferior colliculus (solid lines) compared to the far-field BAEP (dashed lines). A, Low-pass filtered waveforms. B, Digitally filtered waveforms. Monaural contralateral stimulation. Negativity plotted upward. (*From* Møller AR, Jannetta PJ: Interpretation of brainstem auditory evoked potentials: Results from intracranial recordings in humans. Scand Audiol 12:125–133, 1983; with permission.)

moved rostrally, consistent with propagating action potentials within the ascending brain-stem auditory pathways. Because these recordings were done with binaural stimulation, the relative contributions of crossed and uncrossed fibers cannot be assessed.

Thus, wave IV appears to predominantly reflect activity in ascending auditory fibers within the dorsal and rostral pons. Although the nucleus of the lateral lemniscus has been implicated as a BAEP generator in animal studies,[7, 42] human data are insufficient to confirm its contribution to wave IV.

Wave V

Waves IV and V are the earliest components that are absent, and usually the earliest that are abnormal, in patients with tumors or cerebrovascular accidents of the midpons, rostral pons, or mesencephalon.[89, 90, 93, 97] Occasionally, waves II and III are delayed in latency with rostral brainstem tumors[89, 90] (see Fig. 8). This may be due to pressure on more caudal structures, or perhaps may reflect damage to descending pathways.[36]

With contralateral stimulation, BAEPs recorded over the human inferior colliculus[64] or from depth electrodes near it[16] display a large positivity whose latency matches that of wave V (see Fig. 10); the ipsilateral near-field responses are smaller and do not match the latency of wave V as well.

In a study employing binaural stimulation,[39] a large mesencephalic positivity that overlaps with wave V is noted to invert in polarity over the dorsal pons, in contrast to earlier waves that do not invert (see Fig. 6). The large positivity contains several inflections, suggesting multiple generators. In recordings from electrodes within the human ventricular system,[39] wave V is maximal at the level of the inferior colliculus, and also inverts to a negativity at more caudal recording locations within the fourth ventricle.

These data suggest that wave V predominantly reflects activity of auditory neurons at the mesencephalic level, with activity in the area of the contralateral inferior colliculus making a larger contribution than ipsilateral activity. Clinically, however, unilateral abnormalities of wave V are most often associated with ipsilateral pathology.[5, 28, 105] On the scalp, the maximal amplitude for wave V is found in the midline.[44] Some authors[62, 63] have suggested that the fibers terminating in the inferior colliculus may make a more significant contribution than the activity of collicular neurons themselves. This may be due to the lateral orientation of the brachium of the inferior colliculus, which would reduce its contribution to the vertex waveform.

The largest peak of the monkey BAEP, which closely resembles the human wave V,[54] similarly reflects activity in the mesencephalon contralateral more than ipsilateral.[55] However, it also contains contributions from the medial geniculate nucleus/auditory radiations and the lateral lemniscus; the latter reflects multiple volleys in auditory structures caudal to the inferior colliculus.

The absence of wave V in patients with lesions that destroy the midbrain[89, 90] suggests that more caudal generators may not be clinically important in humans. The presence of a normal wave V in patients with rostral midbrain or supratentorial lesions[38, 93] does not rule out the possibility of geniculate contributions, because the preserved mesencephalic structures could produce a wave V of acceptable amplitude and normal latency. Any lesion that eliminates the mesencephalic contribution will remove the auditory input to the geniculate.

Human depth recordings within the medial geniculate suggest that activity in this structure contributes to wave V. They contain large peaks coincident with surface waves V and VI[15, 39, 102] (see Fig. 11). The positive peaks can be traced continuously to the far field,[39] though the wave V peak has a lower spatial gradient and may in part reflect activity volume conducted to the geniculate from more caudal auditory structures.

Wave VI

Abnormalities of wave VI, with normal waves I through V, have been described[93] in patients with tumors of the rostral midbrain and caudal thalamus (at the level of the medial geniculate and brachium of the inferior colliculus), suggesting that wave VI is generated in the area of the medial geniculate. The clinical-pathologic correlations must be interpreted with caution, because wave VI is absent in vertex-to-ear recordings in many normal people.[12] Depth recordings within the human medial geniculate demonstrate large peaks, either positive[37, 39] (see Fig. 11) or negative,[102] coincident with wave VI. The positivities can be continuously traced to the

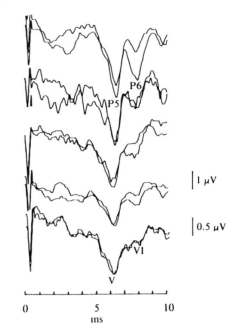

MGB

Figure 11. BAEPs recorded by a depth electrode passed through the human thalamus, through or near the medial geniculate. The two large positive peaks are traced to the scalp (*bottom waveform*). Binaural stimulation. Negativity is plotted upward. (*From* Hashimoto I, Ishiyama Y, Yoshimoto T, et al: Brain-stem auditory evoked potentials recorded directly from human brain stem and thalamus. Brain 104:841–859, 1981; with permission.)

far-field wave VI, with gradients indicating generation within the medial geniculate.[39] Differences in the placement of the electrodes relative to the equivalent dipole may account for the polarity differences of both the wave V and the wave VI peaks within the geniculate.

Topographic data support a geniculate generator of wave VI. Activity propagating along axons of medial geniculate neurons within the auditory radiations produces far-field potentials that are maximal in the direction of propagation.[60, 104] Wave VI is larger at lateral than at midline electrodes,[61, 91] and a detailed topographic study[44] reveals multiple maxima, some on the midline and some far lateral, suggesting multiple generators.

In the monkey, continued activity in the inferior colliculus also contributes to the homologue of wave VI,[55] and in humans a large wave VI peak is recorded from electrodes placed directly on the inferior colliculus, visible when the large slow-wave components generated there are removed by filtering[64] (see Fig. 10). Thus, the inferior colliculus may contribute to the human wave VI.

Wave VII

Wave VII is so often absent in conventionally recorded normal BAEPs[26] that its absence in pathologic conditions cannot be used for generator localization. A normal wave VI but a delayed wave VII was described in a single patient who had "evidence of deep hemispheric damage bilaterally" with absent middle latency auditory evoked potentials and who was clinically unresponsive to sound.[93] This raises the possibility that wave VII reflects activity in the distal portions of the auditory radiations, with separate peaks generated by activity at the initial and terminal parts of the axons, as is the case for the eighth nerve. Waves I through VII were all normal in another cortically deaf patient with bilateral temporal lobe infarctions,[74] however, which argues against a generator at the most distal part of the auditory radiations.

Surface topography supports a predominantly contralateral generator for wave VII near auditory cortex.[44] Published data from subdural, cortical surface, and depth recordings near human primary auditory cortex[8, 32, 52] have not identified BAEP generators there, however, probably because of methodologic factors.

There is also a large near-field peak at the latency of wave VII or its homologue in the region of the inferior colliculus in both humans[64] (see Fig. 10) and monkeys[55]; the latter can be traced continuously to the far field, whereas detailed mapping of the former has not been performed.

Slow Negativity (SN)

Intracranial recordings in the vicinity of the human brain stem record a large negativity that follows wave V in latency and is largest where wave V is largest, at the level of the inferior colliculus[37, 39, 63, 64] (see Fig. 10); it can be traced continuously to the far-field SN. In the monkey, this large negativity inverts in polarity across the outer cellular layers of the inferior colliculus.[55] In both species, its prolonged time course, as compared with the potentials generated within the lateral lemniscus, suggests that it reflects predominantly postsynaptic potentials within the inferior colliculus. Slow potentials derived from synaptic activity in more caudal structures overlap in time with those from the inferior colliculus in the monkey,[55] and may make minor contributions to the surface waveforms in both species. The medial geniculate does not contribute to the slow negativity in either species.[37, 55]

OTHER ASPECTS OF BAEP GENERATION

Action Potentials Versus Synaptic Potentials

BAEPs were initially attributed to propagating action potentials within brain stem auditory pathways,[48] but more recently the possible role of postsynaptic potentials has been stressed.[6] The phasic potentials (waves I through VII) originate in action potentials propagating within the eighth nerve and the central auditory pathways. This is consistent with the duration of the individual peaks, and is confirmed by peak latency shifts when the recording electrode is moved along the human eighth nerve[39, 87] or along the brain stem auditory pathways in both humans[39] and experimental animals.[1, 55] Only the SN derives from postsynaptic potentials.

Effects of Fiber Tract Geometry and Media Inhomogeneities

The vertex-positive phasic BAEPs were initially assumed[45, 48] to be the positive peaks that may be seen in advance of a propagating action potential when the recording electrode is situated distal to the axon terminals.[60, 104] Recently, mathematical models and studies of peripheral nerves have emphasized the role of fiber tract geometry and changes in the impedance

Table 1. *Generators of Human BAEPs*

WAVE	GENERATORS
I	8NCAP (N1) in the distal eighth nerve
	Cochlear summating potential?
IN	8NCAP (N1) at the internal auditory meatus
II	8NCAP (N2) in the distal eighth nerve
	8NCAP (N1) in the proximal eighth nerve
	Cochlear nucleus activity/outflow
IIN	8NCAP (N2) at the internal auditory meatus
III	Activity/outflow of the superior olivary complex, bilateral
	Cochlear nucleus activity/outflow?
IV	Ascending auditory fibers in dorsal and rostral pons
V	Activity in the area of the inferior colliculi (afferent fibers and/or activity/outflow of collicular neurons)
	Activity/outflow of the medial geniculate nuclei
VI	Activity/outflow of the medial geniculate nuclei
	Activity in the area of the inferior colliculi?
VII	Activity in the distal auditory radiations?
	Activity in the area of the inferior colliculi?
SN	Postsynaptic potentials in the inferior colliculi
	Postsynaptic potentials in other brain-stem auditory nuclei?

8NCAP = eighth-nerve compound action potential.

of surrounding tissues in the generation of far-field potentials.[13, 50] This is illustrated by waves IN and IIN, which are produced by the transition of the 8NCAP volleys from the eighth nerve within the bony internal auditory canal to the nerve lying free within the posterior fossa subarachnoid space. Nonetheless, peak latency shifts in intracranial recordings have confirmed that far-field potentials may be generated by action potentials propagating within brain stem parenchyma without impedance discontinuities.

Role of Descending Inhibitory Pathways

With lesions of the rostral brain stem, waves I and II are often quite large (for example, see Fig. 8). Although BAEP amplitudes are variable across subjects, growth of wave I concurrently with attenuation of later waves in the same subject has been observed in preterminal patients who subsequently developed brain death[30, 35] and in a monkey with a rostral brain-stem lesion.[53] Wave I decreased while wave V increased in amplitude following removal of an extra-axial tumor that was compressing the brain stem in another patient.[71]

The enlarged wave I most likely reflects loss of descending inhibitory pathways.[30, 69] Although absolute amplitudes are generally not used as criteria for classification of BAEPs, the V/I amplitude ratio is of clinical utility.[3] Growth of I concurrent with attenuation of V may therefore enhance the sensitivity of this measure in the detection of rostral brain-stem damage.

SUMMARY

The generators of human BAEPs, as summarized in Table 1 and Figure 12, are more complex than has often been presumed. Most peaks reflect

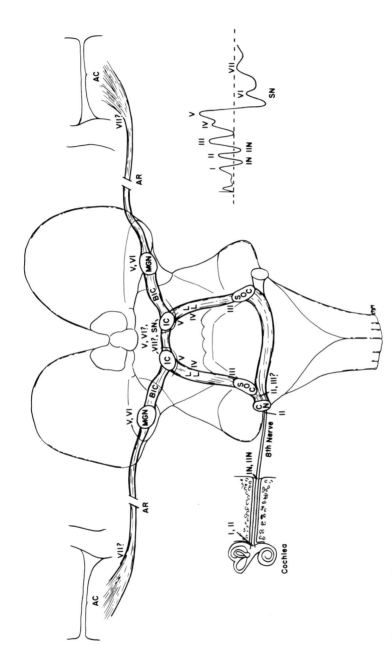

Figure 12. Summary diagram showing the probable generators of the human BAEPs, as recorded between the vertex and the stimulated ear. The slow negativity (SN) originates in postsynaptic potentials, but the other labeled peaks reflect action potentials within the subcortical auditory pathways. AC = auditory cortex; AR = auditory radiations; BIC = brachium of the inferior colliculus; CN = cochlear nucleus; IC = inferior colliculus; LL = lateral lemniscus; MGN = medial geniculate nucleus; SOC = superior olivary complex.

Figure 13. BAEPs were recorded at several sites along a depth pass through auditory cortex in a monkey. *A*, The grand average of the far-field BAEPs recorded simultaneously from the vertex. *B*, The average of the BAEPs recorded by the depth electrode. As the electrode was at different positions, this does not represent the BAEP waveform seen at any physical location. Rather, it serves to indicate the average latencies of the components for comparison to *C*, which is the standard deviation among the set of depth-recorded BAEP waveforms. The peaks corresponding to monkey waves 7b and 8 indicate that they were near-field potentials, which changed considerably during the depth pass, whereas the earlier BAEP components did not. Contralateral click stimulation. Monkey wave 7b usually overlaps with wave 7 in the far field, and waves 7 and 8 are most likely homologous to human waves V and VI. Positivity plotted upward. (*Adapted from* Legatt AD, Arezzo JC, Vaughan HG Jr: Short-latency auditory evoked potentials in the monkey. II. Intracranial generators. Electroencephalogr Clin Neurophysiol 64:53–73, 1986; with permission.)

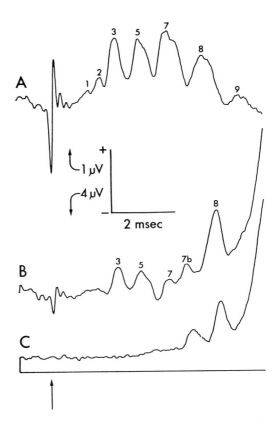

activity in several structures, though patterns of BAEP abnormality can be correlated with abnormalities in general areas of the brain stem. The phasic peaks originate in action potentials, whereas the SN reflects postsynaptic potentials within brain-stem auditory nuclei.

FUTURE DIRECTIONS

Waves VI and VII are not present in conventionally recorded BAEPs in many normal individuals,[12, 26] which limits their clinical utility. Electrodes off the midline may record larger waves VI[44, 61, 91] and VII[44] than those at the vertex. Changes in filter settings may increase the prevalence of an identifiable wave VII.[26] Because the BAEP components are differentially affected by changes in stimulus parameters like rate,[20, 83] alterations in stimulus paradigms may also yield more consistent waves VI and VII and permit testing of the subcortical auditory pathways rostral to the inferior colliculi.

A possible wave VII generator in the distal auditory radiations has not heretofore been confirmed by intracranial recordings in humans, probably because of methodologic factors. Analysis of spatial gradients of such data can identify locally generated components[55] (see Fig. 13), and may allow identification of such a generator in the future.

The phasic peaks I through VII are identified in a standard vertex-to-ipsilateral ear recording configuration. In the future, analysis of three-channel Lissajous's trajectories or detailed topographic mappings, as well as modifications of recording techniques, may permit recording of BAEP components that more accurately represent the patterns of activity of the underlying generators. After validation with intracranial recordings and clinical correlations, these may permit a more detailed understanding of the genesis of human BAEPs and further increase their clinical utility and specificity.

REFERENCES

1. Achor LJ, Starr A: Auditory brain stem responses in the cat. I. Intracranial and extracranial recordings. Electroencephalogr Clin Neurophysiol 48:154–173, 1980
2. Achor LJ, Starr A: Auditory brain stem responses in the cat. II. Effects of lesions. Electroencephalogr Clin Neurophysiol 48:174–190, 1980
3. American Electroencephalographic Society: Guidelines for clinical evoked potential studies. J Clin Neurophysiol 1:3–53, 1984
4. Arezzo J, Legatt AD, Vaughan HG Jr: Topography and intracranial sources of somatosensory evoked potentials in the monkey. I. Early components. Electroencephalogr Clin Neurophysiol 46:155–172, 1979
5. Brown RH Jr, Chiappa KH, Brooks E: Brain stem auditory evoked responses in 22 patients with intrinsic brain stem lesions: Implications for clinical interpretations. Electroencephalogr Clin Neurophysiol 52:38P, 1981
6. Buchwald JS: Generators. *In* Moore EJ (ed): Bases of Auditory Brain-Stem Evoked Responses. New York, Grune and Stratton, 1983, pp 157–195
7. Buchwald JS, Huang C-M: Far-field acoustic response: Origins in the cat. Science 189:382–384, 1975
8. Celesia GG: Organization of auditory cortical areas in man. Brain 99:403–414, 1976
9. Chatrian GE, Wirch AL, Edwards KH, et al: Cochlear summating potential recorded from the external auditory meatus of normal humans. Amplitude-intensity functions and relationships to auditory nerve compound action potential. Electroencephalogr Clin Neurophysiol 59:396–410, 1984
10. Chiappa K: The use of evoked potentials in clinical practice with special reference to the diagnosis of multiple sclerosis. Neurol Clin 6:861–880, 1988
11. Chiappa K: Evoked Potentials in Clinical Medicine. New York, Raven Press, 1983
12. Chiappa K, Gladstone KJ, Young RR: Brain stem auditory evoked responses. Studies of waveform variations in 50 normal human subjects. Arch Neurol 36:81–87, 1979
13. Chimento TC, Williston JS, Jewett DL, et al: The 3-channel Lissajous' trajectory of the auditory brain-stem response. VIII. Isolated frog sciatic nerve in a volume conductor. Electroencephalogr Clin Neurophysiol 68:380–385, 1987
14. Cohen D, Sohmer H: Comparison of earlobe and promontorium recording sites in electrocochleography. Audiology 16:462–468, 1977
15. Cohen J, Harner RN, Sussman NM, et al: Origin of late components of the brain-stem auditory evoked response (BAER). Electroencephalogr Clin Neurophysiol 61:22P, 1985
16. Curio G, Oppel F: Intraparenchymatous ponto-mesencephalic field distribution of brain-stem auditory evoked potentials in man. Electroencephalogr Clin Neurophysiol 69:259–265, 1988
17. Curio G, Oppel F, Scherg M: Peripheral origin of BAEP wave II in a case with unilateral pontine pathology: A comparison of intracranial and scalp recordings. Electroencephalogr Clin Neurophysiol 66:29–33, 1987

18. Davis H, Hirsh SK: A slow brain stem response for low-frequency audiometry. Audiology 18:445–461, 1979

19. De Moura LFP: Inner ear pathology in acoustic neurinoma. Arch Otolaryngol 85:125–133, 1967

20. Don M, Allen AR, Starr A: Effect of click rate on the latency of auditory brain stem responses in humans. Ann Otol Rhinol Laryngol 86:186–195, 1977

21. Eggermont JJ, Don M: Mechanisms of central conduction time prolongation in brainstem auditory evoked potentials. Arch Neurol 43:116–120, 1986

22. Engström H, Rexed B: Über die Kaliberverhältnisse der Nervenfasern im N. stato-acusticus des Menschen. Z Mikr-anat Forsch 47:448–455, 1940

23. Epstein C: The use of brainstem auditory evoked potentials in the evaluation of the central nervous system. Neurol Clin 6:771–790, 1988

24. Erwin CW, Radtke R: The use of somatosensory and brainstem auditory evoked potentials in monitoring brain stem function intraoperatively. Neurol Clin 6:899–916, 1988

25. Evans EF, Nelson PG: On the functional relationship between the dorsal and ventral divisions of the cochlear nucleus of the cat. Exp Brain Res 17:428–442, 1973

26. Fabiani M, Casini A, Marullo T: Wave VII recognizability in brainstem auditory-evoked potentials. Acta Neurol Scand 67:312–315, 1983

27. Fabiani M, Sohmer H, Tait C, et al: A functional measure of brain activity: Brain stem transmission time. Electroencephalogr Clin Neurophysiol 47:483–491, 1979

28. Faught E, Oh SJ: Brainstem auditory evoked responses in brainstem infarction. Stroke 16:701–705, 1985

29. Ferbert A, Buchner H, Bruckmann H, et al: Evoked potentials in basilar artery thrombosis: Correlation with clinical and angiographic findings. Electroencephalogr Clin Neurophysiol 69:136–147, 1988

30. Garcia-Larrea L, Bertrand O, Artru F, et al: Brain-stem monitoring. II. Preterminal BAEP changes observed until brain death in deeply comatose patients. Electroencephalogr Clin Neurophysiol 68:446–457, 1987

31. Gersdorff MCK: Simultaneous recordings of human auditory potentials: Transtympanic electrocochleography (ECoG) and brainstem-evoked responses (BER). Arch Otorhinolaryngol 234:15–20, 1982

32. Goff WR, Allison T, Lyons W, et al: Origins of short latency auditory evoked potentials in man. In Desmedt JE (ed): Auditory Evoked Potentials in Man. Psychopharmacology Correlates of Evoked Potentials. Prog Clin Neurophysiol 2:30–44, 1977

33. Goldie WD, Chiappa K, Young RR: Brainstem auditory evoked responses and short latency somatosensory evoked responses in the evaluation of deeply comatose patients. Acta Neurol Scand 60(suppl 73):71, 1979

34. Grandori F: Field analysis of auditory evoked brainstem potentials. Hearing Res 21:51–58, 1986

35. Hall JW III, Mackey-Hargadine JR, Kim EE: Auditory brain-stem response in determination of brain death. Arch Otolaryngol 111:613–620, 1985

36. Harrison JM, Howe ME: Anatomy of the descending auditory system (mammalian). In Keidel WD, Neff WD (eds): Auditory System. Handbook of Sensory Physiology. Vol 5. Part 1. Berlin, Springer-Verlag, 1974, pp 363–388

37. Hashimoto I: Auditory evoked potentials from the human midbrain: Slow brain stem responses. Electroencephalogr Clin Neurophysiol 53:652–657, 1982

38. Hashimoto I, Ishiyama Y, Tozuka G: Bilaterally recorded brainstem auditory evoked responses: Their asymmetric abnormalities and lesions of the brainstem. Arch Neurol 36:161–167, 1979

39. Hashimoto I, Ishiyama Y, Yoshimoto T, et al: Brain-stem auditory evoked potentials recorded directly from human brain stem and thalamus. Brain 104:841–859, 1981

40. Hausler R, Levine RA: Brain stem auditory evoked potentials are related to interaural time discrimination in patients with multiple sclerosis. Brain Res 191:589–594, 1980

41. Hopf HC: Die Generatoren der AEP-Wellen II–III. Flogerungen aus Befunden bei definierten Hirnstammprozessen. Akt Neurol 12:58–61, 1985

42. Huang C-M, Buchwald JS: Interpretation of the vertex short-latency acoustic response: A study of single neurons in the brain stem. Brain Res 137:291–303, 1977

43. Hughes JR, Fino J: Usefulness of piezoelectric earphones in recording the brain stem auditory evoked potentials: A new early deflection. Electroencephalogr Clin Neurophysiol 48:357–360, 1980

44. Hughes JR, Fino JJ: A review of generators of the brainstem auditory evoked potential: Contribution of an experimental study. J Clin Neurophysiol 2:355–381, 1985
45. Jewett DL: Volume-conducted potentials in response to auditory stimuli as detected by averaging in the cat. Electroencephalogr Clin Neurophysiol 28:609–618, 1970
46. Jewett DL, Martin WH, Sininger Y, et al: The 3-channel Lissajous' trajectory of the auditory brain-stem response. I. Introduction and overview. Electroencephalogr Clin Neurophysiol 68:323–326, 1987
47. Jewett DL, Romano MN, Williston JS: Human auditory evoked potentials: Possible brain stem components detected at the scalp. Science 167:1517–1518, 1970
48. Jewett DL, Williston JS: Auditory-evoked far fields averaged from the scalp of humans. Brain 94:681–696, 1971
49. Kaga K, Shindo M, Tanaka Y: Auditory brain stem responses and nonsense monosyllable perception test findings for patients with auditory nerve and brain stem lesions. Laryngoscope 96:1272–1278, 1986
50. Kimura J, Kimura A, Ishida T, et al: What determines the latency and amplitude of stationary peaks in far-field recordings. Ann Neurol 19:479–486, 1986
51. Lazorthes G, Lacomme Y, Gaubert J, et al: La constitution du nerf auditif. Press Méd 69:1067–1068, 1961
52. Lee YS, Lueders H, Dinner DS, et al: Recording of auditory evoked potentials in man using chronic subdural electrodes. Brain 107:115–131, 1984
53. Legatt AD: Short Latency Auditory Evoked Potentials in the Monkey. Doctoral Dissertation, Albert Einstein College of Medicine, 1981
54. Legatt AD, Arezzo JC, Vaughan HG Jr: Short-latency auditory evoked potentials in the monkey. I. Wave shape and surface topography. Electroencephalogr Clin Neurophysiol 64:41–52, 1986
55. Legatt AD, Arezzo JC, Vaughan HG Jr: Short-latency auditory evoked potentials in the monkey. II. Intracranial generators. Electroencephalogr Clin Neurophysiol 64:53–73, 1986
56. Legatt AD, Pedley TA, Emerson RG, et al: Electrophysiological monitoring of seventh and eighth nerve function during surgery for acoustic neuromas. Electroencephalogr Clin Neurophysiol 64:30P, 1986
57. Legouix JP, Pierson A: Investigations on the sources of whole-nerve action potentials recorded from various places in the guinea pig cochlea. J Acoust Soc Am 56:1222–1225, 1974
58. Lev A, Sohmer H: Sources of averaged neural responses recorded in animal and human subjects during cochlear audiometry (electro-cochleogram). Arch Klin Exp Ohr Nas Kehlk Heilk 201:79–90, 1972
59. Lorente de Nó R: Action potentials of the motoneurons of the hypoglossus nucleus. J Cell Comp Physiol 29:207–287, 1947
60. Lorente de Nó R: Analysis of the distribution of the action currents of nerve in volume conductors. Stud Rockefeller Inst Med Res 132:384–497, 1947
61. Martin ME, Moore EJ: Scalp distribution of early (0 to 10 msec) auditory evoked responses. Arch Otolaryngol 103:326–328, 1977
62. Møller AR, Jannetta PJ: Auditory evoked potentials recorded from the cochlear nucleus and its vicinity in man. J Neurosurg 59:1013–1018, 1983
63. Møller AR, Jannetta PJ: Interpretation of brainstem auditory evoked potentials: Results from intracranial recordings in humans. Scand Audiol 12:125–133, 1983
64. Møller AR, Jannetta PJ: Evoked potentials from the inferior colliculus in man. Electroencephalogr Clin Neurophysiol 53:612–620, 1982
65. Møller AR, Jannetta PJ: Compound action potentials recorded intracranially from the auditory nerve in man. Exp Neurol 74:862–874, 1981
66. Møller AR, Jannetta PJ: Intracranially recorded responses from the human auditory nerve: New insights into the origin of brain stem evoked potentials (BSEPs). Electroencephalogr Clin Neurophysiol 52:18–27, 1981
67. Moore JK: The human auditory brain stem as a generator of auditory evoked potentials. Hearing Res 29:33–43, 1987
68. Moore JK: The human auditory brain stem: A comparative view. Hearing Res 29:1–32, 1987
69. Musiek FE: Neuroanatomy, neurophysiology, and central auditory assessment. Part III: Corpus callosum and efferent pathways. Ear Hearing 7:349–358, 1986

70. Musiek FE, Geurkink NA: Auditory brain stem response and central auditory test findings for patients with brain stem lesions: A preliminary report. Laryngoscope 92:891–900, 1982

71. Musiek FE, Weider DJ, Mueller RJ: Reversible audiological results in a patient with an extra-axial brainstem tumor. Ear Hearing 4:169–172, 1983

72. Natout MAY, Terr LI, Linthicum FH Jr, et al: Topography of vestibulocochlear nerve fibers in the posterior cranial fossa. Laryngoscope 97:954–958, 1987

73. Ornitz EM, Walter DO: The effect of sound pressure waveform on human brainstem auditory evoked responses. Brain Res 92:490–498, 1975

74. Özdamar Ö, Kraus N, Curry F: Auditory brain stem and middle latency responses in a patient with cortical deafness. Electroencephalogr Clin Neurophysiol 53:224–230, 1982

75. Pfeiffer RR: Anteroventral cochlear nucleus: Wave forms of extracellularly recorded spike potentials. Science 154:667–668, 1966

76. Picton TW: Auditory evoked potentials in the assessment of hearing. Neurol Clin 6:791–808, 1988

77. Picton TW, Taylor MJ, Durieux-Smith A, et al: Brainstem auditory evoked potentials in pediatrics. In Aminoff MJ (ed): Electrodiagnosis in Clinical Neurology. Ed 2. New York, Churchill Livingstone, 1986, pp 505–534

78. Plantz RG, Williston JS, Jewett DL: Spatio-temporal distribution of auditory-evoked far field potentials in rat and cat. Brain Res 68:55–71, 1974

79. Portmann M, Cazals Y, Negrevergne M, et al: Transtympanic and surface recordings in the diagnosis of retrocochlear disorders. Acta Otolaryngol 89:362–369, 1980

80. Raudzens PA, Shetter AG: Intraoperative monitoring of brain-stem auditory evoked potentials. J Neurosurg 57:341–348, 1982

81. Rosenhall U: Brain stem electrical responses in cerebello-pontine angle tumours. J Laryngol Otol 95:931–940, 1981

82. Scherg M, Von Cramon D: A new interpretation of the generators of BAEP waves I–V: Results of a spatio-temporal dipole model. Electroencephalogr Clin Neurophysiol 62:290–299, 1985

83. Scott ML, Harkins SW: Amplitude of the brainstem auditory evoked response: The effect of interstimulus interval. Int J Neurosci 8:147–152, 1978

84. Sininger Y, Gardi JN, Martin WH, et al: The 3-channel Lissajous' trajectory of the auditory brain-stem response. VII. Planar segments in humans. Electroencephalogr Clin Neurophysiol 68:368–379, 1987

85. Sohmer H, Feinmesser M: Cochlear action potentials recorded from the external ear in man. Ann Otol Rhinol Laryngol 76:427–435, 1967

86. Sohmer H, Feinmesser M, Szabo G: Sources of electrocochleographic responses as studied in patients with brain damage. Electroencephalogr Clin Neurophysiol 37:663–669, 1974

87. Spire JP, Dohrmann GJ, Prieto PS: Correlation of brainstem evoked response with direct acoustic nerve potential. In Courjon J, Mauguière F, Revol M (eds): Clinical Applications of Evoked Potentials in Neurology. New York, Raven Press, 1982, pp 159–167

88. Starr A: Auditory brain-stem responses in brain death. Brain 99:543–554, 1976

89. Starr A, Achor LJ: Auditory brain stem responses in neurological disease. Arch Neurol 32:761–768, 1975

90. Starr A, Hamilton AE: Correlation between confirmed sites of neurological lesions and abnormalities of far-field auditory brainstem responses. Electroencephalogr Clin Neurophysiol 41:595–608, 1976

91. Starr A, Squires K: Distribution of auditory brainstem potentials over the scalp and nasopharynx in humans. Ann NY Acad Sci 388:427–442, 1982

92. Steinhart CM, Weiss IP: Use of brainstem auditory evoked potentials in pediatric brain death. Crit Care Med 13:560–562, 1985

93. Stockard JJ, Rossiter VS: Clinical and pathologic correlates of brain stem auditory response abnormalities. Neurology 27:316–325, 1977

94. Stockard JJ, Sharbrough FW: Unique contributions of short-latency auditory and somatosensory evoked potentials to neurologic diagnosis. In Desmedt JE (ed): Clinical Uses of Cerebral, Brainstem and Spinal Somatosensory Evoked Potentials. Prog Clin Neurophysiol 7:231–262, 1980

95. Stockard JJ, Stockard JE, Sharbrough FW: Brainstem auditory evoked potentials in

neurology: Methodology, interpretation, and clinical application. *In* Aminoff MJ (ed): Electrodiagnosis in Clinical Neurology, 2nd ed. New York, Churchill Livingstone, 1986, pp 467–503

96. Stockard JJ, Stockard JE, Sharbrough FW: Nonpathologic factors influencing brainstem auditory evoked potentials. Am J EEG Technol 18:177–209, 1978
97. Stockard JJ, Stockard JE, Sharbrough FW: Detection and localization of occult lesions with brainstem auditory responses. Mayo Clin Proc 52:761–769, 1977
98. Strominger NL: The origins, course and distribution of the dorsal and intermediate acoustic striae in the rhesus monkey. J Comp Neurol 147:209–234, 1973
99. Strominger NL, Nelson LR, Dougherty WJ: Second-order auditory pathways in the chimpanzee. J Comp Neurol 172:349–366, 1977
100. Strominger NL, Strominger AI: Ascending brain stem projections of the anteroventral cochlear nucleus in the rhesus monkey. J Comp Neurol 143:217–242, 1971
101. Terkildsen K, Osterhammel P, Huis in't Veld F: Far field electrocochleography electrode positions. Scand Audiol 3:123–129, 1974
102. Velasco M, Velasco F, Almanza X, et al: Subcortical correlates of the auditory brain stem potentials in man: Bipolar EEG and multiple unit activity and electrical stimulation. Electroenceph Clin Neurophysiol 53:133–142, 1982
103. Velasco M, Velasco F, Almanza X, et al: Subcortical correlates of the auditory brain stem potentials in man: Referential EEG responses. Int J Neurosci 15:241–248, 1981
104. Woodbury JW: Potentials in a volume conductor. *In* Ruch TC, Patton HD, Woodbury JW, et al (eds): Neurophysiology, 2nd ed. Philadelphia, W. B. Saunders, 1965, pp 85–91
105. York DH: Correlation between a unilateral midbrain-pontine lesion and abnormalities of brain-stem auditory evoked potential. Electroencephalogr Clin Neurophysiol 65:282–288, 1986
106. Zerlin S, Mowry HJ: Click lateralization and the auditory brain stem response. Audiology 19:346–354, 1980

Department of Neurology, NW-7
Montefiore Medical Center
111 East 210th Street
Bronx, New York 10467-2490

0733–8619/88 $0.00 + .20

The Anatomic and Physiologic Bases of Median Nerve Somatosensory Evoked Potentials

Thoru Yamada, MD*

Following stimulation of the median nerve, a series of potentials are recorded from the arm, shoulder, neck, and scalp. Depending on the montages or selection of references, some potentials may be enhanced and others may be abolished, or the same potential may be registered as either an upgoing or downgoing peak. Different laboratories use different recording techniques, which makes interlaboratory comparison difficult and confusing. Understanding the physioanatomic principles and characteristics of far-field potentials and their related recording technique is important to fully grasp the differences of the recording methods. This in turn gives insight about the possible anatomic origins or related anatomic structures of various potentials elicited after the stimulation of the median nerve.

This chapter describes the basic recording technique, commonly encountered technical problems, and physiologic meanings of various somatosensory evoked potential (SEP) components, along with the discussion of possible anatomic origins and physioanatomic mechanisms of far-field or stationary field potentials.

RECORDING METHOD

Recording Electrodes

Recording electrodes are generally silver-silver chloride cups filled with ECG gel attached to the skin with collodion. It is important to keep the electrode impedance less than 5 KΩ. The high-impedance electrode not only introduces 60-cycle interference, but also increases stimulus-related baseline shift. Lowering the electrode impedance especially at noncephalic electrodes, for example at the hand or knee, is often difficult. Preparing the skin by Omni® prep before placing the electrode helps to reduce the impedance.

---

*Professor of Neurology, Division of Clinical Electrophysiology, Department of Neurology, College of Medicine, University of Iowa Hospitals, Iowa City, Iowa

Stimulation

Stimulation of the median nerve at the wrist is commonly used for clinical tests because this yields a higher amplitude and better-defined response than that recorded with finger stimulation. The median nerve at the wrist includes both motor and sensory fibers, but it is doubtful that the antidromic motor impulse significantly contributes to the SEP waveform. For stimulation of pure sensory fibers, the second and/or third digit are stimulated.[20, 21] The waveforms recorded with pure sensory (finger) and mixed-nerve (wrist) stimulation are essentially the same, but the amplitude of the latter is about twice as large as with finger stimulation. Stimulus electrodes are flat-surfaced disks 7–8 mm in diameter, placed on the skin overlying the median nerve at 3 cm proximal to the distal crease, with the cathode 2 cm proximal to the anode. For finger stimulation, ring electrodes are used.

Stimulus electrodes are placed where the twitch of abductor pollicis brevis is elicited with the smallest stimulus intensity. The optimal stimulus intensity is three to four times sensory threshold or 1.3 times motor threshold, or the sum of motor and sensory thresholds.[21, 50] This intensity is submaximal for peripheral nerve potential, but is close to supramaximal for scalp SEP within 100 msec after the stimulus. With 0.1-msec pulse duration, the intensity generally ranges from 10 to 15 mA for constant current or from 80 to 120 V for a constant-voltage stimulator. The stimulus should be delivered via a stimulus isolation unit, which limits the current around the stimulus electrodes, thus reducing the stimulus artifacts and eliminating possible electric hazards to the subject. The stimulus rate is 3 to 4/sec for recording the SEP within 100 msec after the stimulus. The rate can be increased up to 8/sec without attenuation or latency changes of the SEP components within 25 msec after the stimulus.[3, 69] A rate faster than 3/sec attenuates the components with latency greater than 100 msec. For the study of long-latency SEP (greater than 100 msec after the stimulus), a rate slower than 0.5/sec is necessary to yield a measurable late component (see Fig. 13).[3, 13]

Frequency Filter Setting

Frequency band width may vary from 10 to 30 Hz for a low (high-band pass) and 1 to 3 KHz for a high (low-band pass) frequency filter. Theoretically, it is preferable to record with a wide-open filter setting (1–3000 Hz).[17] However, the technical problems increase with the lower low- and the higher high-frequency filter settings (see the next section). A frequency band of 30 Hz to 3 KHz is generally used for the recording of short-latency SEP (20–30 msec). For middle- and long-latency SEP, the low-frequency filter should be lower than 10 Hz. The latency and amplitude of a given wave differs depending on the filter setting: with the higher low- or high-filter setting, the peak latency becomes shorter but different components shift with different degrees (Fig. 1). With appropriate filter setting, it is possible to enhance a particular component of interest. Digital filtering, in contrast to the analog filtering previously described, causes no latency shift.[27, 36] Thus, the potentials measured in the digitally filtered tracing can be correlated directly with those of the original tracing recorded with wide-open band pass (see Fig. 1).

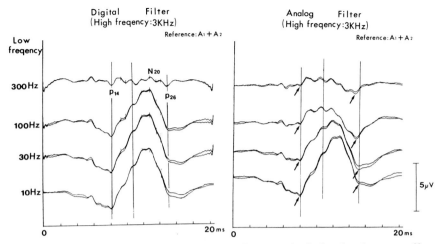

Figure 1. Comparison of digital and analog filtering. The higher low-frequency filter eliminates the slower waves, thus extracting the faster components. The latencies of corresponding peaks are the same among different digital filter settings, but tend to be shorter with the higher low-frequency filter in analog filtering. Note the different degree of latency shift (*arrows*) depending on the component in the analog filter. (*From* Yamada T, Kayamori R: Somatosensory Evoked Potential: Clinical Application. Niigata, Japan, Nishismura Shoten, 1986; with permission.)

Amplification and Summation

The amplification is generally 20×10^3, which is close to the sensitivity of 5 uV/mm pen deflection in EEG instruments. Because the autorejection mode is determined by the amplitude scale (unrealistically large response contaminated by the artifact is rejected from averaging), the amplification may be optimally increased to reject approximately 10 to 15 per cent of total samples. A minimum of 1000 responses should be averaged to yield reliable SEP, including far-field potentials. The test is repeated at least once to confirm the reproducibility of the response.

TECHNICAL PROBLEMS

The most common technical problem encountered in recording SEP is movement or muscle artifact contamination on the responses. This increases particularly with the use of a noncephalic reference. It is essential that the subject lie supine in a comfortable, relaxed posture. Recording during sleep minimizes these artifacts without affecting the responses within 14 to 15 msec after the stimulus. It has generally been thought that sleep affects primarily the middle (30 to 100 msec) or long-latency (greater than 100 msec) peak and has little effect on the short-latency (fewer than 30 msec) components. Recent studies, however, showed slight latency prolongation of the first negative peak, N20, in sleep (see section on physiologic significance for further detail).[30, 82]

The use of a noncephalic reference increases the chances of contamination by 60-Hz interference and physiologic (ECG, for example) or nonphysiologic artifacts. It also tends to accentuate stimulus artifacts causing baseline shift. Following are some considerations to improve the recording technique.

1. Electrode wires and input cable: The longer the interelectrode distance between active (G1) and reference (G2) electrodes, the greater the chance of artifact contamination. The use of shielded wires may minimize the electrical interference. By trial and error, rearranging the location of the wires may eliminate the interference. Avoid placing the input cable near the power line or the stimulus cable.

2. Electrode impedance: Maintaining low impedance of recording, stimulus, and ground electrodes minimizes the interference and stimulus artifacts.

3. Frequency-band pass setting: The use of a narrow band filter with higher low-filter and lower high-filter settings may minimize the contamination of physiologic or nonphysiologic artifacts. The use of a low-frequency filter (less than 10 Hz) in noncephalic reference recording brings about excessive sample rejection due to high-amplitude ECG complexes, particularly T wave. This prolongs the procedure time and makes the test impractical. The higher low-filter setting (for example, 30 Hz) facilitates sample collection by minimizing contamination by T wave of ECG, EEG, and eye movement artifacts. The use of lower high-filter settings, on the other hand, decreases the high-frequency interference and makes the waveforms smoother and clearer. The narrow-band pass filters, however, may cause waveform distortion along with untoward latency shift, and also tend to increase the stimulus-related baseline shift. Finding the optimal filter setting, depending on the wave peaks of interest, is important.

4. 60-Hz notch filter: The use of a 60-Hz filter should be avoided because it not only distorts the wave form, but also increases the stimulus artifact.

5. Stimulus rate and intensity: Avoid using the rate harmonic with 60 Hz. Even if 60-Hz interference exists during the early stage of averaging, this may decrease as the number of averages increases. If 60 Hz or another electrical interference pattern continues or becomes greater during the process of averaging, try the different stimulus rate. Because stimulus artifact is greater with increased stimulus intensity, use the lowest effective intensity.

6. Incompatible stimulator and amplifier: Some amplifiers and stimulators have different grounding systems, which may result in large stimulus artifacts. One can try different stimulators. A fast recovery amplifier,[77] specially designed to eliminate stimulus artifact, is useful.

PHYSIOANATOMIC SUBSTRATES OF FAR-FIELD POTENTIALS

Far-Field Potentials (P9, P11, P13, P14) Recorded from the Scalp

When the SEPs are recorded from the scalp with the use of a noncephalic (knee) reference, four positive potentials—P9, P11, P13, and P14—are registered.[6, 8, 11, 22, 37, 41, 48, 49, 66, 86] These positive potentials have fixed latencies irrespective of the recording site (Fig. 2). In contrast, the later peaks have different latencies depending on the electrode location. Diffuse distribution, fixed latencies, and positive polarity lead to the concept of far-field potential. These presumably represent a volume-conducted field of positivity recorded at a distance from the generator. The potentials are generated when a traveling impulse passes through a certain anatomic site.

Figure 3 illustrates schematic models of generation of far-field potential recorded with referential and bipolar montages (see section on physioanatomic mechanism for further details).

Because of the diffuse distribution of these far-field potentials over the entire scalp, they would be variably canceled if the reference site is close to the scalp. It is preferable to use a noncephalic reference for all SEP recordings, but this often brings out technical problems as discussed earlier and is difficult to apply for routine clinical testing. As a compromise, an Fpz reference has been widely used. With this reference, however, all of the four positive potentials are canceled because of equipotentiality between the two scalp electrodes (Fig. 4). Further, the first negative peak, "N19," recorded with this derivation is an amalgam of the central N19 and frontal

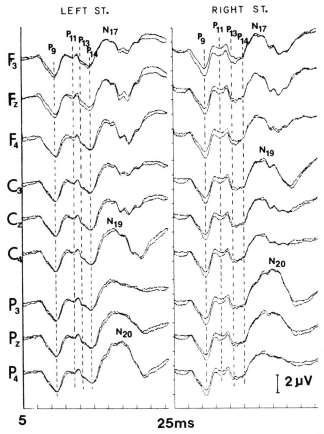

Figure 2. Short-latency SEP recorded with a noncephalic (knee) reference from multiple scalp electrodes. Note the fixed latencies of the P9, P11, P13, and P14 peaks irrespective of recording electrodes. In contrast, the subsequent negative peaks have different latencies depending on the electrode locations.

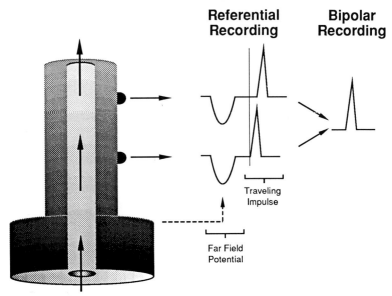

Figure 3. Schematic model of generation of far-field potential and the difference between referential and bipolar recordings. Far-field potential (rounded positive potential) is generated when an impulse crosses at a site where the geometry surrounding the nerve fiber changes. Referential recording registers both far-field and traveling impulse (pointed negative potential), whereas far-field potential is cancelled with bipolar recording because of equipotentiality between the two electrodes.

P20 peak and is not a "true" N19 peak (see the next section for further details). We routinely use a linked-ear (A1 + A2) reference for clinical application because the ear provides a relatively "quiet" reference without causing troublesome technical problems. The ear is equally active with the scalp electrode for the P9 and P11 peaks, and P9 and P11 are not registered from the scalp with the use of the ear reference. However, the ear is not active or at least is less active with the P13–P14 or P14 potential as compared with the scalp electrodes. Thus, the responses recorded with the ear reference consistently register P14 or P13–P14 complex and N19 peaks (see Fig. 4). P9 and P11 can be recorded as N9 and N11 from the neck electrode referenced to the ear, as is discussed below.

Relationship Between Scalp-Recorded Far-Field Potentials and Cervical-Recorded Short-latency Potentials

P9–N9. SEP recorded from the neck referenced to the knee consists of positive-negative diphasic waves. The positive peak (P9) extends from the scalp to the neck, becoming progressively smaller caudally (Fig. 5). When recorded from the neck referenced to the ear or scalp (Fpz), P9 becomes the upgoing peak "N9" owing to greater positivity at the ear or scalp than at the neck (Fig. 6). The latency of P9 (N9) slightly but always precedes the negative peak of Erb's potential; thus, it has generally been agreed that P9 (N9) arises from the distal part of the brachial plexus.[6, 8–11, 25, 27, 31, 35, 43, 49, 66, 86] As opposed to the far-field potential, a negative potential recorded near the generator source is customarily referred to as a near-field potential. In this sense, Erb's potential is a near-field potential that closely relates to the far-field potential of P9 recorded at a distance. It should be remembered that N9 recorded from the neck referenced to the ear or scalp is not a near-field potential; N9 is an instrumentally inverted P9 potential (see section on physioanatomic mechanism for further discussion of positive far-field and negative stationary field potentials).

P11–N11. From the neck with a knee reference, N11 is inconsistently registered as a small notch over the rising phase of the major negative peak, N13 (see Fig. 5). Cervical N11 and scalp P11 appear to have the same generator. This generator, near the neck, produces negative near-field potential (N11) at the neck. Simultaneously at a distance electrode (scalp), positive far-field potential (P11) is generated. Cervical N11 and scalp P11 thus represent vertically oriented dipole fields.[23, 86] N11 is better defined and most consistent when referenced to the ear or scalp (Fpz) owing to the additive effect of P11 far-field potentials on N11 near-field potential (see Figs. 6 and 7). An estimated conduction time measured by the F and M waves from the wrist to the neck is close to 11 msec.[26, 47] Also, the shorter refractory period of N11 than the subsequent N13 peak suggests that N11 is of presynaptic origin.[39] These findings imply that N11 arises presynaptically from the dorsal root entry zone.[41, 53, 87] Alternatively, a dorsal horn[55, 70] or dorsal column origin[6, 9, 22] has been suggested.

Figure 4. Short-latency SEP peaks with different montage derivations. Because of the equipotentiality of P9, P11, P13, and P14 between C4 and Fpz, it cancels these far-field potentials. The notched peak of N17 is also eliminated, and N19 from C4 and P20 from Fpz creates a new potential, "N19." With the ear reference recording, P9 and P11 that are equipotential between the scalp (C4) and ear (A1 + A2) are not registered, but the P14 and N19 peaks are consistent components. (*From* Yamada T, Machida M, Tippen J: Somatosensory evoked potential. *In* Owen JM, Davis H (eds): Evoked Potential Testing: Clinical Application. Orlando, Florida, Grune and Stratton, 1985; with permission.)

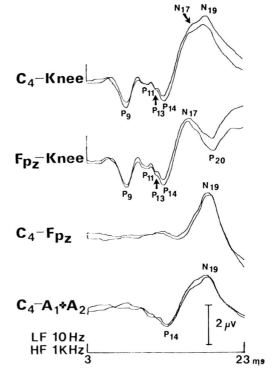

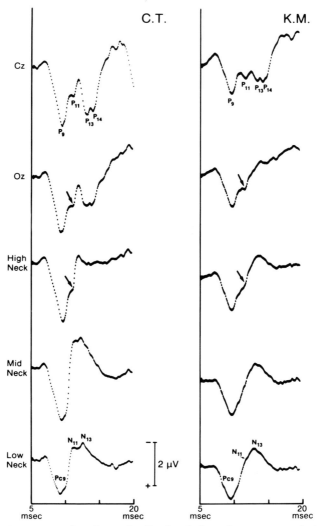

Figure 5. Responses from longitudinally placed electrodes at Cz, Oz, high, mid-, and low cervical region with a knee reference in two subjects. Note the progressive decrease in amplitude of P11 from Cz to the high cervical electrode (*arrows*) and corresponding negativity, N11, at the low cervical electrode. In contrast, the positive field of P9 extends from Cz to the low cervical electrode (Pc9). (*From* Yamada T, Kimura J, Nitz DM: Short latency somatosensory evoked potentials following median nerve stimulation. Electroencephalogr Clin Neurophysiol 48:367–376, 1980; with permission.)

P13–N13. Similar to the cervical N11 and scalp P11, a close latency relationship between cervical N13 and scalp P13 suggests a common generator producing a vertically oriented dipole with negativity at the neck and positivity at the scalp[56] (see Fig. 6). However, Desmedt and co-workers[19] recorded a positive field (P13) in the anterior neck and proposed a horizontally oriented dipole arising from postsynaptic excitatory potential in the interneuron of the dorsal horn. In the experimental study using the cat, Kaji and co-workers[42] found that N13 was fractionated into two peaks, N13a and N13b: N13a had a positive field (P13a) with ventrodorsal dipole orientation, and N13b accompanied P13b oriented rostrocaudally.

Cervical N13 was proposed to be generated from the dorsal column at the level of high[8, 51, 75] or midcervical cord[82, 87] or at the foramen magnum.[34, 53] An origin at the cuneate nucleus was also suggested.[8, 19, 38, 41, 49] N13 is considered to be a near-field potential with little or no latency shift from low to high cervical cord[29, 47] (see Figs. 5 and 17). Recording of N13 from the neck with a noncephalic reference often yields a broad negative wave without distinct separation between N11 and N13; thus, the measurement of the peak is often difficult. Cervical N13 is better defined when referenced to the ear or the scalp. "N13" thus recorded is an amalgam of N13 from the cervical and P13 from the ear or the scalp electrode.

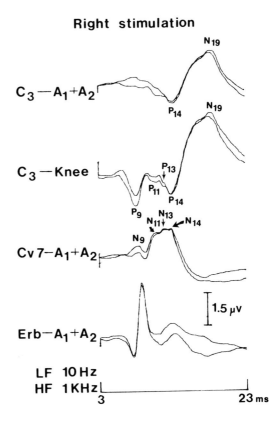

Figure 6. Short-latency SEPs recorded from scalp, neck, and Erb's points. From the scalp referenced to the knee, P9, P11, P13, and P14 are registered, whereas only P14 is recorded when referenced to the ear. N9, N11, N13, and N14 from the Cv7 referenced to the ear correspond to P9, P11, P13, and P14 from the scalp with the knee reference, respectively. The N9 or P9 peak slightly precedes the negative peak of Erb's potential. (*From* Yamada T, Machida M, Tippin J: Somatosensory evoked potential. *In* Owen JM, Davis H (eds): Evoked Potential Testing: Clinical Application. Orlando, Florida, Grune and Stratton, Inc, 1985; with permission.)

Right Unilatlateral Stimulation
(REFERENCE: A₁+ A₂)

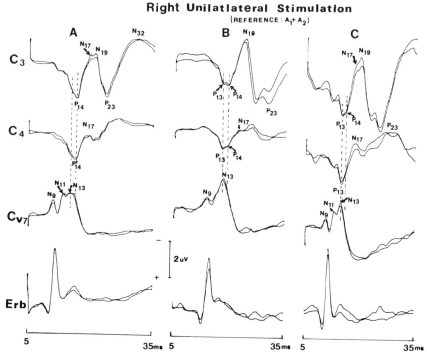

Figure 7. Examples of short-latency SEPs recorded with a linked-ear reference in three normal subjects from C3, C4 scalp, cervical (Cv7), and Erb's point. From the cervical electrode (Cv7), N9 and N13 are consistently recorded. The P14 peak, which is slightly preceded by the cervical N13, is identified as the onset peak of N19 (A). When P13 is present, it coincides in latency with cervical N13 (B and C). In some, P13 may be more prominent than P14, and P14 appears as a small notched peak over the rising phase of N19 (C). P14 is often better identified at the contralateral scalp electrode, C3 (B and C). (*From* Yamada T, Ishida T, Kudo Y, et al: Clinical correlates of abnormal P14 in median SEPs. Neurology 36:765–771, 1986; with permission.)

N14–P14. Unlike N11 or N13, near-field potentials recorded from the neck, an equivalent negative near-field potential for positive far-field potential (P14), can rarely be recorded. The potential designated "N14" recorded from the neck referenced to the ear or scalp exclusively or predominantly consists of the far-field potential of P14 derived from the reference electrode (see Fig. 6). Because P14 is more active with the scalp than with the ear, "N14" is better defined with the neck to scalp than with the neck to ear recording, but this recording makes it difficult to distinguish N13 and N14 that arise from the two distant anatomic generators. The author recommends recording from the scalp and neck, both referenced to the ear, in two separate channels. With this recording we can easily distinguish cervical N13 and scalp P14 (see Figs. 6 and 7).

Because scalp P14 or P13–P14 complex was the first positive potential distributed diffusely in ear reference recording, earlier studies suggested that P14 arises from the thalamus.[3, 33] However, Nakanishi and colleagues[64] observed a normal P14 peak in patients with thalamic lesions, indicating that P14 arises caudal to the thalamus. This was later confirmed by others.[20, 58, 80, 84] It has generally been agreed that P14 originates from the brain stem, probably the medial lemniscus.[19, 23, 37, 40, 73, 81, 87] Origin at the cervicomedullary junction,[53] cuneate nucleus,[61] or thalamus was also proposed. Scalp P14 has often been considered together with P13 as a P13–P14 complex, but P13 and P14 likely originate from two different generators.[11, 19, 59] Although anatomic distinction for the origins of scalp P13 and P14 peaks remains uncertain, scalp P14 and cervical N13 should be treated as distinct components originating above and below the foramen magnum, respectively.[59, 81]

Four-Channel Short-Latency SEP Recording

Recordings from the neck and scalp in separate channels with the use of an ear (A1 + A2) reference register all four short-latency potentials previously described; N9, N11, and N13 from the neck and P14 from the scalp (see Fig. 7). We routinely use C3 (C3'), C4 (C4'), Cv7, and Erb's points, all referenced to the linked ear as shown in Figure 7. These four channel recordings mutually assist in identifying short-latency SEP components: The negative peak of Erb's potential slightly but consistently follows N9 and precedes the N11 peak. N13 from Cv7 slightly precedes P14 from the scalp. P14 is identified bilaterally at the scalp as the onset peak of N17 or N19. N17, which is best recorded ipsilaterally to the side of stimulation, may also be registered contralaterally as a small notch preceding the N19 peak. The N19 peak appears only contralaterally to the side of stimulation.

PHYSIOANATOMIC SUBSTRATES OF SCALP-RECORDED SEP

Topographic Characteristics of Early SEP

In contrast to P9, P11, P13, and P14, which have fixed latencies irrespective of recording sites, subsequent negative-positive-negative potentials show progressive latency delay from frontal to parietal electrode on the hemisphere contralateral to the side of stimulation; they are N17–P20–N29 at frontal, N19–P23–N32 at central, and N20–P26–N34 at parietal electrodes (Fig. 8). The commonly used C3' or C4' (2 cm behind C3 or C4) electrode for clinical testing usually registers the same response as of P3 or P4. Of the first negative peaks (N17, N19, and N20), parietal N20 is the largest, whereas the frontal N29 is often the largest of the second negative peaks (N29, N32, and N34). The out-of-phase relationship between frontal P20 and parietal N20 led to the theory that they are of the same origin and oriented in a dipole across the central sulcus.[4, 7, 74] However, the slight latency difference,[20, 67, 80, 84] dissociate changes in patients with parietal lobe lesions,[57] and the nonparallel latency shift in sleep between P20 and N20[82] contradicted the dipole theory. The recent studies by Desmedt and Bourguet[16] and Deiber and colleagues[15] have found an additional positive peak in the frontal region, which is consistent with the dipole theory.

In contrast to the central and parietal peaks, which are registered only over the contralateral hemisphere, frontal peaks (N17–P20–N29) are distributed bilaterally (see Fig. 8). They are also recorded at ipsilateral central

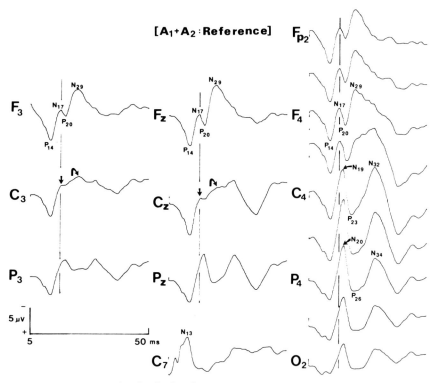

Figure 8. Topographically displayed SEPs to the left median nerve stimulation. N17–P20–N29 are distributed widely over the contralateral (*right column*), ipsilateral (*left column*), and midline (*middle column*) frontal regions (vertical lines indicate N17 latency). N19–P23–N32 are localized to the contralateral central region. The parietal N20–P26–N34 peaks are also recorded at the occipital region. (*From* Yamada T, Kayamori R: Somatosensory Evoked Potential: Clinical Application. Niigata, Japan, Nishimura Shoten, 1986; with permission.)

and vertex electrodes. Of these, N17 (equivalent to N16 by Tsuji and Murai[74] and to N18 by Desmedt and co-workers[20] and Mauguiere and colleagues[58]) has been studied in the most detail. Because of diffuse distribution, N17 is believed to arise subcortically, possibly from the thalamus[20, 75, 80] or just caudal to the thalamus.[58] In our experience,[80, 84] the topographically analyzed SEP in patients with thalamic lesions involving primary sensory nuclei showed the total absence of responses after P14 far-field potentials (Fig. 9). This indicates that all SEP components after P14 including ipsilateral response within 100 msec after the stimulus are mediated through the primary sensory nuclei in the thalamus contralateral to the side of stimulation.

Anatomic substrates of N19 or N20 have been in much dispute. Parietal N20 has been suggested to have a thalamic,[8, 9, 34] thalamocortical, or cortical origin.[2, 21, 22, 38, 53, 57, 75, 84, 87] The localization of N20 at the contralateral post-Rolandic region suggests that this potential relates directly to the primary sensory projection system. In our topographic SEP studies,[80, 84] however, central N19 is found to be discretely localized to the central region, whereas parietal N20 extends to the occipital region (see Fig. 8). Furthermore, central N19 and parietal N20 can be affected independently in patients

Left Stimulation

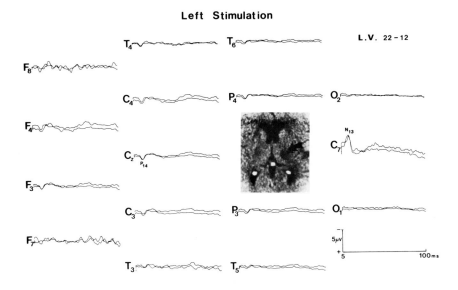

Right Stimulation

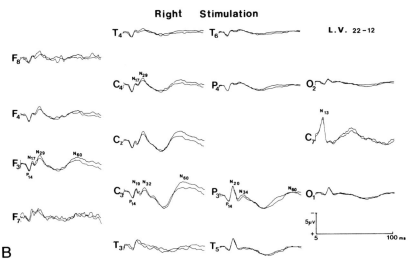

Figure 9. *A*, A patient with a lesion in the right posterolateral thalamus probably involving primary sensory nuclei. *B*, With the affected limb stimulation (*A*) only N13 from the neck (C7) and P14 from the scalp were recorded. SEPs elicited by right-sided stimulation were normal. For example, compare P4 (*A*) with P3 (*B*) responses. (*From* Yamada T, Graff-Radford NR, Kimura J, et al: Topographic analysis of somatosensory evoked potentials in patients with well-localized thalamic infarction. J Neurol Sci 68:31–46, 1985; with permission.)

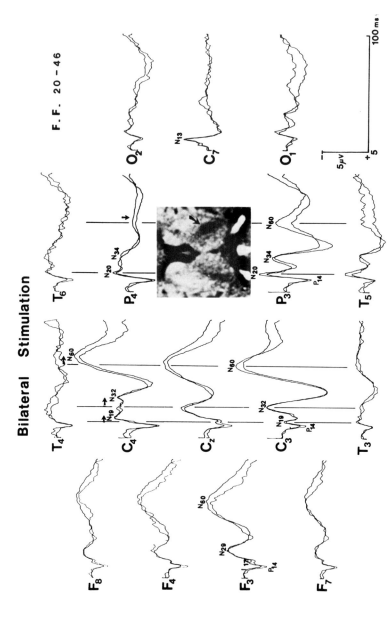

Bilateral Stimulation

F.F. 20-46

Figure 10. A patient with a lesion in the right internal capsule. Bilateral stimulation revealed delayed central N19–N32–N60 (C4) and poorly defined parietal N34–N60 (P4). The middle peak between N19 and N32 at C4 was probably an extension of N32 from the intact hemisphere. Note the dissociated alteration with delayed central N19 and normal parietal N20. Also note depressed parietal N60 in contrast to the well-defined central N60. (*From* Yamada T, Graff-Radford NR, Kimura J, et al: Topographic analysis of somatosensory evoked potentials in patients with well-localized thalamic infarction. J Neurol Sci 68:31–46, 1985; with permission.)

with localized cerebral lesions, suggesting that they are two distinct components of independent origins (Fig. 10). Further details of their anatomic substrates or relationship remain to be elucidated.

Late SEP Peaks

Much less is known concerning the anatomic substrates of the latter peaks, P40–N60, which are seen predominantly over the contralateral hemisphere. The clinical application of these peaks is difficult because of considerable intertrial variabilities (Fig. 11). Their amplitude or latency changes depending on the level of consciousness, habituation, or cognitive functions.[3, 24, 32, 76] For example, sleep affects P40–N60 peaks, producing latency prolongation and decreased amplitude[31] (Fig. 12). In fact, P40–N60 peaks cannot be assessed reliably if the left- and right-side responses after two separate trials in different time domains are compared. To circumvent this difficulty, we routinely use bilateral stimulation.[79] Bilateral stimulation theoretically results in an amalgam of ipsi- and contralateral responses in each hemisphere, but practically the responses recorded resemble the contralateral responses. SEPs including P40–N60 by bilateral stimulation are normally symmetric between homologous electrodes (Figs. 13A and B); thus, the asymmetric peaks are determined to be abnormal.[79, 80, 84, 87, 91] As long as the stimulus is delivered via a stimulus isolation unit, the procedure is safe. In addition to the conventional unilateral stimulation, we recommend bilateral stimulation in clinical testing, especially for evaluation of P40–N60 peaks.

Figure 11. A and B, Repeated trials of contralateral SEP in two normal subjects. The responses in A were consistently repeatable. In contrast, the responses in B were inconsistent, particularly in P40–N60. (*From* Yamada T, Dickens QS, Machida M, et al: SEPs to bilateral simultaneous median nerve stimulation in man: Method and clinical application. Front Clin Sci 3:58–67, 1985; with permission.)

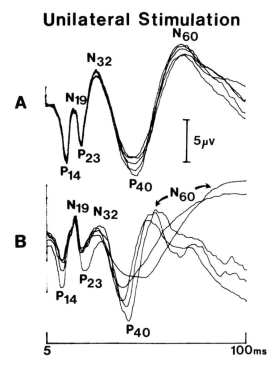

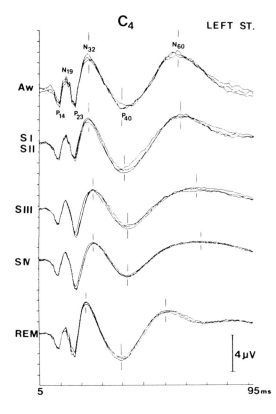

Figure 12. Serial SEPs recorded in sleep. Latency prolongation and amplitude reduction is most prominent in N60, although there is less degree of changes in other peaks. In REM sleep, SEP wave form becomes similar to that of the waking state. Although change of the N19 peak is hardly visible with this time scale, the wave form becomes smoother in sleep. (See Figs. 18A and B and 19A and B and section on physioanatomic substrates of scalp-recorded SEP for further detail.)

In contrast to the earlier peaks that show characteristic anterior-posterior latency shift, the latency relationships of P40–N60 from different regions are inconsistent. An abnormality limited to P40–N60 peaks has been observed in patients with multiple sclerosis[91] or with deep subcortical lesions, including a lesion involving thalamic nuclei other than the primary sensory nuclei (VPL, VPM).[80] We further found that the P40–N60 at a certain electrode can be selectively affected while leaving P40–N60 at other electrodes intact (see Fig. 10). Patients with selective abnormality of P40–N60, with normal short-latency peaks, generally have no sensory deficit clinically. These findings suggest that the P40–N60 peaks at different electrodes are mediated through independent and regionally specific thalamocortical projection systems, possibly via relay or nonspecific thalamic nuclei.

The subsequent triphasic positive-negative-positive waves—P100–N150–P250–N350—are distributed bilaterally and are maximum at the vertex region (Fig. 14). This is in contrast to the preceding peaks, which are dominant over the contralateral hemisphere. Because these late peaks are the largest of all SEP components, reaching 10 to 40 uV, it requires

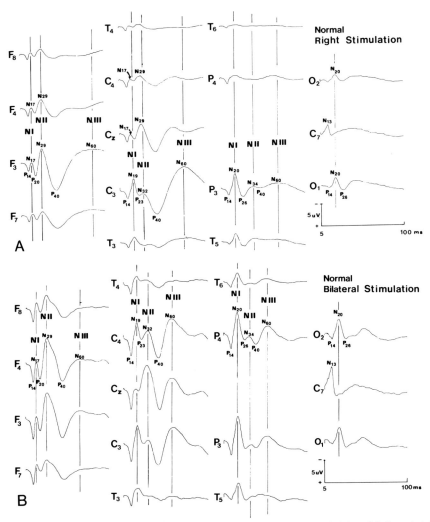

Figure 13. Topographically displayed SEPs after right unilateral (A) and bilateral (B) stimulation of the median nerve. Bilateral stimulation (B) yields symmetric responses between homologous electrodes, which are similar to those elicited by contralateral stimulation (A). (*From* Yamada T, Kayamori R, Kimura J, et al: Topography of somatosensory evoked potentials after stimulation of the median nerve. Electroencephalogr Clin Neurophysiol 59:29–43, 1984; with permission.)

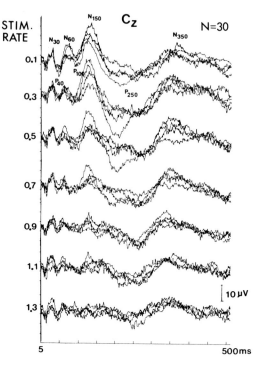

Figure 14. Long-latency SEP with different stimulus rates. Each response was obtained with 30 summations. With the faster rate of stimuli, P100–N150–P250 peaks are abolished. Less degree of amplitude reduction is seen in P40–N60 peaks.

fewer than 50 summations to yield measurable responses. However, they have a recovery time of several seconds[3, 5]; thus the stimulus rate faster than one/sec markedly attenuates the response, particularly P100–N150 peaks (see Fig. 14).

Similar potentials have been recorded by auditory or visual stimuli. These late peaks have been thought to be related to the nonspecific thalamocortical diffuse projection system.[13, 60] Underlying neuropsychologic functions that influence these peaks are poorly understood, but may relate to habituation, adaptation, or attentiveness to the stimuli.

PHYSIOANATOMIC MECHANISM OF FAR-FIELD AND STATIONARY-FIELD POTENTIALS

Four positive far-field potentials—P9, P11, P13, and P14—recorded from the scalp with the use of a noncephalic reference have been considered to be volume-conducted potentials reflecting the approaching field of positivity in advance of a propagating impulse.[52, 78] However, it is uncertain why the traveling nerve impulse in the absence of fixed neural discharges gives rise to a stationary positive field (that is, a diffusely distributed potential with the same latency irrespective of the recording sites). Several investigators have approached this problem using different methods. Using "fluid electrodes" to study action potentials, Nakanishi[62] has shown that stationary peaks occur where the resistance of the conduction media changes abruptly. Kimura and co-workers[44-46] have demonstrated that stationary potentials are generated at a boundary between two adjacent conducting media when an approaching traveling impulse causes sudden change in the current density. Using a computer model, Cunningham and colleagues[12] and Stegman and co-workers[72] predicted the existence of stationary far-field potentials associated with changes in the volume conductor (see Fig. 3).

In our recent study,[89] we demonstrated three stationary negative peaks—N3, N6, and N9—which are recorded over the stimulated arm referenced to the knee (Fig. 15). Other investigators have also found equivalent peaks to our N3, N6, and N9.[27, 31] These stationary potentials appeared to be generated when the traveling impulse passed a site where the arm significantly changed shape: N3 at the forearm muscle, N6 at the distal end of the deltoid muscle, and N9 at the acromion. N9 matched in latency with the scalp-recorded P9. In contrast, the N6 negative field appeared to extend to the scalp (see Fig. 15). This N9 is not the same as the "N9" recorded from the neck with an ear reference.

Emerson and colleagues[29] recently described two additional stationary potentials (N10 and N12) that have fixed latencies from the low cervical spine to the scalp. N10 is recorded from the lateral neck ipsilateral to the side of stimulation and coincides in timing with the traveling impulse reaching the cervical roots proximal to Erb's point. N12 corresponds to a traveling wave, possibly dorsal column volley, at the first cervical level

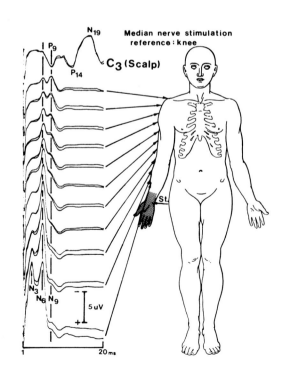

Figure 15. Stationary-field potentials recorded (with knee reference) from the lateral aspect of the arm, avoiding the actual median nerve pathway (to avoid contamination of the traveling impulse). This revealed "pure" stationary peaks, N3, N6, and N9. N9 is prominent near the shoulder, N6 near the arm, and N3 near the forearm. (*From* Yamada T, Machida M, Oishi M, et al: Stationary negative potentials near the source versus positive far-field potentials at a distance. Electroencephalogr Clin Neurophysiol 60:509–524, 1985; with permission.)

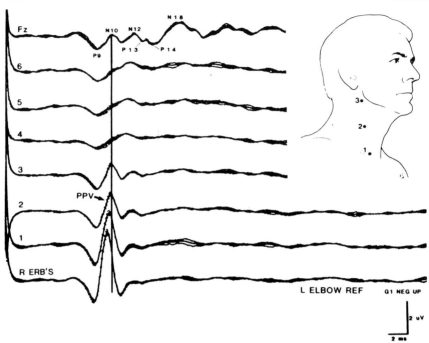

Figure 16. Right median SEPs recorded simultaneously from a scalp electrode (Fz) and from electrodes placed vertically along the anterior borders of both sternocleidomastoid muscles. (Electrode positions 4–6 are not shown, but are on the left side corresponding to positions 1–3 illustrated here.) The scalp N10 far field is recorded during passage of the afferent volley through the proximal brachial plexus. (*From* Emerson RG, Pedley TA: Generator sources of median somatosensory evoked potentials. J Clin Neurophysiol 1:203–218, 1984; with permission.)

(Fig. 16). The cervical recorded N13 described more than a decade ago has some similar characteristics with these stationary potentials; this negative potential shows little or no latency shift from low to high cervical spine[29, 86] (see Fig. 5). Similar characteristics were found in lumbar-recorded N24, which has a fixed latency from L1 to L4 spine after stimulation of the tibial nerve.[85, 88]

There has been much debate regarding factors that determine the polarity and latency of the far-field or stationary potentials. For an impulse moving from a smaller to a larger volume, Cunningham and coworkers[12] believe that the propagating impulse crossing the geometric junction always makes initial positivity, regardless of the type of dimensional change. Nakanishi and colleagues[65] observed polarity inversions of far-field potentials when changing arm positions in the cat. Desmedt and coworkers[25] reported a latency shift of the P9 onset peak by raising the shoulder. We also observed latency changes of the N3, N6, and N9 peaks depending on the arm position.[43]

Stegman and colleagues[72] examined the potential distribution in cylinders of infinite length with an impulse propagating along the center line. Variable conditions included (1) an abrupt change in conduction with uniform geometry, (2) an abrupt change in cylinder diameter with uniform conductivity, and (3) a change in the direction of propagation without changes in geometry and conduction. All three conditions produced stationary potential peaks in the cylinder between points on opposite sides of, and distant from, the site of change. The latency and duration of these peaks correspond to the time when the traveling impulse crosses the site of change. In the case of conductivity change with uniform geometry, the models show a positive peak when the impulse crosses from a greater conductive medium into a smaller conductive medium and a negative peak with the reverse order. When an impulse crosses from a large volume into a smaller volume (with uniform conductivity), positive stationary potential is generated. They further demonstrated a stationary negative potential when the propagating nerve impulse reversed its direction within a homogeneous conductive medium.

Determining the polarity of a stationary potential would be much more complex in humans because the nerve impulse traverses various regions with differing impedance and shape and with nonhomogeneous conductive medium surrounding the nerve. The question then arises, what is the relationship between positive stationary far-field potentials recorded at a distance (scalp) and negative stationary far-field potentials recorded near the generator sources (stimulated arm)? For example, are scalp-recorded P9 and arm-recorded N9 independent or related to each other? Our recent study demonstrated that abduction of the arm at the shoulder prolonged latencies of P9 and N9 in parallel fashion.[43] This suggests that they are the same potentials oriented in a dipole with a negative field near the generator and the positive field at a distance. The same positive far-field and negative stationary-field relationship may apply to cervical N13, which has a positive counter far field at the scalp[42, 86] or at the anterior neck.[19, 29] Similarly, lumbar N24 after tibial nerve stimulation accompanies P24 recorded at the scalp[85, 88] or at the abdomen.[18] These findings suggest that the negative stationary fields generated when a traveling impulse passes a certain anatomic structure are a prerequisite for the generation of a positive far-field potential at a distance and that they represent dipole-oriented field potentials distributed throughout the entire body.

PHYSIOLOGIC SIGNIFICANCE OF MULTIPLE WAVELETS OVER THE RISING AND DESCENDING PHASES OF THE NEGATIVE PEAK

Cracco and Cracco[11] and Allison and co-workers[2, 4] found one or two inflections over the rising phase of the initial negative peak, "N20," following stimulation of the median nerve. The use of a restricted filter band pass with a high-pass filter greater than 100 Hz enhanced these small wavelets by attenuating the slower-frequency components. With the use of the restricted filter band pass, Maccabee and colleagues[54] found that parietal "N20" was consistently fractionated into three distinct subcomponents—N16, N19, and N20. However, an analog high-pass filter is known to cause a phase shift (see Fig. 1) and may even create spurious peaks.

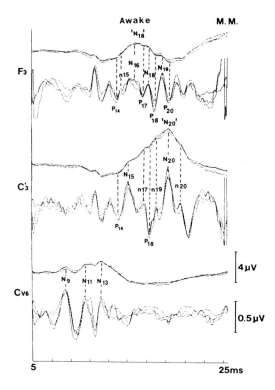

Figure 17. Major negative waves, "N18" and "N20," recorded from F3 and C'3 electrodes, respectively, and cervical peaks (N9, N11, and N13) with the use of linked-ear reference following right median nerve stimulation. The subject was awake. The upper and lower tracings from each electrode were responses with open band pass (30–3000 Hz) and restricted digital filtering (250–2500 Hz), respectively. Series of wavelets (FFP) over the rising and descending phases of slow negative waves were enhanced by digital filtering. N or P were capitalized for major FFP. Note the out-of-phase relationship between frontal N17, N18, and P20 and parietal n17, P18, and N20, respectively. (*From* Yamada T, Kameyama S, Fuchigami Y, et al: Changes of short latency somatosensory evoked potential in sleep. Electroencephalogr Clin Neurophysiol, 70:126–136, 1988; with permission.)

Responses recorded with a restricted analog band pass filter are, therefore, not easily comparable with those recorded with an open band pass. Digital zero-phase shift filtering eliminates these problems, and the response recorded with an open band pass and restricted filter can be correlated directly. Using the digital filtering, Eisen and co-workers[28] and Green and colleagues[36] identified several subcomponents superimposed on the slow major negative peak of N20. These fast-frequency potentials (FFP) were thought to represent multiple generators through thalamocortical radiations.

In our study[82] frontal FFP consists of N16, P17, N18, P18, N19, and P20 and a small n15. Parietal FFP consists of N15, P18, and N20 with additional small FFP n17, n19, and n20 (Fig. 17). Frontal P17, N18, P18, and P20 and parietal n17, P18, n19, and N20, respectively, tended to have out-of-phase relationships. These FFPs were most consistently and best recorded while the subject was awake.

During NREM sleep, the waveforms became smoother with attenuation of the overriding FFP components at both frontal (Figs. 18A and B) and parietal electrodes (Figs. 19A and B). In fact, we were able to predict correctly whether the subject was awake or asleep by observing the response during the process of averaging. The attenuated FFP reappeared in REM sleep. The changes were more prominent in frontal than in parietal responses. Additional change was the latency prolongation of frontal P20 and parietal N20 in sleep with greater prolongation of P20 than N20.

Digitally filtered tracings even more clearly and dramatically expressed the progressive attenuation of FFP in NREM and their recovery in REM sleep (see Figs. 18B and 19B).

These findings raise questions about some of the previously assumed or proposed concepts of SEP. The first is the effect of sleep on SEP. It has generally been thought that sleep primarily affects middle (30 to 100 msec) or long-latency (greater than 100 msec) peaks, with prolongation of latencies and/or attenuation or augmentation of amplitude, and that it has little effect on short-latency peaks. Whether the subject is awake or asleep has not been considered important for the clinical application of short-latency SEP. In fact, it is a common practice to record the SEP during sleep because this yields a clearer response owing to reduced muscle artifact. The N20 latency prolongation in sleep has implications for clinical SEP studies, during which level of consciousness has customarily been ignored, although these changes were most prominent in deeper NREM sleep. Nonparallel prolongation of frontal P20 and parietal N20 would further complicate this problem if recorded with commonly used Fpz or Fz reference.

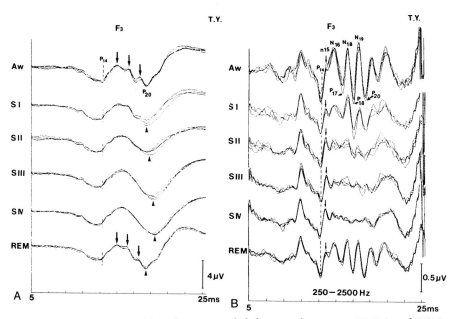

Figure 18. A, Series of frontal SEP recorded during waking state, NREM, and REM sleep. There were three negative inflections (arrows) corresponding to N16, N18, and N19 FFP over the main negative wave during the waking state (AW). They disappeared during NREM sleep and reappeared in REM sleep. Note progressive prolongation of P20 latencies (solid triangle) in NREM and its return in REM sleep. B, Series of frontal FFP tracings extracted by digital filtering from the original responses shown in A. Note progressive attenuation of all FFP except for n15 (downward arrows) during deepening of sleep stages and their recovery in REM sleep. (From Yamada T, Kameyama S, Fuchigami Y, et al: Changes of short latency somatosensory evoked potential in sleep. Electroencephalogr Clin Neurophysiol, 70:126–136, 1988; with permission.)

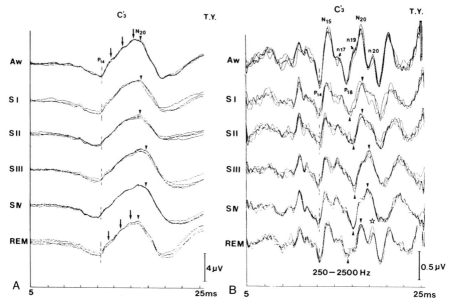

Figure 19.A, Series of parietal SEPs recorded during waking state, NREM, and REM sleep. Three negative wavelets (*arrows*), corresponding to N15, n17, and n19 FFP, appeared over the rising phase of the main negative wave. They became less conspicuous during NREM sleep and reappeared in REM sleep. The N20 peak, measured by the last negative peak before the descending phase (*solid triangle*), was prolonged in latency during stage III and IV sleep and returned to the waking value in REM sleep. B, Series of parietal FFP tracings extracted by digital filtering from the original responses shown in A. All FFP amplitude reduced in sleep, but major deflections P14–N15–P18–N20 remained. More conspicuous changes were progressive latency prolongation of P18 (*upward triangle*) and N20 (*downward triangle*) in NREM sleep. In REM sleep, FFP amplitude was smaller, but the morphology and latencies were similar to those of waking state. *Star* indicates reappearance of n20 in REM sleep. (*From* Yamada T, Kameyama S, Fuchigami Y, et al: Changes of short latency somatosensory evoked potential in sleep. Electroencephalogr Clin Neurophysiol 70:126–136, 1988; with permission.)

The second quandary provoked is the relationship between frontal P20 and parietal N20. The close latency relationship between frontal P20 and parietal N20 has suggested that they are dipole-oriented potentials arising from the same generator.[4, 7, 74] Although both frontal P20 and parietal N20 latencies were prolonged in sleep, the P20 latency shift was significantly greater than that of N20. The discrepancy of latency shift between these two peaks suggests that they are independently generated potentials.

Finally, we can no longer view the first negative wave (N17 or N19) as a product of the primary sensory system alone. Yingling and Skinner[93] and Skinner and Yingling[71] demonstrated that mesencephalic reticular formation and mediothalamic-frontocortical systems regulate neuronal activity in the reticular nuclei of the thalamus, which in turn impose an inhibitory influence on the thalamic relay nuclei. They suggested that the enhancement of evoked potential amplitude produced by mesencephalic reticular formation activation is the result of general inhibition of reticular cells, thus releasing the thalamic relay nuclei from inhibition.[93] Also, there is descending influence on the reticular nuclei from the frontal granular cortex.[71, 92, 93] This frontocorticoreticular system, by regulating thalamic inhibition, may relate to our findings (that is, appearance and disappearance of FFP, more prominently at the frontal region, depending on the level of consciousness).

Our findings indicate that the first frontal and parietal waves following P14 represent composites of multiple physioanatomic functions reflected by regionally specific thalamocortical sensory pathways and their interaction with relay, reticular, and possibly other thalamic nuclei.

ACKNOWLEDGMENT

The author wishes to thank Drs. R. Dagli, L. Krain, and A. Leis for reviewing the manuscript.

REFERENCES

1. Albe-Tessard D, Tasker R, Yamashiro K, et al: Comparison in man of short latency averaged evoked potentials recorded in thalamic and scalp hand zones of representation. Electroencephalogr Clin Neurophysiol 65:405–415, 1986
2. Allison T: Scalp and cortical recordings of initial somatosensory cortex activity to median nerve stimulation in man. Ann NY Acad Sci 388:671–678, 1982
3. Allison T: Recovery functions of somatosensory evoked response in man. Electroencephalogr Clin Neurophysiol 14:331–343, 1962
4. Allison T, Goff WR, Williamson PD, et al: On the neural origin of early components of the human somatosensory evoked potentials. In Desmedt JE (ed): Progress in Clinical Neurophysiology, vol. 7, Clinical Uses of Cerebral, Brainstem and Spinal Somatosensory Evoked Potentials. Basel, Karger, pp 51–68, 1980
5. Angel RW, Quick WM, Boylls CC, et al: Decrement of somatosensory evoked potentials during repetitive stimulation. Electroencephalogr Clin Neurophysiol 60:335–342, 1985
6. Anziska B, Cracco RQ: Short latency SEPs to median nerve stimulation: Comparison of recording methods and origin of components. Electroencephalogr Clin Neurophysiol 52:531–539, 1981
7. Broughton RJ: Discussion. In Donchin E, Lindsley DB (eds): Average Evoked Potentials. Washington, D.C., U.S. Government Printing Office, pp 79–84, 1969
8. Chiappa KH: Short-latency somatosensory evoked potentials: Methodology. In Evoked Potentials in Clinical Medicine. New York, Raven Press, pp 296–308, 1983
9. Chiappa KH, Choi SK, Young RR: Short-latency somatosensory evoked potentials following median nerve stimulation in patients with neurological lesions. In Desmedt JE (ed): Clinical Uses of Cerebral, Brainstem and Spinal Somatosensory Evoked Potentials, Progress in Clinical Neurophysiology. Basel, Karger, 7:205–230, 1980
10. Cracco RQ, Anziska B, Cracco JB, et al: Short-latency somatosensory evoked potential to median and peroneal nerve stimulation: Studies in normal subjects and patients with neurological disease. Ann NY Acad Sci 388:412–425, 1982
11. Cracco RQ, Cracco JB: Somatosensory evoked potentials in man: Far field potentials. Electroencephalogr Clin Neurophysiol 41:460–466, 1976
12. Cunningham K, Halliday AM, Jones SJ: Simulation of "stationary" SAP and SEP phenomena by 2-dimensional potential field modeling. Electroencephalogr Clin Neurophysiol 65:416–428, 1986
13. Davis H, Mast T, Yosie N, et al: The slow vertex potentials: Interaction among auditory, tactile, electric and visual stimuli. Electroencephalogr Clin Neurophysiol 33:537–545, 1972
14. Dawson GD, Scott JW: The recording of nerve action potentials through skin on man. Neurol Neurosurg Psychiatry 12:259–267, 1949

15. Deiber MP, Giard MH, Mauguiere F: Separate generators with distinct orientation for N20 and P22 somatosensory evoked potentials to finger stimulation. Electroencephalogr Clin Neurophysiol 65:321–334, 1986

16. Desmedt JE, Bourguet M: Color imaging of parietal and frontal somatosensory potential fields evoked by stimulation of median or posterior tibial nerve in man. Electroencephalogr Clin Neurophysiol 62:1–17, 1985

17. Desmedt JE, Brunko E, Debecker J, et al: The system bandpass required to avoid distortion of early component when averaging somatosensory evoked potential. Electroencephalogr Clin Neurophysiol 37:407–410, 1974

18. Desmedt JE, Cheron G: Spinal and far-field components of human somatosensory evoked potentials to posterior tibial nerve stimulation analyzed with oesophageal and noncephalic recording. Electroencephalogr Clin Neurophysiol 56:635–651, 1983

19. Desmedt JE, Cheron G: Prevertebral (esophageal) recording of subcortical somatosensory evoked potentials in man: The spinal P13 component and the dual nature of spinal generators. Electroencephalogr Clin Neurophysiol 52:257–275, 1981

20. Desmedt JE, Cheron G: Non-cephalic reference of early somatosensory potentials to finger stimulation in adult or aging normal man: Differentiation of widespread N18 and contralateral N20 from the prerolandic P22 and N30 components. Electroencephalogr Clin Neurophysiol 52:553–570, 1981

21. Desmedt JE, Cheron G: Somatosensory evoked potentials to finger stimulation in octogenarians and in young adults: Wave forms, scalp topography and transit time of parietal and frontal components. Electroencephalogr Clin Neurophysiol 50:404–425, 1980

22. Desmedt JE, Cheron G: Central somatosensory conduction in man: Neural generators and interpeak latencies of far-field components recorded from neck and right or left scalp and ear lobes. Electroencephalogr Clin Neurophysiol 50:382–403, 1980

23. Desmedt JE, Huy NT: Bit-mapping colour imaging of the potential fields of propagated and segmental subcortical components of somatosensory evoked potential in man. Electroencephalogr Clin Neurophysiol 58:481–497, 1981

24. Desmedt JE, Huy NT, Bourguet M: The cognitive P40, N60 and P100 components of somatosensory evoked potential and the earliest electrical signs of sensory processing in man. Electroencephalogr Clin Neurophysiol 56:272–282, 1983

25. Desmedt JE, Huy NT, Carmeliet J: Unexpected latency shift of the stationary P9 somatosensory evoked potential far field with changes in shoulder position. Electroencephalogr Clin Neurophysiol 56:628–634, 1983

26. Dorfman LJ: Indirect estimation of spinal cord conduction velocity in man. Electroencephalogr Clin Neurophysiol 42:26–34, 1977

27. Eisen A, Odusote K, Bozek C, et al: Far-field potentials from peripheral nerve: Generated at sites of muscle mass changes. Neurology 36:815–818, 1986

28. Eisen A, Roberts K, Low M, et al: Questions regarding the sequential neural generator theory of the somatosensory evoked potential raised by digital filtering. Electroencephalogr Clin Neurophysiol 63:384–388, 1986

29. Emerson RG, Pedley TA: Generator sources of median somatosensory evoked potentials. J Clin Neurophysiol 1:203–218, 1984

30. Emerson RG, Sgro JA, Pedley TA, et al: State dependent change in the N20 component of the median nerve somatosensory evoked potential. Neurology 88:64–67, 1988

31. Frith RW, Benstead TJ, Daube JR: Stationary waves recorded at the shoulder after median nerve stimulation. Neurology 36:1458–1464, 1986

32. Goff WR, Allison T, Shapiro A, et al: Cerebral somatosensory responses evoked during sleep in man. Electroencephalogr Clin Neurophysiol 21:1–9, 1966

33. Goff WR, Rosner BS, Allison T: Distribution of cerebral somatosensory evoked responses in normal man. Electroencephalogr Clin Neurophysiol 14:697–713, 1962

34. Goldie WD, Chiappa KH, Young RR, et al: Brainstem auditory and short-latency somatosensory evoked responses in brain death. Neurology 31:248–256, 1981

35. Green JB, McLeod S: Short latency somatosensory evoked potentials in patients with neurological lesions. Arch Neurol 36:846–851, 1979

36. Green JB, Nelson AV, Michael D: Digital zero-phase shift filtering of short-latency evoked potentials. Electroencephalogr Clin Neurophysiol 63:384–388, 1986

37. Hashimoto I: Somatosensory evoked potentials from human brainstem: Origins of short latency potentials. Electroencephalogr Clin Neurophysiol 57:221–227, 1984

38. Hume AL, Cant BR: Conduction time in central somatosensory pathway in man. Electroencephalogr Clin Neurophysiol 45:361–375, 1978
39. Iragui VJ: The cervical somatosensory evoked potential in man: Far field, conducted and segmental components. Electroencephalogr Clin Neurophysiol 57:228–235, 1984
40. Jacobson GP, Tew JM: The origin of the scalp recorded P14 following electrical stimulation of the median nerve: Intraoperative observation. Electroencephalogr Clin Neurophysiol 71:73–76, 1988
41. Jones SJ: Short latency potentials recorded from the neck and scalp following median nerve stimulation in man. Electroencephalogr Clin Neurophysiol 43:853–863, 1977
42. Kaji R, Tanaka R, Kawaguchi S, et al: Origin of short latency somatosensory potentials to median nerve stimulation in the cat. Brain 109:443–468, 1986
43. Kameyama S, Yamada T, Matsuoka H, et al: Stationary potentials after median nerve stimulation: Change with arm position. Electroencephalogr Clin Neurophysiol 1988, in press
44. Kimura J, Kimura A, Ishida T, et al: What determines the latency and the amplitude of stationary peaks in far-field recordings? Ann Neurol, 19:479–486, 1986
45. Kimura J, Mitsudome A, Beck DO, et al: Field distributions of antidromically activated digital nerve potentials: Models for far-field recording. Neurology 33:1164–1169, 1983
46. Kimura J, Mitsudome A, Yamada T, et al: Stationary peaks from a moving source in far-field recording. Electroencephalogr Clin Neurophysiol 58:351–361, 1984
47. Kimura J, Yamada T, Kawamura H: Central latencies of somatosensory cerebral evoked potential. Arch Neurol 35:683–688, 1978
48. King DW, Green JB: Short latency somatosensory potentials in humans. Electroencephalogr Clin Neurophysiol 46:702–708, 1979
49. Krichevsky M, Wiederholt WC: Short latency somatosensory evoked responses in man. Arch Neurol 35:706–711, 1978
50. Lesser RP, Koehle R, Lueder H: Effect of stimulus intensity on short latency somatosensory evoked potentials. Electroencephalogr Clin Neurophysiol 47:377–382, 1979
51. Lesser RP, Lueder H, Hahn J, et al: Early somatosensory potentials evoked by median nerve stimulation: Intraoperative monitoring. Neurology 31:1519–1523, 1983
52. Lorente de No R: A study of nerve physiology. New York, Rockefeller Institute, Studies from Rockefeller Institute, 1947
53. Lueder H, Lesser R, Hahn J, et al: Subcortical somatosensory evoked potentials to median nerve stimulation. Brain 106:341–372, 1983
54. Maccabee RJ, Pinkhasow EI, Cracco RQ: Short latency somatosensory evoked potentials median nerve stimulation: Effect of low frequency filter. Electroencephalogr Clin Neurophysiol 55:34–44, 1983
55. Mathews WB, Beauchamp M, Small DG: Cervical somatosensory evoked responses in man. Nature (London) 252:230–232, 1974
56. Mauguiere F, Courjon J, Schott B: Dissociation of early SEP components in unilateral traumatic section of the lower medulla. Ann Neurol 13:309–313, 1983
57. Mauguiere F, Desmedt JE, Courjon F: Asteroegnosis and dissociated loss of frontal and parietal components of somatosensory evoked potentials in hemispheric lesions. Brain 106:271–311, 1983
58. Mauguiere F, Desmedt JE, Courjon J: Neural generators of N18 and P14 far field somatosensory evoked potentials studied in patients with lesion of thalamic or thalamocortical radiations. Electroencephalogr Clin Neurophysiol 59:493–499, 1983
59. Mauguiere F, Ibanez V: The dissociation of early SEP components in the cervical lesions of the cervico-medullary junction: A use for routine interpretation of abnormal cervical responses to median nerve stimulation. Electroencephalogr Clin Neurophysiol 62:406–420, 1985
60. Megela AL, Teyler TJ: Habituation and the human evoked potential. J Comp Physiol Psychol 93:1154–1170, 1979
61. Møller AR, Jannetta PJ, Burgers J: Neural generators of the somatosensory evoked potentials: Recording from the cuneate nucleus in man and monkeys. Electroencephalogr Clin Neurophysiol 65:241–248, 1986
62. Nakanishi T: Origin of action potential recorded by fluid electrodes. Electroencephalogr Clin Neurophysiol 55:114–115, 1983
63. Nakanishi T: Action potentials recorded by fluid electrodes. Electroencephalogr Clin Neurophysiol 53:343–345, 1982

64. Nakanishi T, Shimada Y, Sakuta M, et al: The initial positive component of the scalp-recorded somatosensory evoked potentials in normal subjects and in patients with neurological disorders. Electroencephalogr Clin Neurophysiol 45:26–34, 1978

65. Nakanishi T, Tamaki M, Kudo K: Possible mechanism of generation of SEP far-field component in the brachial plexus in cat. Electroencephalogr Clin Neurophysiol 63:68–74, 1986

66. Nakanishi T, Tamaki M, Ozaki Y, et al: Origin of short latency somatosensory evoked potentials to median nerve stimulation. Electroencephalogr Clin Neurophysiol 56:74–85, 1983

67. Papakostopoulos D, Crow HJ: Direct recording of the somatosensory evoked potentials from the cerebral cortex of man and the difference between precentral and postcentral potentials. In Desmedt JE (ed): Clinical Uses of Cerebral, Brainstem and Spinal Somatosensory Evoked Potentials. Prog Clin Neurophysiol. Basel, Karger, 7:15–26, 1980

68. Phillips LH, Daube JR: Lumbosacral spinal evoked potentials in humans. Neurology 30:1175–1183, 1980

69. Pratt H, Starr A: Mechanically and electrically evoked somatosensory evoked potentials in human: Effect of stimulus presentation rate. Electroencephalogr Clin Neurophysiol 49:240–249, 1980

70. Sedgwich EM, El-Negamy E, Frankel H: Spinal cord potentials in traumatic paraplegia and quadriplegia. J Neurol Neurosurg Psychiatry 43:823–830, 1980

71. Skinner JE, Yingling CD: Regulation of slow potential shifts in nucleus reticularis thalamus by the mesencephalic reticular formation and the frontal granular cortex. Electroencephalogr Clin Neurophysiol 40:288–296, 1976

72. Stegman DF, Van Oosterom A, Colon EJ: Far-field evoked potential components induced by a propagating generator: Comparative evidence. Electroencephalogr Clin Neurophysiol 67:176–187, 1987

73. Suzuki I, Mayanagi Y: Intracranial recording of short latency somatosensory evoked potentials in man: Identification of origin of each component. Electroencephalogr Clin Neurophysiol 59:286–296, 1984

74. Tsuji S, Murai Y: Scalp topography and distribution of cortical somatosensory evoked potential to median nerve stimulation. Electroencephalogr Clin Neurophysiol 65:429–439, 1986

75. Tsuji S, Shibasaki H, Kato M, et al: Subcortical, thalamic and cortical somatosensory evoked potentials to median nerve stimulation. Electroencephalogr Clin Neurophysiol 59:465–476, 1984

76. Velasco M, Velasco F: Differential effect of task relevance on early and late components of cortical and subcortical somatic evoked potential in man. Electroencephalogr Clin Neurophysiol 39:353–364, 1975

77. Walker DD, Kimura J: A fast-recovery electrode amplifier for electrophysiology. Electroencephalogr Clin Neurophysiol 45:789–792, 1978

78. Woodbury JW. In Ruch TC, Patton HD, Woodbury JW, et al (eds): Neurophysiology. Philadelphia, WB Saunders, pp 85–91, 1965

79. Yamada T, Dickins QS, Machida M, et al: SEPs to bilateral simultaneous median nerve stimulation in man: Method and clinical application. In Cracco RQ, Bodis-Wollner I (eds): Frontiers of Clinical Science "Evoked Potentials," 3:58–67. New York, Alan R. Liss, 1985

80. Yamada T, Graff-Radford NR, Kimura J, et al: Topographic analysis of somatosensory evoked potentials in patients with well-localized thalamic infarction. J Neurol Sci 68:31–46, 1985

81. Yamada T, Ishida T, Kudo Y, et al: Clinical correlates of abnormal P14 in median SEPs. Neurology 36:765–771, 1986

82. Yamada T, Kameyama S, Fuchigami Y, et al: Changes of short latency somatosensory evoked potential in sleep. Electroencephalogr Clin Neurophysiol 70:126–136, 1988

83. Yamada T, Kayamori R: Somatosensory Evoked Potential: Clinical Application (in Japanese). Niigata, Japan, Nishimura Shoten, 1986

84. Yamada T, Kayamori R, Kimura J, et al: Topography of somatosensory evoked potentials after stimulation of the median nerve. Electroencephalogr Clin Neurophysiol 59:29–43, 1984

85. Yamada T, Kimura J, Machida M: Scalp-recorded far-field potentials and spinal potentials after stimulation of the tibial nerve. *In* Nodar RH, Barber C (eds): Evoked Potentials II, The Second International Evoked Potential Symposium. Boston, Butterworth, pp 353–362, 1984

86. Yamada T, Kimura J, Nitz DM: Short latency somatosensory evoked potentials following median nerve stimulation. Electroencephalogr Clin Neurophysiol 48:367–376, 1980

87. Yamada T, Kimura J, Wilkinson JT, et al: Short- and long-latency median somatosensory evoked potentials. Findings in patients with localized neurological lesions. Arch Neurol 40:215–220, 1983

88. Yamada T, Machida M, Kimura J: Far-field somatosensory evoked potential after stimulation of the tibial nerve. Neurology 32:1151–1158, 1982

89. Yamada T, Machida M, Oishi M, et al: Stationary negative potentials near the source vs positive far-field potentials at a distance. Electroencephalogr Clin Neurophysiol 60:509–524, 1985

90. Yamada T, Machida M, Tippin J: Somatosensory Evoked Potential. *In* Owen JM, Davis H (eds): Evoked Potential Testing: Clinical Application. Orlando, Fla., Grune & Stratton, 1985

91. Yamada T, Shivapour E, Wilkinson JT, et al: Short- and long-latency somatosensory evoked potential in multiple sclerosis. Arch Neurol 39:88–94, 1982

92. Yingling CD, Skinner JE: Selective regulation of thalamic sensory relay nuclei by nucleus reticularis thalami. Electroencephalogr Clin Neurophysiol 41:476–482, 1976

93. Yingling CD, Skinner JE: Regulation of unit activity in nucleus reticularis thalami by mesencephalic reticular formation and the frontal granular cortex. Electroencephalogr Clin Neurophysiol 39:635–642, 1975

Division of Clinical Electrophysiology
Department of Neurology
University of Iowa Hospitals
Iowa City, Iowa 52242

0733–8619/88 $0.00 + .20

Anatomic and Physiologic Bases of Posterior Tibial Nerve Somatosensory Evoked Potentials

Ronald G. Emerson, MD*

NEURAL GENERATORS OF SOMATOSENSORY EVOKED POTENTIALS

Somatosensory evoked potentials (SEPs) following posterior tibial nerve (PTN) stimulation reflect the activation of the white and gray matter structures of the large-fiber afferent sensory system.

White Matter Generators

White matter fiber tracts generate propagated compound action potentials. Triphasic (positive-negative-positive) waveforms are recorded as regenerative depolarization approaches, reaches, and passes a recording electrode. When recorded from a series of electrodes overlying the fiber pathways, the latency of the propagated action potential increases at recording sites located progressively more distant from the point of stimulation. These signals are usually recordable only in the vicinity of the fiber tract itself and are termed "near-field" potentials. As an example, electrodes at the popliteal fossa or overlying the spine record near-field signals reflecting the afferent volley following PTN stimulation.

White matter fiber tracts also generate another class of evoked potentials called "far-field" potentials. Unlike propagated action potentials, these are widely distributed, and their latency is independent of electrode position. For example, following median nerve stimulation, the afferent volley in the medial lemniscus generates the P14 potential,[15, 16] recordable in nearly identical form at widespread scalp locations. These far-field potentials appear to be generated when the propagated action potential reaches or traverses certain fixed points along the course of the nerve. Far-field potentials were classically thought to reflect the approaching volley

*Neurological Institute of New York, Columbia University College of Physicians and Surgeons, New York, New York

recorded beyond the point of termination of an active fiber.[34, 52] More recently, these have also been attributed to the effects of abrupt changes in the geometry[29, 30] or conductive properties[35, 40] of tissue surrounding the nerve.

Gray Matter Generators

Graded postsynaptic potentials generated in gray matter structures also contribute to surface-recorded evoked potentials. Scalp-recorded EEG primarily reflects extracellular current flow resulting from summated excitatory and inhibitory postsynaptic potentials generated in parallel rows of vertically oriented cortical pyramidal neurons and their dendrites.[17, 31, 50] Similar postsynaptic activity is likely responsible for cortical components of somatosensory evoked potentials. Some subcortical nuclei also generate postsynaptic potentials that are volume conducted to the body surface. Examples include postsynaptic activity in the central gray matter of cervical[14, 20, 35] and lumbar[46] spinal cords and the cochlear nuclear complex.[32]

GENERATOR SOURCES OF THE POSTERIOR TIBIAL SEP

This section reviews the specific generators of the somatosensory evoked potential following stimulation of the posterior tibial nerve at the ankle (PTN SEPs). Common peroneal nerve stimulation, utilized clinically in some laboratories, produces similar but nonidentical responses.[41] The reader is cautioned that there are no standard waveform designations, and that terminology differs considerably among laboratories. For example, the initial localized scalp-recorded response following posterior tibial nerve stimulation, which corresponds to the activation of the primary sensory cortex, is designated P38 in this article and by Seyal and colleagues,[45] but P36 by Kakigi and Shibasaki,[27] and P2 by Cruse[11] and colleagues. Understanding of the current SEP literature requires the reader to carefully note each author's definition of terms.

PTN SEPs are the result of activation of the large-fiber afferent sensory pathways. The afferent signals that produce the PTN SEP traverse the dorsal columns of the spinal cord,[12, 23, 25] although the dorsolateral funiculus may also play a role.[8, 49]

Spinal Components

Following PTN stimulation, electrodes over the lower spine record two distinct potentials (Fig. 1). The earliest one, labeled PV (propagated volley), has characteristics of a propagated volley, increasing in latency at progressively more rostral electrode sites. PV represents the afferent volley in the cauda equina at caudal lumbar sites, and the gracile tract more rostrally.[46]

A second distinct potential, the N22, is recorded over the lower spine. In contrast to PV, N22 is a stationary potential. Its latency remains constant, but its amplitude attenuates at sites rostral and caudal to the point of maximum voltage. N22 is maximal over the lower thoracic spine (T10 to L1), and is accompanied by a synchronous but phase-opposite waveform,

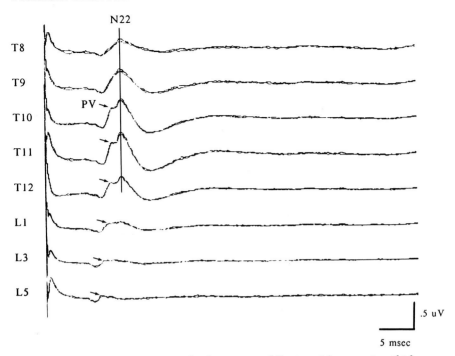

Figure 1. SEP recorded over the lower spine following right posterior tibial nerve stimulation. Left iliac crest reference.

P22, recordable from electrodes in the upper gastrointestinal tract[13] or over the anterior abdominal wall[46] (Fig. 2). Recordings following closely paired stimuli demonstrate that N22 has a long refractory period characteristic of a synaptically dependent signal.[46]

It is probable that N22/P22 represents postsynaptic activity in the gray matter of the lumbar cord generated in response to inputs from axon collaterals. The N22/P22 in humans seems to correspond to the N wave in experimental animals,[46] which is generated by interneurons in the dorsal horn of the spinal cord. It appears as a long duration negativity recordable over the dorsum of the spinal cord, reversing polarity between dorsal and ventral horns.[4, 6, 7, 9, 22] The N22/P22 is analogous to the N13/P13 recorded from cervical electrodes following median nerve stimulation, which probably reflects postsynaptic activity in the gray matter of the cervical spinal cord.[14, 20]

Bipolar electrode derivations have been recommended for recording spinal evoked potentials by the American Electroencephalographic Society,[2] presumably to facilitate recording of the afferent volley. The most prominent component of the spinal SEP is usually not PV, but rather N22. In some recordings, N22 is the only spinal component identifiable. N22 is characteristically widely distributed over the lower spine and is therefore subject to in-phase cancellation in bipolar spinal recordings. It is more effectively recorded referentially, for example, between a spinal electrode and the

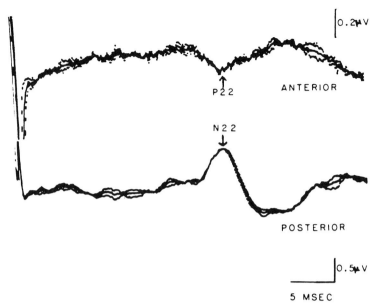

Figure 2. PTN SEPs recorded from a dorsal electrode 10 cm rostral to the L4 spine (*lower trace*) and a ventral electrode on abdominal wall at the same rostral caudal level (*upper trace*). The ventral P22 is temporally coincident with the dorsal N22. (*From* Seyal M, Gabor AJ: The human posterior tibial somatosensory evoked potential: Synapse dependent and synapse independent spinal components. Electroencephalogr Clin Neurophysiol 62:323–331, 1985; with permission.)

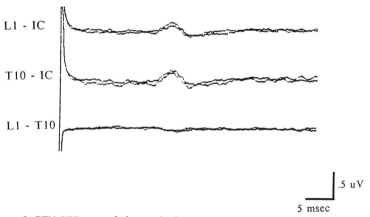

Figure 3. PTN SEPs recorded over the lower spine using referential (*upper two traces*) and bipolar (*lower trace*) techniques. The lumbar potential is well recorded using an iliac crest (IC) reference, but is nearly absent in the L1-T10 bipolar derivation, owing to in-phase cancellation.

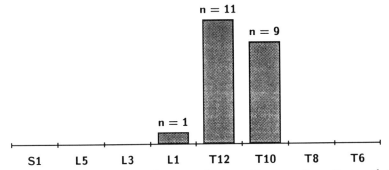

Figure 4. Vertebral level of peak N22 amplitude in 21 consecutive patients with PTN SEP studies interpreted as normal.

iliac crest (Fig. 3). Note that the latency of N22 is independent of the exact location of the spinal electrode (see Fig. 1).

The location of the N22 peak voltage may be used as an indication of the rostrocaudal position of the lumbar enlargement of the spinal cord. Figure 4 depicts the vertebral level of the peak amplitude of N22 in 21 consecutive adult patients referred for SEPs. The observation that N22 is typically maximal between the T10 and T12 vertebral levels is anticipated from the termination of the conus medullaris at L1 or L2.[5] In patients with tethered cord syndromes,[26, 43, 44] the N22 is diplaced caudally or absent (Fig. 5). Table 1 delineates spinal SEP findings in 11 consecutive patients referred for evaluation of possible tethered cord syndrome. In five patients, the normal location of the N22 corresponded to a normally positioned spinal cord, confirmed radiologically or at surgery. In six patients, lumbar recordings were abnormal, reflecting caudal displacement or absence of the lumbar potential.[19]

Seyal and colleagues[47] have described a second stationary potential, N29, with a spatial distribution restricted to the upper cervical spine. It is low amplitude and has a long refractory period, and they suggest that it reflects postsynaptic activity in the gracile nucleus (Fig. 6).

Subcortical Scalp-Recorded Components

Recordings from scalp electrodes using a noncephalic reference, such as shoulder or lower cervical spine, initially demonstrate a widely distributed response characterized by a small positive inflection, the P31, followed by a longer duration negativity, N34 (Figs. 7A and B). Sometimes a second inflection, P28, precedes P31. At sites away from the vertex, N34 returns gradually to baseline.

There are limited direct data regarding the specific generators of subcortical components of the PTN SEP, and the best information comes from analogy to the better-studied median nerve SEP. The N34 potential is strikingly similar to the N18 potential recorded following median nerve stimulation[28] in polarity as well as temporal and topographic characteristics, and most likely reflects subcortical postsynaptic activity in thalamus and/or brain stem.[15, 38] For similar reasons, the preceding P31 following PTN

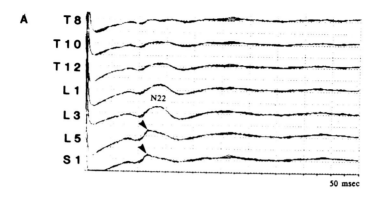

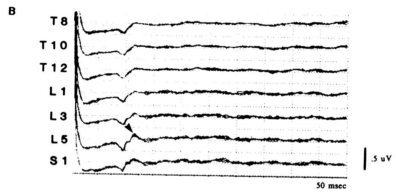

Figure 5. Spinal recordings in a 7-year-old patient with a lumbosacral lipoma and tethering of the spinal cord. To right PTN stimulation (A), the N22 is cadually displaced. To left PTN stimulation, the N22 is absent, leaving only the PV component of the lumbar response (*arrow*). Contralateral iliac crest reference.

stimulation is probably analogous to the P14 far-field component recorded following median nerve stimulation[28] and may therefore arise from the caudal medial lemniscus.[1, 3, 15, 16, 37]

Cortical Components

At the scalp vertex and adjacent areas ipsilateral to the stimulated limb, N34 is terminated by the onset of a large but topographically restricted potential, P38 (see Figs. 7A and B). On noncephalic reference recordings, Fpz is nearly inactive for potentials occurring after 34 msec, and is therefore a convenient reference site for recording subsequent localized scalp activity. Figures 8A and B demonstrate almost complete in-phase cancellation of P28, P31, and P34, with preservation of localized activity near Cz using an Fpz reference.

P38 is the first localized scalp-recorded component of the PTN SEP. It is asymmetrically distributed about Cz. Its exact topographic distribution varies considerably from subject to subject, with maximal positivity at or

Table 1. *Spinal SEP Findings in 11 Patients Referred for Evaluation of Possible Tethered Cord Syndrome*

AGE (YEARS)	DIAGNOSIS/CLINICAL PRESENTATION	LUMBAR POTENTIAL MAXIMUM	ANATOMICALLY CONFIRMED END OF CONUS	
Normally Positioned Spinal Cords				
3	Lumbosacral lipoma	R:L1 L:L1	L1	[SURG]*
8	S/P meningomyelocele repair Neurogenic bladder	R:T12 L:T12	L1	[MRI]
14	Neurogenic bladder	R:T10 L:T10	L1	[MRI]
34	Back pain and urinary urgency	R:T12 L:T12	T12-L1	[MRI]
62	Arachnoiditis with back pain and leg weakness	R:T10 R:T10	L1	[SURG]*
Tethered Spinal Cords				
5	S/P meningomyelocele repair Progressive gait disturbance	R:L5 L:L5	S1	[MRI, SURG]
7	Lumbosacral lipoma Lower extremity weakness Urinary tract infections	R:L3 L:L5	L5-S1	[MYL, SURG]
8	S/P meningomyelocele repair Progressive scoliosis	R:L4 L:L4	L3	[MYL, SURG]
14	Lumbosacral lipoma Lower extremity weakness	R:Absent L:Absent	L5-S1	[MYL, SURG]
16	Neurogenic bladder	R:Absent L:Absent	L5	[MYL, SURG]
28	Progressive leg weakness Sphincter dysfunction	R:L5 L:L5	L5	[MYL, SURG]

Legend: MRI = magnetic resonance imaging, MYL = myelogram, SURG = surgery, R = right, L = left.

The normal and tethered groups are statistically significantly different ($p < 0.005$) using the Poisson statistic.

*In these cases, myelography was misleading or ambiguous.

lateral to Cz ipsilateral to the stimulated limb (see Figs. 8A and B). In the midsagittal plane, P38 is of greatest amplitude at or just posterior to Cz. In most subjects, an approximately simultaneous negative potential, N38, is recorded over the parasagittal scalp contralateral to the stimulated limb. N38 is generally of lower voltage than P38.[11, 27, 45]

This "paradoxical" scalp distribution of the PTN SEP, with the most prominent localized component (P38) occurring *ipsilateral* to the side of stimulation, results from the location of the primary sensory cortex for leg and foot on the mesial aspect of the postcentral gyrus within the interhemispheric fissure. PTN stimulation depolarizes pyramidal cells of layer IV in the cortical receiving area. This generates an active sink in the cortical depths and a corresponding positivity (from the superficial passive source) on the cortical surface.[24] P38 reflects the ipsilaterally oriented cortical surface positivity, whereas the negative end of this "dipole" produces the

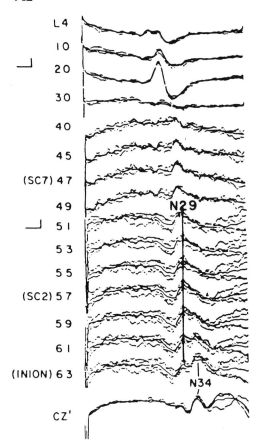

Figure 6. Spinal recordings to simultaneous bilateral PTN stimulation. SC2 and SC7 are recording sites over the second and seventh spinal vertebra. Numbers indicate distance in centimeters rostral to the L4 vertebral level. Cz' is midway between Cz and Pz (International 10–20 System). Left elbow reference. Calibration: 5 msec, 0.2 μV for upper four tracings, and 5 msec, 0.4 μV for lower tracings. (*From* Seyal M, Kraft LW, Gabor AJ: Cervical synapse-dependent somatosensory evoked potential following posterior tibial stimulation. Neurology 37:1417–1421, 1987; with permission.)

contralateral N38.[11, 45] This has been demonstrated by intraoperative cortical surface recordings that show a localized initial positivity on the mesial cortical surface following stimulation of the contralateral PTN accompanied by a simultaneous but lower voltage negativity on the lateral cortex of the same hemisphere, with latencies corresponding to the scalp-recorded P38/N38 response.[33]

It is likely that intersubject variability in scalp topography of the P38/N38 response reflects the known anatomic differences in the location of the primary sensory area for the leg.[42] If the leg area is located at the superior edge of the interhemispheric fissure, the cortical generator for P38 would be vertically oriented, and one would expect it to be maximal at or about the vertex. On the other hand, if the leg area is located deeper in the interhemispheric fissure, the cortical generator would be more horizontally oriented, and the P38 would project ipsilaterally.[33, 45] The rare situation where the leg area is located *lateral* to the superior lip of the interhemispheric fissure would explain occasional reports of P38 maximum amplitude *contralateral* to the stimulated limb.[33, 51]

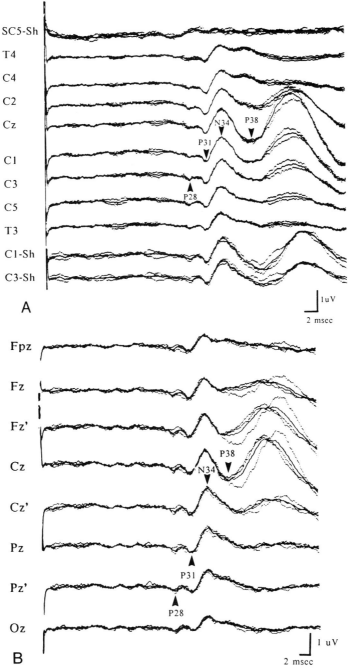

Figure 7. *A*, Left PTN SEP recorded in the coronal plane through Cz to a reference over the fifth cervical vertebra (SC5) *(middle channels)*. Absence of P28, P31, N34, and P38 on an SC5 to shoulder (Sh) recording *(top channel)* and presence of identical waveforms on scalp to shoulder recordings *(bottom two channels)* confirm the relative inactivity of SC5 with respect to these potentials. *B*, Left PTN SEP recorded in the midline sagittal plane using an SC5 reference. Note that Fpz is nearly inactive for events occurring after 35 msec.

743

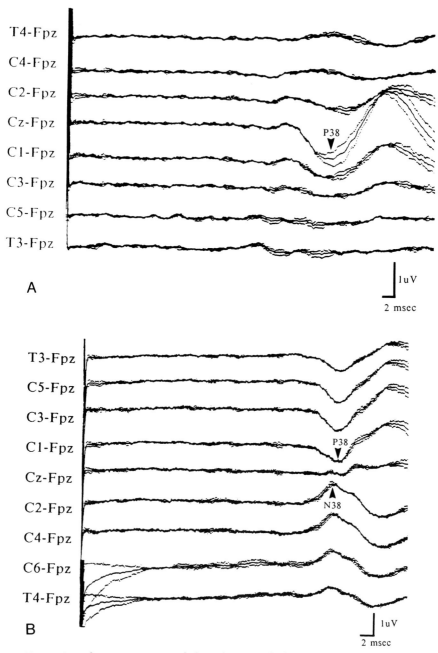

Figure 8. Left PTN SEPs recorded in the coronal plane through Cz using an Fpz reference in two different subjects (*A* and *B*) demonstrating the range of normal variability of the scalp topography of the cortical response.

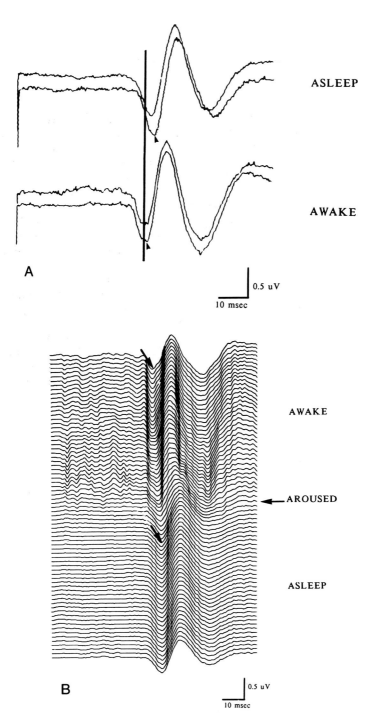

ASLEEP

AWAKE

A

0.5 uV

10 msec

AWAKE

←AROUSED

ASLEEP

B

0.5 uV

10 msec

Figure 9. State-dependent changes of the P38 latency. *A*, The upper tracing was recorded with the subject asleep following sedation with diazepam. The lower tracing was recorded immediately following arousal. *B*, Transition from sleep to wake illustrated using the two-dimensional filtering technique.[48] Each line represents 32 averaged sequential responses.

Although this model of a single dipole in the cortical leg area producing the P38/N38 is appealing, it is undoubtedly an oversimplification. In many subjects, the P38 peaks after, rather than simultaneously with, the N38. This is inconsistent with a single "dipole" cortical generator, and contributions from multiple generators have been proposed.[10, 27, 44] Multiple cortical generators are likely from investigations of median nerve SEP. Following median nerve stimulation, several inflections are often present in the N20 primary cortical response, which likely reflect the contribution of multiple generators[18, 36, 38, 39] to a composite N20 complex. Differential effects on separate cortical generators have been invoked as the basis for a recently described state-dependent change in the morphology of the N20.[21] It is likely that the P38/N38 complex reflects nearly simultaneous activation of several regions within the primary sensory receiving area for leg and foot.

Latencies of the P38/N38 complex are affected by alterations in the level of subject arousal. In normal adults, stage II sleep prolongs the P38 by up to 2.4 msec (mean 1.4 msec) and the N38 by up to 4.8 msec (mean 2.1 msec)[48] (see Figs. 9A and B). It may be that these peak latency shifts result from downward modulation during sleep of specific generators contributing to the P38/N38. Subjects and patients are generally encouraged to sleep during SEP recording, and in many laboratories it is standard practice to administer sedative drugs. Indeed, sedation is often required to obtain high-quality SEP recordings. In view of significant latency shifts of the P38/N38 complex with changes in the level of arousal, caution is warranted in the clinical interpretation of small latency "abnormalities" in SEPs obtained without controlling for state.

SUMMARY

Following stimulation of the posterior tibial nerve, lumbar electrodes record a response that is the composite of two signals, one (PV) corresponding to the afferent volley in the cauda equina and gracile tract, and another (N22) generated postsynaptically in the gray matter of the lumbar cord.

Subcortical structures generate two distinct, widely distributed signals, recordable from scalp electrodes using a noncephalic reference, P31 and N34. P31 is most likely generated by the afferent volley in the caudal medial lemniscus. N34 probably reflects subcortical postsynaptic activity in brain stem and/or thalamus, respectively.

The "primary" cortical response, P38/N38, has a complex scalp distribution reflecting the location of the leg area on the mesial apect of the postcentral gyrus, within the interhemispheric fissure. It is most likely a composite waveform with multiple cortical generators.

REFERENCES

1. Allison T, Hume AL: A comparative analysis of short-latency somatosensory evoked potentials in man, monkey, cat and rat. Exp Neurol 72:592–611, 1981

2. American Electroencephalographic Society: Guidelines for clinical evoked potential studies. J Clin Neurophysiol 1:3–53, 1984
3. Arezzo J, Legatt AD, Vaughn HG: Topography and intracranial sources of somatosensory evoked potentials in the monkey. I. Early components. Electroencephalogr Clin Neurophysiol 52:531–539, 1979
4. Austin GM, McCouch GP: Presynaptic components of intermediary cord potential. J Neurophysiol 18:441–451, 1955
5. Barson AJ: The vertebral level of termination of the spinal cord during normal and abnormal development. J Anat 106:489–497, 1970
6. Beall JE, Applebaum AE, Foremann RD, et al: Spinal cord potentials evoked by cutaneous afferents in the monkey. J Neurophysiol 40:199–211, 1977
7. Bernhard CG: The spinal cord potentials in leads from the cord dorsum in relation to peripheral source of afferent stimulation. Acta Physiol Scand 29(suppl 106):1–29, 1953
8. Burke D, Gandevia SC: Muscle afferent contribution to the cerebral potentials of human subjects. In Cracco RQ, Bodis-Wollner I (eds): Evoked Potentials. New York, Alan R. Liss, 1986, pp 262–268
9. Campbell B: The distribution of potential fields within the spinal cord. Anat Res 91:77–88, 1945
10. Cracco RQ: Traveling waves of the human scalp-recorded somatosensory evoked response: Effects of differences in recording technique and sleep on somatosensory and somatomotor responses. Electroencephalogr Clin Neurophysiol 33:566–577, 1972
11. Cruse R, Klem G, Lesser RP, Lueders H: Paradoxical lateralization of cortical potentials evoked by stimulation of posterior tibial nerve. Arch Neurol 39:222–225, 1982
12. Cusick JF, Myklebust JB, Larson SJ, Sance A Jr.: Spinal cord evaluation by cortical evoked responses. Arch Neurol 36:140–143, 1979
13. Desmedt JE, Cheron G: Spinal and far-field components of the human somatosensory evoked potentials to posterior tibial nerve stimulation analysis with oesophageal derivations and non-cephalic reference recording. Electroencephalogr Clin Neurophysiol 56:635–651, 1983
14. Desmedt JE, Cheron G: Prevertebral (oesophageal) recording of subcortical somatosensory potentials in man: The spinal P13 component and the dual nature of the spinal generators. Electroencephalogr Clin Neurophysiol 52:257–275, 1981
15. Desmedt JE, Cheron G: Non-cephalic reference recording of early somatosensory potentials to finger stimulation in adult or aging normal man: Differentiation of widespread N18 and contralateral N20 from the prerolandic P22 and N30 components. Electroencephalogr Clin Neurophysiol 52:553–570, 1981
16. Desmedt JE, Cheron G: Central somatosensory conduction in man: Neural generators and interpeak latencies of the far-field components recorded from neck and right or left scalp electrodes. Electroencephalogr Clin Neurophysiol 50:382–403, 1980
17. Eccles JC: Interpretation of action potentials evoked in the cerebral cortex. Electroencephalogr Clin Neurophysiol 3:449–464, 1951
18. Eisen A: The somatosensory evoked potential. Can J Neurol Sci 9:65–77, 1982
19. Emerson RG, Pavlakis SG, Carmel PC, DeVivo DC: Use of spinal somatosensory evoked potentials in the diagnosis of tethered cord. Ann Neurol 20:443–444, 1986
20. Emerson RG, Seyal M, Pedley TA: Somatosensory evoked potentials following median nerve stimulation. I. The cervical components. Brain 107:169–182, 1984
21. Emerson RG, Sgro JA, Pedley TA, et al: State dependent changes in the N20 component of the median nerve somatosensory evoked potential. Neurology 38:64–68, 1988
22. Gasser HS, Graham HT: Potentials produced in the spinal cord by stimulation of dorsal roots. Am J Physiol 103:303–320, 1933
23. Giblin DR: Somatosensory evoked potentials in healthy subjects and in patients with lesions of the nervous system. Ann NY Acad Sci 112:93–142, 1964
24. Goff WR, Allison T, Vaughan HG Jr.: The functional neuroanatomy of event related potentials. In: Callaway E, Tueting P, Koslow SH (eds): Event Related Brain Potentials in Man. New York, Academic Press, 1978, pp 1–79
25. Halliday AM: Changes in the form of certain evoked responses in man associated with various lesions of the nervous system. Electroencephalogr Clin Neurophysiol Suppl 25:178–192, 1967
26. Hoffman HJ, Hendrick EB, Humphreys RP: The tethered spinal cord: Its protean manifestations, diagnosis and surgical correction. Child Brain 2:145–155, 1976

27. Kakigi R, Shibasaki H: Scalp topography of the short latency somatosensory evoked potentials following posterior tibial nerve stimulation in man. Electroencephalogr Clin Neurophysiol 56:430–437, 1983

28. Kimura J, Kimura A, Machida M, et al: Model for far-field recordings of SEP. In: Cracco RQ, Bodis-Wollner I (eds): Evoked Potentials. New York, Alan R. Liss, 1986, pp 246–261

29. Kimura J, Mitsudome A, Beck DO, et al: Field distribution of antidromically activated digital nerve potentials: Model for far-field recordings. Neurology 33:1164–1169, 1983

30. Kimura J, Mitsudome A, Yamada T, et al: Stationary peaks from a moving source in a far-field recording. Electroencephalogr Clin Neurophysiol 58:351–361, 1984

31. Klee M, Rall W: Computed potentials of cortically arranged population of neurons. J Neurophysiol 40:647–666, 1977

32. Legatt AD, Arezzo JC, Vaughan HG: Short-latency auditory evoked potentials in the monkey. II. Intracranial generators. Electroencephalogr Clin Neurophysiol 64:53–73, 1986

33. Lesser RP, Lueders H, Dinner DS, et al: The source of "paradoxical lateralization" of cortical evoked potentials to posterior tibial stimulation. Neurology 37:82–88, 1987

34. Lorente De No, RA: A study of nerve physiology. Studies from the Rockefeller Institute 132:384–477, 1947

35. Lueders H, Lesser RP, Hahn J, et al: Subcortical somatosensory evoked potentials to median nerve stimulation. Brain 106:341–372, 1983

36. Maccabee PJ, Pinkhasov EI, Cracco RQ: Short latency somatosensory evoked potentials to median nerve stimulation: Effect of low frequency filters. Electroencephalogr Clin Neurophysiol 55:34–44, 1983

37. Mauguiere F, Courjon J: The origin of short latency somatosensory evoked potentials in humans. Ann Neurol 9:606–611, 1981

38. Mauguiere F, Desmedt JE, Courjon J: Neural generators of N18 and P14 far-field somatosensory evoked potentials studied in patients with lesions of thalamus or thalamocortical radiations. Electroencephalogr Clin Neurophysiol 56:283–292, 1983

39. Mauguiere F, Desmedt JE, Courjon J: Astereognosis and dissociated loss of frontal or parietal components of somatosensory evoked potentials in hemispheric lesions. Brain 206:271–311, 1983

40. Nakanishi T: Action potentials recorded by fluid electrodes. Electroencephalogr Clin Neurophysiol 53:343–345, 1982

41. Pelosi L, Cracco JB, Cracco RQ, et al: Comparison of scalp distribution of SSEPs to stimulation of different nerves in the lower extremity. Electroencephalogr Clin Neurophysiol, 1988, in press

42. Penfield W, Rasmussen T: The Cerebral Cortex of Man: A Clinical Study of Localization of Function. New York, Macmillan, 1950

43. Rossini PM, Cracco, RQ, Cracco JB, et al: Short latency somatosensory evoked potentials to peroneal nerve stimulation: Scalp topography and effect of different frequency filters. Electroencephalogr Clin Neurophysiol 52:540–552, 1981

44. Roy MW, Gilmore R, Walsh JW: Evaluation of children and young adults with tethered cord syndrome. Utility of spinal and scalp recorded somatosensory evoked potentials. Surg Neurol 26:241–248, 1986

45. Seyal M, Emerson RG, Pedley TA: Spinal and early scalp-recorded components of the somatosensory evoked potential following stimulation of the posterior tibial nerve. Electroencephalogr Clin Neurophysiol 55:320–330, 1983

46. Seyal M, Gabor AJ: The human posterior tibial somatosensory evoked potential: Synapse dependent and synapse independent spinal components. Electroencephalogr Clin Neurophysiol 62:323–331, 1985

47. Seyal M, Kraft LW, Gabor AJ: Cervical synapse-dependent somatosensory evoked potentials following posterior tibial nerve stimulation. Neurology 37:1417–1421, 1987

48. Sgro JA, Emerson RG, Pedley TA: State dependent non-stationarity of the P38 cortical response following posterior tibial nerve stimulation. Electroencephalogr Clin Neurophysiol 69:77, 1988

49. Snyder BGE, Holliday TA: Pathways of ascending evoked spinal cord potentials in dogs. Electroencephalogr Clin Neurophysiol 58:140–154, 1984

50. Towe AL: On the nature of the primary evoked response. Exp Neurol 15:113–139, 1966

51. Vas GA, Cracco JB, Cracco RQ: Scalp-recorded short latency cortical and subcortical

somatosensory evoked potentials to peroneal nerve stimulation. Electroencephalogr Clin Neurophysiol 52:1–8, 1981

52. Woodbury WJ: Potentials in a volume conductor. *In* Ruch TC, Patton HD, Woodbury JW, et al (eds): Neurophysiology, 2nd ed. Philadelphia, W. B. Saunders, 1965, pp 85–91

Neurological Institute
710 West 168 Street
New York, New York 10032

0733–8619/88 $0.00 + .20

The Anatomic and Physiologic Bases of Motor-Evoked Potentials

Paolo M. Rossini, MD

The introduction of noninvasive transcranial stimulation (TCS) of the brain has recently permitted a direct approach to the assessment of function of the central motor pathways in healthy and diseased humans.[31, 33–35, 44, 45]

METHODOLOGIC ASPECTS

Different types of technical approaches and methods for assessment of conduction time have been developed. Two kinds of electric TCS have been utilized for unanesthetized subjects testing: (1) bifocal TCS, which utilizes two stimulating electrodes, placed on the scalp region that roughly overlies the motor strip, connected to special stimulators capable of discharging elevated amounts of current; (2) unifocal TCS, which needs a lower amount of current than the bifocal one,[20, 44, 45] consisting of a pericranial cathode of six to eight interconnected electrodes and a unique anode placed on the scalp area to be stimulated (Fig. 1). In both methods, anodal stimulation demonstrates a lower threshold than does cathodal stimulation in eliciting motor-evoked potentials (MEPs), presumably by hyperpolarizing the apical dendrites of the pyramidal neurons and by indirectly depolarizing the initial segment of their axons either in the deepest gray matter layers or at the immediate subcortical level.[14, 19, 40] When analyzing differences between bifocal and unifocal TCS, we should consider that in the former, the axis of the electric field is mainly tangentially oriented and distributed along the scalp surface. If we consider the skull to act as a poor dielectric, we can identify media with high conductivity around it (skin and muscles on one side, meninges and CSF on the other). Therefore, with bifocal TCS, high amounts of current are required to distort the electric fields between anode and cathode at a level that penetrates the skull and excites the underlying brain structures. With unifocal TCS, the

---

Clinical Neurophysiology, Department of Public Health, The University of Rome "Tor Vergata," Rome, Italy

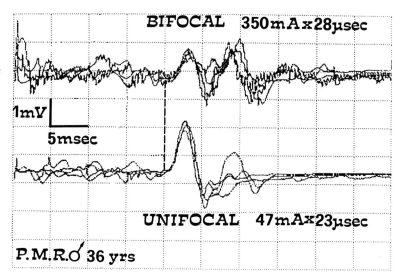

Figure 1. MEPs to electric TCS with bifocal *(upper traces)* and unifocal *(lower traces)* stimulation recorded in the same subject during the same session. Notice that onset latencies and general morphology are similar, whereas the amount of current delivered to the subject is approximately seven times lower during unifocal compared with bifocal TCS.

electric fields are maximally focused beneath the anode, and current flows from the surface circumscribed by the array of pericranial electrodes with an orientation perpendicular to the brain surface. This fact assumes paramount importance in view of the observation that—because of their radial orientation—large pyramidal cells, dendrites, and axons are preferentially penetrated and excited by parallel-flowing current paths. Therefore—at least for pyramidal neurons on the brain convexity—current paths perpendicularly oriented to the brain surface are optimal. Also with TCS of varying intensities, the amount and depth to which current penetrates pyramidal neurons are regulated by the anisotropy that they display to radial versus tangential current flow.[9] Counteracting these effects is the tendency of current injected at the surface to spread laterally rather than penetrating white matter, given the low resistance of the gray matter as compared with the summed resistance of white matter.[24]

If we compare the amplitude of the MEPs to TCS with that of motor action potentials (MAPs) to peripheral nerve stimulation, we find the former ranging between one half to one fifth of the latter in leg and foot muscles, whereas the ratio is three fourths to one fourth for the hand and arm muscles (Fig. 2). MEPs to bifocal stimulation are larger in amplitude than those to unifocal TCS, whereas they do not significantly differ in latency.

Three years ago magnetic TCS was introduced.[8, 21, 41] In this technique the discharge of a bank of capacitors through a copper coil gives rise to a time-varying and robust magnetic field that generates a net current flow proportional to the conductivity of the tissue through which it passes (Fig. 3). If the induced current reaches adequate intensity and duration, it can produce a neuronal depolarization with characteristics similar to those of a conventional electric TCS. Therefore, several aspects related to electric

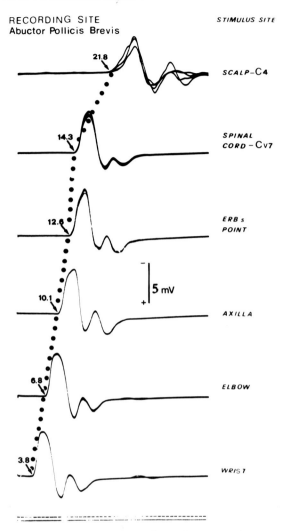

Figure 2. MEPs to bifocal electric TCS and spinal root stimulation *(top pair of traces)* and motor action potentials to median nerve stimulation at different districts. All recordings are carried out from the abductor pollicis brevis muscle; each trace is the superimposition of three responses. Notice the lower amplitude and higher variability of MEPs to TCS compared with cervical MEPs and MAPs. The motor CCT in this subject can be calculated during relaxation by subtracting the latency of cervical MEP *(second trace)* from the scalp MEP *(first trace)*; that is, 21.8 − 14.3 or 7.5 msec.

TCS, including safety, can be extended to magnetic TCS.[1, 8] The volume of tissue affected by the magnetically induced electric field has an annular, donutlike shape that is maximal just underneath the coil's circumference. This partly limits the possibility for selective activation of small brain regions, at least with the present coil shapes.

By progressively increasing the intensity of TCS while recording from a relaxed muscle, a threshold level is reached where the probability of

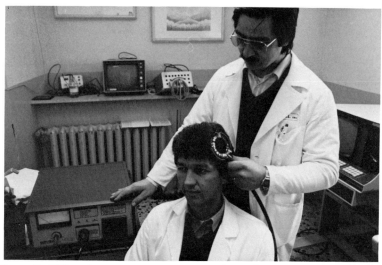

Figure 3. TCS with magnetic time-varying pulses. The examiner is maintaining the stimulator coil on the scalp area overlying the motor cortex for the right hand.

evoking a MEP is as low as 0.1 to 0.3 (Fig. 4). Stimuli about 20 per cent above the threshold level are sufficient to raise the probability to 0.8 to 0.9 as well as to decrease MEP onset latency and to increase its amplitude, shape complexity, and total duration.[20, 45, 47]

Mapping of the brain motor areas has been carried out by means of electric[42, 43] and magnetic TCS (in preparation) by separately stimulating up to 24 different scalp sites overlying the motor strip and by recording MEPs from proximal and distal muscles of the contralateral upper limb during relaxation and contraction. The area with lowest threshold for hand muscles has been localized 6.5 to 7.5 cm lateral to the scalp vertex, and up to 1.5 cm frontal to the line connecting it to the earlobe (Fig. 5). The best sites for forearm and shoulder muscles were, respectively, placed 5 cm lateral to the vertex and 1 cm frontal to the vertex–ear line, and 3 cm lateral to the vertex along the vertex–ear line. The surface of the hand "hot spot" was larger than the one for the forearm and shoulder muscles.[6, 51, 53] By increasing the TCS intensity to suprathreshold levels, or by slightly contracting the target muscles (TMs), a remarkable enlargement of the scalp area from which MEPs were elicited has been observed (see Fig. 5). TCS of the scalp vertex elicits bilateral MEPs in lower limb and pelvic muscles, which probably reflect stimulus spread to both motor cortices across the interhemispheric fissure. The steeper decrement of MEPs' amplitude when TCS is delivered frontally to the "hot spot" compared with TCS on more posterior sites may reflect different densities of large pyramidal cells in the cortical layer.[59] In fact, such giant pyramidal cells decline more rapidly in size and number at the anterior border of area 4 than at its posterior border. Alternatively, more frontally placed TCS might activate the suppressor motor area 4S,[22] which is interposed between areas 4 and 6, and yields inhibition of muscular contraction of the hemibody contralateral to the stimulated cerebral site. However, this brain district is interposed in a

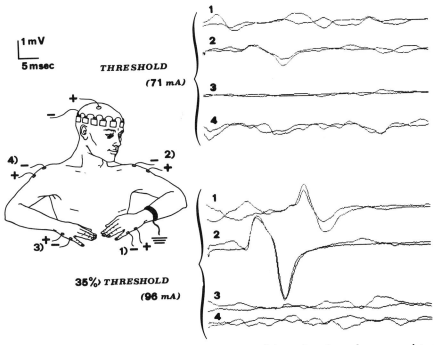

Figure 4. MEPs elicited by unifocal electric TCS delivered to the scalp area overlying the left shoulder muscles. Recording simultaneously gathered from contralateral (*upper pair in each group*) and ipsilateral shoulder and hand muscles. Notice that when threshold intensities are employed, MEPs are limited to the contralateral shoulder muscles (*trace 2 of the upper group*). In contrast, by increasing the stimulus strength by about 35 per cent above threshold (*lower group*) larger MEPs are elicited from the shoulder muscles and spread to the hand muscles is also evident. Notice that despite the subject's "facilitating" the four tested muscles at a similar degree (as judged by background EMG), MEPs are elicited only in the hemibody contralateral to the stimulus.

MAGNETIC STIMULATION

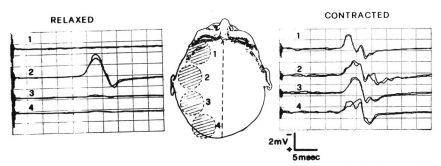

Figure 5. MEPs to magnetic TCS recorded from the right thenar muscles during relaxation (*left*) and during contraction (*right*) at numbered sites. Notice that during relaxation, MEPs are elicited only when the coil is overlapping the scalp area over the hand motor strip (2). In contrast, during moderate contraction, MEPs were invariably evoked regardless of the position of the coil over the scalp.

nonpyramidal cortico-bulbo-reticular pathway that has an elevated excitability threshold and, therefore, is probably unaffected by the type of TCS
currently employed.[32] Also the pyramidal cells buried in the primary sensory
cortex might contribute to MEPs' elicitation. However, the relatively larger
Betz cells of area 2 mainly generate slow pyramidal tract neurons (SPTNs),
which act primarily as modulators of the afferent input at the dorsal horn
and the ascending spinal tracts nuclei and of the efferent flow at the level
of the red nucleus.[6, 26, 39]

The MEPs' amplitude is generally larger in hand and forearm muscles
than in the truncal, leg, foot, and pelvic ones. This rule partly stems from
the different thresholds shown by such muscles during TCS. These—on
their own—might reflect difficulty in recruiting fibers deeply positioned
within the interhemispheric fissure and/or might be related to the fact that
in the human, the cervical cord receives several times as many pyramidal tract fibers per unit of muscle mass than does the rest of the spinal
cord.[28, 29] Moreover, it should be considered that corticospinal (CS) fibers
can directly govern only the spinal motoneurons (MNs) to distal arm and
leg muscles, whereas those for more proximal and axial musculature act
indirectly via spinal interneurons. Such adjunctive synaptic relays are known
to increase the threshold for MNs' excitation. Finally, progressively larger
temporal dispersion for descending impulses might also account for less
synchronous recruitment of the spinal MNs at progressively more caudal
levels.

Since the pioneering studies on brain stimulation, it has been observed
that one can lower the excitability threshold of the stimulated central
motor tracts and can increase to 1 the probability of eliciting a MEP by
performing a voluntary contraction of the TM immediately prior to and
during TCS.[34, 35, 45] This maneuver provokes a remarkable amplitude enlargement that reflects the decrement of excitability threshold of the "system"
activated by TCS. In parallel, a MEPs anticipation can be observed that—at
least in the hand muscle—can extend to 6 msec the difference between
"relaxed" and "contracted" MEPs (Figs. 6 and 7). One possible explanation
lies in the fact that voluntary muscle contraction "facilitates" a large
population of spinal MNs through group I reafferent activity from muscles
and tendon receptors, as well as via an intense excitatory firing descending
the CS tracts. The impact of two main mechanisms on this scenario has
been invoked to explain amplitude/latency changes between "contracted"
and "relaxed" MEPs. One is based on the observation that individual
stimuli delivered to brain motor areas elicit a sequence of repetitive
descending waves, separated by very short (about 1 msec) intervals. The
earliest of such wavelets has been labeled *D-wave* because, in relation to
its fast recovery cycle and to its resistance to synaptic blocking agents and
to asphyxia, it probably reflects *Direct* (= synapse-free) excitation of the
CS fibers. The following waves have been labeled *I-waves* because, being
less stable and less resistant to the aforementioned procedures, they are
considered the result of *Indirect* (= synapse-mediated) depolarization of
the same CS fiber previously propagating the D-wave.[2, 38] In brief, during
relaxation the early D- and progressively following I-waves might gradually
drive a small proportion of spinal MNs to their firing threshold. During

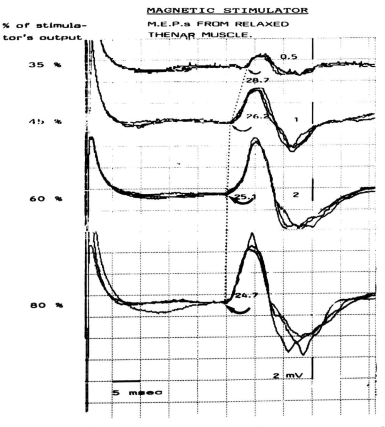

Figure 6. MEPs to TCS with magnetic pulses of increasingly stronger intensity. Recordings from relaxed thenar muscles. Notice that with more intense stimuli, MEPs of progressively larger amplitude, longer duration, and shorter latency onset are evoked (note the different calibration bars). Latency shifts mainly affect the response onset and, to a lesser extent, the following peaks.

contraction, a fringe of MNs being already close to threshold for excitation, the arrival of the D- and early I-waves is sufficient to fire an excitatory post-synaptic potential (EPSP) in a large population of spinal MNs. This explains the small amplitude and long latency of the "relaxed" MEPs, and the amplitude increments and latency decrements of the "contracted" MEPs[42, 43, 46, 49] (Figs. 7 and 8). A second mechanism underlying MEPs' facilitation is based on the "size principle" of motoneuronal recruitment, which states that at the initiation of a voluntary contraction—whether or not it provokes a ballistic or a ramp movement—relatively slow PTNs, small spinal alpha MNs, and small motor units are recruited first. In other words, a "slow" system from brain to muscle is initially activated, and only the small motor units are fired. This has been ascribed to the lower excitability threshold that both the SPTNs and the small spinal MNs display compared with FPTNs and large spinal MNs. As the contraction continues, higher threshold MNs are also recruited both at cortical and spinal levels. A "fast" system from brain to muscle, which fires large motor units in the

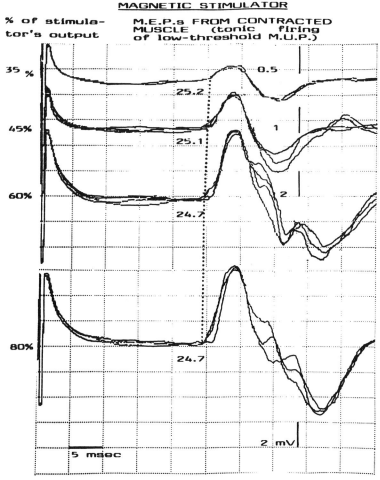

Figure 7. MEPs to TCS with magnetic pulses of increasingly higher intensity recorded during slight contraction of the examined muscles. With threshold intensities, onset latencies are close to their minimal value. Amplitudes are enhanced by more intense stimuli.

TM, is now taken into operation. On this basis small and long-latency MEPs are replaced by large and short-latency ones.[43] As previously noted, the intensity of TCS can also influence the latency and amplitude of MEPs elicited in the relaxed TM; however, the shortest latency of a MEP onset is achieved only during contraction of the TM. Such a parameter does not vary in conjunction with the amount of muscle effort.

Besides the aforementioned phenomena, voluntary contraction of the TM during TCS produces a significant enlargement of the area of the scalp from which TCS can elicit a MEP (see Fig. 5).

Continuous vibration of the TM's tendon facilitates MEPs' amplitude and latency after about 30 sec of application. Such an effect presumably follows the vibration-induced reflex tonic contraction. MEPs elicited during

Single Fiber MEPs

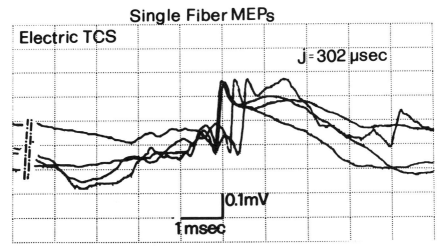

Figure 8. Single-fiber EMG (SFEMG) recordings from thenar muscles during electric unifocal TCS. Jitter (j) was calculated after collecting four responses to TCS in complete relaxation. (Poststimulus delay of 20 msec.)

vibration are smaller in amplitude but show the same latency compared with those obtained during voluntary contraction of the same TM.[42, 43] When the two maneuvers are carried out together (voluntary contraction with vibration), amplitude decrements are observed in comparison with MEPs recorded during contraction alone. This might be ascribed to the fact that vibration interferes at presynaptic levels with the facilitation exerted by group I afferents on the spinal MNs and possibly cortical MNs during contraction without vibration. When TCS is performed with paired shocks separated by an extremely short interstimulus interval (ISI) (that is, < 0.5 msec), MEPs can be facilitated up to 20 to 30 per cent with respect to those obtained with single stimuli.[42, 43] By analyzing the recovery cycle, it was noticed that MEPs to "test" stimuli fully recover the amplitude of those to "conditioning" stimuli with interstimulus intervals as brief as 3.6 msec. Such an ISI is the same at which test MAPs recover the amplitude of the conditioning MAPs during direct nerve stimulation with paired shocks.[43] This indicates that MEPs elicited in a contracted muscle by electrical unifocal TCS are mediated by a neuronal network capable of responding to elevated rates of stimulation and therefore probably contain fast and large myelinated fibers with few synaptic interruptions. Such an observation does not mean that the same pool of spinal MNs is responsible for "conditioning" and "test" MEPs—this would be unlikely with an ISI of 3 msec, owing to the partial or total refractoriness for depolarization after having fired an action potential—but it should be explained by the presence of a "fringe" of spinal MNs driven close to firing threshold by the conditioning TCS, which is discharged by the impact of the test TCS.[42] That only few synapses are interposed between the site of electrical stimulation on the scalp and the recording site on the TM has recently been confirmed by measuring the jitter of single muscle fiber discharges during consecutive TCS. Jitter values were 250 to 800 microsec during electric TCS and 300 to 2000 microsec during magnetic TCS (Figs. 8 and

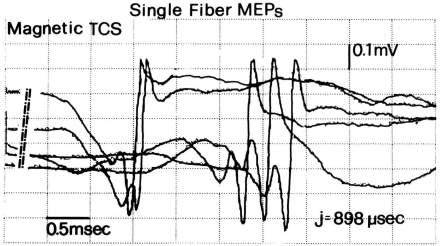

Figure 9. Same paradigm as in Figure 8 obtained during magnetic TCS with threshold intensities. Notice that the jitter is larger than the one measured during electric TCS.

9). This suggests that the former may travels a less complex circuit than the latter.[43, 60] Jitter during cervical stimulation is of the same order for electric and magnetic stimuli, approximately 150 μsec, being slightly less than that for the H-reflex but larger than that measured during direct nerve stimulation. This suggests that during cervical stimulation the MN is postsynaptically excited.[36]

The evidence previously mentioned demonstrates that the longer latencies of magnetic MEPs at least in part originate in the larger number of synaptic delays processed at cortical and/or at subcortical and/or at spinal levels on the way to the spinal MNs.

Prestimulation of the hemiscalp ipsilateral to the TM enhances the amplitude of MEPs elicited by TCS of the contralateral hemiscalp. Such facilitation becomes evident with intervals separating the ipsi- from the contra-TCS of approximately 4 msec; it remains evident for ISIs of up to 20 to 30 msec. This phenomenon, with very brief ISIs, is compatible with transcallosal facilitation of the arm motor area.[15] Such an effect is more evident in forearm than in hand muscles presumably because the precentral motor strip containing the representation of the distalmost limb muscles does not project to homotopic cortices of the opposite hemisphere.[25, 37, 50] Findings in some respect corresponding to our observations have been recently presented by Amassian and Cracco,[4] who recorded scalp potentials possibly mediated by transcallosal transmission after TCS of the opposite side of the head. When TCS utilizes threshold intensities, MEPs are limited to muscles of the hemibody contralateral to the hemiscalp undergoing TCS. The number of uncrossed CS tracts might be too small or they might be poorly excitable to threshold stimuli. When employing suprathreshold TCS, small ipsilateral MEPs can be recorded, especially from proximal muscles. In this case, however, one should be aware of the possibility that this may reflect unwanted current spread to the opposite motor cortex either through volume conduction or via callosal connections.

By utilizing an experimental protocol in which different patterns of muscle contractions were carried out in response to a warning signal, the earliest facilitation was apparent well in advance of movement initiation in the TM acting as a prime mover for the motor program, whereas only a few msec before the onset of muscle contraction other muscles acting as agonists were also facilitated (Fig. 10). This observation fits well with the known presence of pyramidal cell clusters in the motor cortex whose CS fibers distribute collaterals to different spinal cord levels to achieve a comprehensive excitatory/inhibitory control of agonist and antagonist muscles for the intended movement.[51–53] In fact, virtually all the CS tracts from forelimb or hindlimb motor areas send several branches to widely separated segments in the cervical, upper thoracic, and lumbosacral cord. Conduction velocities of such axon collaterals are remarkably slower than those of stem axons, being as slow as 1 m/sec in a FPTN and 0.4 m/sec in a SPTN; late modulatory effects on a large population of spinal MNs can be expected to be mediated by these collaterals.[52] Besides premovement facilitation, MEPs also show premovement inhibition in muscle antagonists for the programmed movement. By adopting TCS with suprathreshold intensities, a drop of MEPs' amplitude has been found in muscles acting as antagonists for the intended movement before it had actually begun (Fig. 11). However, facilitation of the agonists usually precedes inhibition of the antagonists.[41]

It is certainly not easy to establish a correlation between a muscle contraction to a voluntary order and to a nonphysiologic TCS. However, data gathered from intracortical microstimulation in primates show that the two situations share some common mechanisms. Both the voluntary command and the electrical stimulation involve the same column of PTNs inducing the related CS fibers to fire repeatedly. Moreover, both conditions affect the same group of muscles that participate as agonists and antagonists to the programmed movement.[12, 13, 16] Intracortical microstimulation facilitates muscle activity to a higher extent than the spike propagated by a voluntary command along the same CS fiber, and the type of "specificity" is about the same. In fact, the TM that is most strongly facilitated by the order to move also shows the maximal facilitation after intracortical stimulation. Single CS fibers may "call-up" a set of spinal MNs in various combinations before and during movement execution, some of which do not receive peripheral nerve inputs, and therefore represent a sort of "private pathway" for cortical effects on MNs.[12, 13] It is worth reminding here that electrical microstimulation of white matter usually displays a higher threshold than stimulation of gray matter. This favors a primary effect of TCS—at least with threshold intensities—on the cortical layers.[7]

CENTRAL CONDUCTION TIME OF MOTOR TRACTS

A central conduction time (CCT) can be calculated by subtracting the spine-to-TM time from the scalp-to-TM time (see Figs. 2 and 12). Because direct spine stimulation is believed to excite the MNs either at their axonal

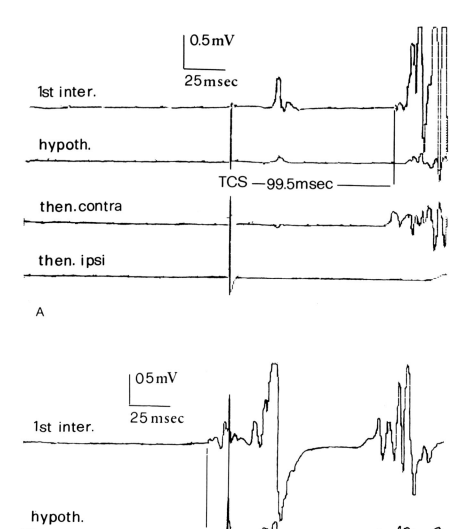

Figure 10. A, Recordings from four muscles in a reaction time (RT) paradigm in response to a flashing light. The subject was instructed to react as fast as possible by moderately contracting the first dorsal interosseus muscle. Traces start with the flash. This is followed after 125 msec (*vertical bar*) by TCS that precedes the onset of the EMG activity by 99.5 msec. The RT in this trial is 224.5 msec. The intensity of TCS was adjusted to below threshold for eliciting MEPs in complete relaxation. B, In this trial, with identical intensities of magnetic TCS, the subject was much faster (RT = 110 msec). In fact, EMG activity anticipated by approximately 15 msec the instant of TSC (*vertical bar*). Notice that MEP amplitude is several times larger in the first interosseus muscle compared with that in Figure 10A.

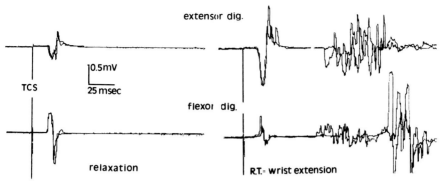

Figure 11. MEPs recorded from wrist extensors *(upper traces)* and flexors during relaxation *(left column)* and immediately before the initiation of a voluntary movement in a RT paradigm, the subject having being instructed to extend the wrist in response to a flashing light. The stimulator output was approximately 20 per cent above threshold for MEP elicitation in relaxed forearm muscles. Each trace represents a superimposition of two trials. Note that well in advance of the initiation of the intended movement, there is a clear facilitation in the muscle group acting as prime mover (the extensors), while a partial inhibition of MEPs in antagonists (flexors) was evident.

hillocks or at the ventral roots as they exit the vertebral foramina,[36, 47] this type of CCT measurement is not entirely central, being "contaminated" by a short peripheral time. F-wave measurements have been utilized for calculating the spine-to-TM time.[43, 47] The F-wave is a late muscular response reflecting backfiring of a small contingent of large alpha spinal MNs (about 5 to 10 per cent of the total one controlling the TM) to antidromically propagated impulses along the motor fibers of a supramaximally stimulated nerve.[4] The group of spinal MNs mediating the early part of MEPs in a contracted TM has been suggested to significantly overlap the one responsible for short-latency F-waves.[43] Therefore, by adopting the following equation:

$$CCT \text{ (msec)} = MEP - ([F - MAP - 1]/2 + MAP)$$

(in which MEP is the latency of responses in the TM to TCS, F is the latency of the earliest of 20 F-waves, and MAP is the latency of the motor

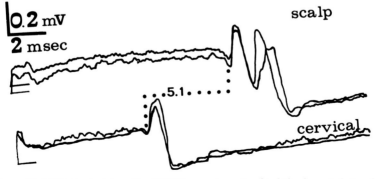

Figure 12. MEPs to electric unifocal TCS *(upper traces)* and to bifocal cervical stimulation. The CCT of the central motor fibers is 5.1 msec.

Table 1. *Motor conduction times (CCTs) of central motor tracts for shoulder (CCT-S), hand (CCT-H), foot (CCT-F), and pelvic (CCT-P) muscles in healthy controls*

	CCT-S	CCT-H	CCT-F	CCT-P	CCT C-LS	D-APB	RA-FHB	
All	4.25	5.17	13.40	13.80	7.54	9.85	20.10	M
	(12)	(49)	(22)	(10)	(22)	(11)	(15)	S.D.
	0.46	0.48	1.00	1.2	0.96	0.65	3.4	
Males		4.92	12.70		7.15			
		(9)	(9)		(9)			
		0.38	0.87		0.81			
Females		4.98	12.50		7.08			
		(9)	(9)		(9)			
		0.35	0.74		0.69			
Tall*		5.67	14.42		8.17			
		(10)	(10)		(10)			
		0.42	0.99		1.02			
Short*		4.81	12.42		7.03			
		(14)	(14)		(14)			
		0.39	0.77		0.66			
Young		5.07	13.04		7.72			
		(10)	(10)		(10)			
		0.32	0.89		0.90			
Old		5.04						
		(4)						
		0.39						

Cervical-to-lumbosacral intraspinal CCT (CCT C-LS) and intervals separating MEPs in axial and distal muscles are also indicated. Numbers ( ) represent the size of the control population.

When gender and age were compared, selected populations of homogeneous heights were utilized (range 167 to 173 cm). CCT-F and CCT-P were obtained with magnetic TCS, and to equalize them to the CCT-H and CCT-S where electric TCS was employed, the plotted values have been subtracted from 1.2 msec. D = deltoid; APB = abductor pollicis brevis; RA = recti abdomini; FHB = flexor hallucis brevis.

*Height/CCT-H corr. coeff. = r = 0.684 (p = 0.001).

response in the TM to direct peripheral nerve stimulation), one can calculate a scalp-to-spine CCT of the motor pathways. We examined this index in a large control population (Table 1) and found it to be correlated with subject height. The scalp-to-cervical cord propagation time seems slightly slower than that to the lumbosacral cord (Table 1), presumably because the latter mainly reflects the recruitment of the largest Betz cells and related uninterrupted FPTNs governing the lumbosacral MNs.[29, 43]

Direct recording via epidural electrodes and indirect measurements during MEPs recordings suggested that the central motor pathways in healthy human beings propagate with a velocity that ranges between 50 and 70 m/sec.[10, 23, 44, 43, 57, 58] This confirms that TCS mainly engages FPTNs, which—as experimentally defined—include neurons with conduction velocities between 21 and 90 m/sec.[14, 18, 54] FPTNs are particularly numerous in primate's cord, where a robust contingent of uninterrupted corticospinal neurons can be traced. They display dense terminal arborization on the apical dendrites projecting toward the most superficial cortical layers. Such arborizations are extremely rich in shafts; this renders them particularly

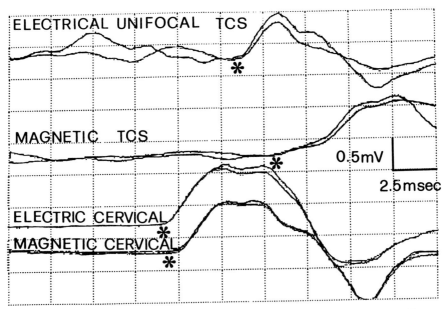

Figure 13. MEPs to electric (upper trace in each pair) and magnetic stimulation of brain (top pair) and cervical roots. Recordings obtained during slight contraction of the examined muscles. Traces cover 5 to 30 msec post-stimulus interval. Notice that cervical MEPs display a nearly identical latency onset in the two stimulating conditions, whilst scalp MEPs to magnetic TCS are delayed by about 1.7 msec with respect to the electric ones. The central CCT was 4.6 msec and 5.9 msec respectively during electric and magnetic TCS.

susceptible to excitation when a depolarizing current reaches the brain surface.[19, 27, 56]

In a group of healthy volunteers, CCTs during unifocal electric and magnetic TCS were obtained and compared (in preparation). Magnetic CCTs were longer than the electric ones by an average of 1.2 msec (Fig. 13). Such a difference has been found by others[21] and ascribed to the fact that magnetic brain TCS might indirectly excite after one or two synaptic delays the same population of corticospinal FPTNs directly excited by electric TCS or might activate the spinal MNs after one or two spinal interneurons. This agrees with our findings in jitter studies, but alternative explanations should include the possibility that "magnetic" MEPs could be generated by corticospinal fibers propagating at a somewhat slower velocity with respect to those mediating electric MEPs. Because collision techniques might help elucidate such a hypothesis, we have performed experimental protocols in which both the motor areas and the nerve governing the same TM were simultaneously stimulated. A higher amount of collision was found in the electric MEPs compared with the magnetic MEPs. If it is considered that the nerve was stimulated at motor threshold to selectively recruit the large-diameter, fast-propagating motor fibers, one might argue that—at least in the nerve—magnetic MEPs are mediated by motor fibers propagating at a slightly slower velocity than those mediating the electric MEPs. However, currently available data are insufficient to draw any definite conclusion.

With suprathreshold intensities of TCS and nerve stimulation, the "tail" of the MEP usually escapes collision. This has been ascribed to repetitive firing of the same spinal motoneuronal pool to the arrival of the discharge descending along FPTNs.[49] However, the possibility that slower PTNs are responsible for the late motor response that escapes collision and eventually reflects delayed spinal MN activation has not been ruled out yet. Slow PTNs might even include those controlling the gamma MNs known to need a lower amount of CS discharge than those of the alpha MNs;[17] this type of contribution would be mostly evident with large MEPs that provoke a muscle twich that—on its own—might elicit a segmental reflex response "contaminating" the tail of the MEP.

At the peripheral nerve level, MEPs to unifocal electric TCS are mediated by rapidly propagating motor fibers when the TM is slightly contracted, as has been substantiated by utilizing near-nerve needle recordings.[11]

Safety aspects are worth noting. Thus far, no adverse effects in several hundred healthy volunteers and patients affected by neurologic disease have been reported using these protocols. To my knowledge, this is also the case in laboratories utilizing the TCS all over the world. In about 10 per cent of the examined subjects, a transient headache in the hours following the protocol has been reported. This has been interpreted as being based on muscular contraction mechanisms. Others have noticed somnolence after stimulation combined with "better sleeping" the following night. Cortisol serum levels were reported not to be modified by electric TCS in healthy volunteers. EEG recording performed immediately before, during, and after TCS did not manifest focal or diffused abnormalities.[30, 31] No changes in the EEG spiking activity as well as in the frequency of seizures in epileptic patients undergoing TCS were noted. This should be considered together with the fact that the frequency of stimulation is far below that known to be associated with kindling. It is worth mentioning that a promising application of TCS is the one that permits the definition of how "excitable" are the structures directly connected with the motor system. We expect a lower than normal threshold in epileptic neurons. This might represent an interesting approach for clinical and pharmacologic testing. Reaction times were not significantly modified concurrently with TCS.[48]

With impulse durations of 150 μsec and intensities of about 100 mA, a current density of 70 μC/cm^2 • pH with an anodal area of 1 cm is produced, which is far from levels of possible neural damage (courtesy of Dr. W. F. Agnew).[3] However, it is very hard to measure the amount of current actually reaching the cerebral structures with electric TCS, because the majority of it is absorbed by the skull and the other extracellular layers that can greatly vary in their thickness and physical characteristics (that is, water content, etc.) from subject to subject. Conversely, magnetic TCS bypasses the extracerebral layers and, therefore, the influence of extracerebral layers on the amount of current induced in the brain is negligible. Consequently, it becomes possible to measure with a good approximation the threshold of TCS intensity necessary for eliciting MEPs in a region, and to define a range of values in a control population. Therefore—once again—the threshold intensity of TCS might result in clinical relevance because lesions predominantly or exclusively affecting the upper motoneuron might initially provoke a selective elevation in the excitability threshold of a given TM to brain, but not to roots and nerve stimulation. When the excitability of the stimulated cerebral areas was tested by stimulating a peripheral nerve close to the TM and by recording somatosensory-evoked potentials in a time interval between 80 and 120 msec after TCS (earlier stimulation was technically difficult because of the TCS artifact), no evident change in amplitude and latency of these responses was observed.

The same standards of electrical safety used for testing so-called "electrically sensitive patients" with other neurophysiologic procedures should be maintained for brain and spine stimulation (that is, patients with a cardiac pacemaker). Furthermore, subjects with metallic objects in cephalic structures (that is, clips for aneurysms) or with skull discontinuities (that is, after craniotomies) should be examined only if strongly suggested by the clinical context and with threshold TCS. Magnetic TCS should be avoided in the former group because displacement or damage of the metallic objects (consider also wearers of hearing-aids) might occur, whereas electric TCS should not be employed in the latter group because the electric current path—which invariably flows through the site of lower resistance—might create an unwanted and potentially dangerous elevated density in the brain area beneath craniotomy.[41]

ACKNOWLEDGMENTS

The author wants to acknowledge the invaluable help of Drs. Caramia, Zarola, Traversa, Pardal, Lecce, Paradiso, Martino, and Mariorenzi in collecting and organizing data; the technical support of Mr. Lavaroni; and the continuous encouragement of Prof. Bernardi.

REFERENCES

1. Adey WR: Tissue interactions with nonionizing electromagnetic fields. Physiol Rev 61:435–499, 1981
2. Adrian ED, Moruzzi G: Impulses in the pyramidal tract. J Physiol 97:153–199, 1939
3. Agnew WF, McCreery B: Considerations for safety in the use of extracranial stimulation for motor evoked potentials. Neurosurgery 20:143–147, 1987
4. Amassian VE, Cracco RQ: Human cortical responses to contralateral transcranial stimulation. Neurosurgery 20:148–155, 1987
5. Amassian VE, Steward M, Quick GJ, et al: Physiological basis of motor effect of a transient stimulus to cerebral cortex. Neurosurgery 20:74–93, 1987
6. Armand J, Aurenty R: Dual organization of motor corticospinal tract in the cat. Neurosci Lett 6:1–7, 1977
7. Asanuma H, Arnold A, Zarzecki P: Further study on the excitation of pyramidal tract cells by intracortical microstimulation. Exp Brain Res 26:443–461, 1976
8. Barker AT, Jalinour R, Freeston IL: Non-invasive magnetic stimulation of the human motor cortex. Lancet 1:1106–1107, 1985
9. BeMent SL, Ranck JB Jr: A quantitative study of electrical stimulation of central myelinated fibers with monopolar electrodes. Exp Neurol 24:147–170, 1969
10. Boyd SG, Rothwell JC, Cowan JMA, et al: A method of monitoring function in corticospinal pathways during scoliosis surgery with a note on motor conduction velocities. J Neurol Neurosurg Psychiatry 49:251–257, 1986
11. Buchtal F, Rosenfalk A: Evoked action potentials and conduction velocity in human sensory nerves. Brain Res 3:1–22, 1966

12. Cheney PD, Fetz E: Comparable patterns of muscle facilitation evoked by individual corticomotoneuronal (CM) cells and by single intracortical microstimuli in primates: Evidence for functional groups. J Neurophysiol 53:706–804, 1985

13. Cheney PD, Fetz E: Patterns of facilitation and suppression of antagonist forelimb muscles from motor cortex in the awake monkey. J Neurophysiol 53:805–820, 1985

14. Deschenes M, Labelle A, Landry P: Morphological characteristics of slow and fast pyramidal tract cells in the cat. Brain Res 178:251–274, 1979

15. Eidelberg E: Callosal and non-callosal connections between the sensory-motor cortices in cat and monkey. Electroencephalogr Clin Neurophysiol 26:557–564, 1969

16. Fetz E, Cheney PD: Muscle field of primate corticomotoneuronal cells. J Physiol 74:239–245, 1978

17. Fidone SJ, Preston JB: Patterns of motor cortex control of flexor and extensor fusimotor neurons. J Neurophysiol 32:103–115, 1969

18. Gorman ALF: Differential patterns of activation of the pyramidal system elicited by surface anodal and cathodal cortical stimulation. J Neurophysiol 29:547–564, 1966

19. Hamada I, Sakai M, Kubota K: Morphological differences between fast and slow pyramidal tract neurons in the monkey motor cortex as revealed by intracellular injection of horseradish peroxidase by pressure. Neurosci Lett 22:233–238, 1981

20. Hassan NF, Rossini PM, Cracco RQ, et al: Unexposed motor cortex activation by low voltage stimuli. In Morocutti C, Rizzo PA (eds): Evoked Potentials: Neurophysiological and Clinical Aspects. Amsterdam, Elsevier, pp 107–113, 1985

21. Hess CW, Mills KR, Murray MMF: Responses in small hand muscles from magnetic stimulation of the human brain. J Physiol 388:397–419, 1987

22. Hines M: The motor cortex. Bull Johns Hopkins Hosp 60:313–336, 1937

23. Inghilleri M, Berardelli A, Cioni B, et al: The conduction velocity of cortico-spinal tract in man. Electroencephalogr Clin Neurophysiol 66:S47, 1987

24. Jankowska E, Padel Y, Tanaka R: The mode of activation of pyramidal tract cells by intracortical stimuli. J Physiol 249:617–636, 1975

25. Jenny AB: Commissural projections of the cortical hand area in monkeys. J Comp Neurol 188:113–136, 1979

26. Jones EC, Coulter JD, Hendry SHC: Intracortical connectivity of architectonic field in the somatic sensory, motor and parietal cortex of monkeys. J Comp Neurol 181:291–296, 1978

27. Landgren S, Phillips CG, Porter R: Cortical fields of origin of the monosynaptic pyramidal pathways to some alpha motononeurons of the baboon's hand and forearm. J Physiol 161:112–125, 1962

28. Lassek AM: The pyramidal tract of the monkey. A Betz cells and pyramidal tract enumeration. J Comp Neurol 74:193–202, 1941

29. Lassek AM: The human pyramidal tract. II. A numerical investigation of the Betz cells of the motor area. Arch Neurol Psychiatry 44:718–724, 1940

30. Levy WJ, McCaffrey M, Hagichi S: Motor evoked potential as a predictor of recovery in chronic spinal cord injury. Neurosurgery 20:138–142, 1987

31. Levy WJ, York DM, McCaffrey M, et al: Motor evoked potentials from transcranial stimulation of the motor cortex in humans. Neurosurgery 15:287–302, 1984

32. McCulloch WC: Cortico-cortical connections. In The Precentral Motor Cortex. Champagne, Illinois, University of Illinois Press, pp 271–311, 1944

33. Merton PA, Morton HB, Hill DK, et al: Scope of a technique for electrical stimulation of human brain, spinal cord and muscle. Lancet ii:597–600, 1982

34. Merton PA, Morton HB: Stimulation of the cerebral cortex in the intact human subject. Nature 285:227, 1980

35. Merton PA, Morton HB: Electrical stimulation of human motor and visual cortex through the scalp. J Physiol 305:9–10, 1980

36. Mills KR, Murray NMF: Electrical stimulation over the human vertebral column: Which elements are excited? Electroencephalogr Clin Neurophysiol 63:582–589, 1985

37. Pandy DN, Vignolo LA: Intra- and interhemispheric projections of the precentral, premotor and arcuate areas in the rhesus monkey. Brain Res 26:217–233, 1971

38. Patton HD, Amassian VE: Single and multiple unit analysis of cortical stage of pyramidal tract activation. J Neurophysiol 17:345–363, 1954

39. Phillps CG, Porter R: Corticospinal neurones, their role in movement. Monographs of the Physiological Society. London, Academic Press, 34:77–175, 1977

40. Ranck JB Jr: Which elements are excited in electrical stimulation of mammalian central nervous system: A review. Brain Res 98:417–440, 1975

41. Rossini PM, Caramia MD: Methodological and physiological considerations on electric and magnetic transcranial stimulation. *In* Rossini PM, Marsden CD (eds): Non-invasive Stimulation of Brain and Spinal Cord: Fundamentals and Clinical Applications. New York, Alan R. Liss, 1988, in press

42. Rossini PM, Caramia M, Zarola F: Mechanisms of nervous propagation along central motor pathways: Non-invasive evaluation in healthy subjects and in patients with neurological disease. Neurosurgery 20:183–191, 1987

43. Rossini PM, Caramia M, Zarola F: Central motor tract propagation in man: Studies with non-invasive, unifocal scalp stimulation. Brain Res 415:211–225, 1987

44. Rossini PM, Di Stefano E, Stanzione P: Nerve impulse propagation along central and peripheral fast conduction motor and sensory pathways in man. Electroencephalogr Clin Neurophysiol 60:320–334, 1985

45. Rossini PM, Gambi D, Di Stefano E, et al: Analisi della conduzione della via motoria centrale mediante stimolazione con elettrodi di superficie. *In* Moglia A, Arrigo A (eds): Soc It EEG Neurofisiol Clin, Corso di Aggiornamento Milano, EMI-Ras, Pavia, pp 71–90, 1984

46. Rossini PM, Gigli GL, Marciani MG, et al: Noninvasive nervous propagation along "central" motor pathways in intact man: Characteristics of motor responses to "bifocal" and "unifocal" spine and scalp noninvasive stimulation. Electroencephalogr Clin Neurophysiol 66:88–100, 1987

47. Rossini PM, Marciani MG, Caramia M, et al: Noninvasive evaluation of input-output characteristics of sensorimotor cerebral areas in healthy humans. Electroencephalogr Clin Neurophysiol 61:272–286, 1985

48. Rossini PM, Zarola F, Stalberg E, et al: Pre-movement facilitation of motor evoked potentials in man during transcranial stimulation of the central motor pathways. Brain Res, 1988, 458:20–30, 1988

49. Rothwell JC, Day BL, Thompson PD, et al: Some experiences of techniques for stimulation of the human cerebral motor cortex through the scalp. Neurosurgery 20:156–163, 1987

50. Schieppati M, Musazzi M, Nardone A, et al: Interhemispheric transfer of voluntary motor commands in man. Electroencephalogr Clin Neurophysiol 57:441–447, 1984

51. Shinoda Y, Arnold A, Asanuma H: Spinal branching of corticospinal axons in the cat. Exp Brain Res 26:215–234, 1976

52. Shinoda Y, Yamaguchi T, Futami T: Multiple axon collaterals of single corticospinal axons in the cat spinal cord. J Neurophysiol 55:425–448, 1986

53. Shinoda Y, Yokota J, Futami T: Divergent projection of individual corticospinal axons to motoneurons of multiple muscles in the monkey. Neurosci Lett 23:7–12, 1981

54. Takahashi K: Slow and fast groups of pyramidal tract cells and their respective membrane potentials. J Neurophysiol 28:908–924, 1965

55. Tanji J, Kurata K: Contrasting neuronal activity in supplementary and precentral motor cortex of monkeys. I. Responses to instructions determining motor responses to forthcoming signals of different modalities. J Neurophysiol 53:121–141, 1985

56. Thach WT: Correlation of neural discharge with pattern and force of muscular activity, joint position, and direction of next movement in motor cortex and cerebellum. J Neurophysiol 41:654–676, 1978

57. Tsubokawa T: Corticospinal D response in humans: Physiological characteristics and clinical value. Electroencephalogr Clin Neurophysiol 67:64P, 1987

58. Ugawa Y: Physiologic analysis of the central motor pathways. Electroencephalogr Clin Neurophysiol 67:64P, 1987

59. Weinrich M, Wise SP, Mauritz KH: A neurophysiological study of the pre-motor cortex in the rhesus monkey. Brain 107:385–414, 1984

60. Zarola F, Caramia MD, Paradiso C, et al: Single fiber EMG jitter analysis of motor responses to brain, roots and nerve stimulation with electric and magnetic impulses. Abstr Soc It EEG Neurophysiol Clin, Sirolo 23–25 June 1988

Neurofisiologia Clinica
Dipartamento di Sanitá Publica
Il Università di Roma "Tor Vergata"
Via Raimondo, 00173
Rome, Italy

The Use of Brain Stem Auditory Evoked Potentials in the Evaluation of the Central Nervous System

Charles M. Epstein, MD*

Brain-stem auditory evoked potentials (BAEPs) are sensitive to anatomic disturbances of the brain-stem auditory pathways, especially those caused by disruption of myelin. They are influenced by temperature, but are practically unaffected by level of consciousness, drugs, and metabolic disequilibrium. These properties make BAEPs useful in evaluating many posterior fossa disorders.

Interpretation of BAEPs requires careful attention to technique and a knowledge of normal variants. BAEPs have a complex three-dimensional electric field at the scalp, which explains the variation in waveform configuration between different recording derivations.

BAEP RECORDING TECHNIQUES

At present techniques for producing, recording, and displaying BAEPs are probably more uniform across laboratories than for other evoked potentials. The classic five to seven peaks are seen within 10 msec of an auditory stimulus. By convention, vertex positivity is usually displayed as an upward deflection, and the individual waves are labeled by their positive peaks (Fig. 1).

Stimulus Parameters

The most frequently used stimulus for BAEP testing is a square-wave click of 100 μsec duration, delivered from a shielded headphone. A compression click moves the diaphragm toward the ear, and a rarefaction click moves it away. Somewhat surprisingly, the rarefaction click tends to fire the acoustic nerve a fraction of a millisecond earlier, and generally produces a better separation of the first five waves in the evoked potential.[55]

---

*Associate Professor of Neurology, Emory University School of Medicine, Atlanta, Georgia

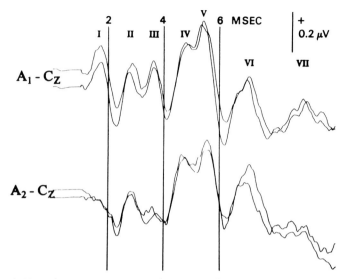

Figure 1. Normal BAEP in conventional ear-vertex derivations. Roman numerals refer to peak component. Arabic numerals refer to msec after stimulation. For this and all other two-channel figures the stimulated ear is above. With the contralateral ear derivation (bottom), wave II is often larger, III is smaller, IV is earlier, and V is later. (*From* Epstein CM, Andriola MR: Introduction to EEG and Evoked Potentials. Philadelphia, JB Lippincott Co, 1983; with permission.)

Clicks of uniform polarity are preferred,[1] but at higher stimulus levels electrostatic artifact from the headphones may obliterate the early waves. This artifact tends to be a problem with conventional earphones above 80 to 90 dB* HL, and can be reduced by alternating click polarity between rarefaction and compression. Stimulus artifact may also be reduced by piezoelectric earphones and by tubular insert phones that separate the transducer from the head with a thin plastic tube. Some laboratories routinely use masking noise in the ear that is not receiving the click stimulus. Masking does not significantly alter the range of normal values, and it is probably unnecessary except when the ear being tested hears at least 40 dB HL worse than the other one. Masking the good ear at 20 to 40 dB HL below the stimulus intensity prevents it from picking up clicks generated on the opposite side.

Latencies of the various waves depend heavily on the amplitude of the

---

*dB = decibels. The decibel is a logarithmic unit of sound intensity, and may be measured in three different systems. Decibels HL (hearing level) is derived from measurements on normal-hearing young adults tested in a quiet, soundproof room, and sets a "zero" level based on their average response across the acoustic spectrum. Decibels SPL (sound pressure level) is a physical measurement of sound wave pressure, with "zero" defined as 0.0004 dynes/square cm. Zero dB SPL is significantly lower than 0 dB HL. It is recommended as the best basis for calibrating BAEPs but is seldom used. As a consequence, "zero" may be somewhat different in different systems. In any case, on the logarithmic decibel scale, every increase of 20 dB means that the sound is ten *times* more intense. (Intensities below "0" dB HL are perfectly possible, but few people hear them.) Decibels SL (sensation level) is the difference between the point at which a given subject first hears the sound and some higher level at which he or she is then tested.

click. Up to about 60 dB above the subject's auditory threshold, the absolute latencies of the first five waves shorten progressively with increasing stimulus intensity. That of wave I may shift abruptly between 40 and 60 dB SL. To minimize the interaction of this amplitude effect and the different levels of hearing in patient populations, many laboratories measure the auditory threshold separately in each ear, and then stimulate monaurally 60 to 70 dB higher (60 to 70 dB SL). The most common rate of stimulation is around 10 per second. Lower rates require a long recording period to give an acceptable average; higher rates produce a less well-defined response and especially tend to attenuate wave I. As a compromise between sensitivity and waveform definition, a click rate of 30/sec may be slightly superior to the commonly used 10/sec, but requires collecting a separate set of normative data.[12] As with other EPs, the exact stimulus rate must be offset fractionally a bit above or below the integer 10 to avoid harmonic interactions with 60 Hz background noise.

Recording Parameters

The tiny size of BAEPs requires exquisite attention to technique for adequate recording. The skin must be prepared carefully and the impedances maintained below 5000 ohms. Placing the ear electrode at the back of the earlobe gives slightly better results than locating it on the mastoid bone or anterior earlobe. Despite averaging and "artifact rejection" options, the evoked potential can easily be overwhelmed by artifact from cranial muscle contraction or from nearby electrical equipment, such as fluorescent lights. Relaxation is best achieved by having the patient lie supine, with the neck supported on a pillow. Small children and tense or uncooperative adults usually require sedation in order to obtain an interpretable record. During the course of the recording, it is important to watch the raw input signal for extraneous artifacts (which might then be recognized and corrected), rather than just staring ineffectually at the average as it develops. If one is available, an audio monitor (with earphones) is an even better way to recognize muscle and electromagnetic artifacts.

Two recording channels are considered mandatory for neurologic applications. Almost universally these are stimulated ear-vertex and unstimulated ear-vertex. A third channel from ear to ear is occasionally useful and is easily incorporated. Well-defined responses that are noise-free and easily interpreted require only two runs to demonstrate that they are reproducible. IF THE BAEP IS AMBIGUOUS OR POORLY DEFINED, IT SHOULD BE REPEATED WITH ATTEMPTS TO REDUCE NOISE AND WITH DIFFERENT STIMULUS PARAMETERS AS OFTEN AS NECESSARY UNTIL REPRODUCIBLE AND INTERPRETABLE RESPONSES ARE RECORDED, OR UNTIL IT IS CLEAR THAT AN INTERPRETABLE STUDY CANNOT BE OBTAINED.

REFLECTION OF BAEP GENERATORS AT THE SCALP

By analogy with other neurophysiologic studies, it is easy to assume that the BAEP waves recorded in a left-ear derivation come from the left

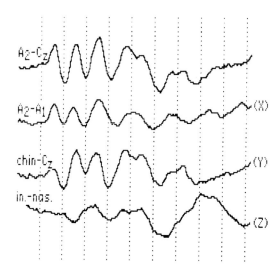

Figure 2. Normal BAEP recorded in conventional ear-vertex (top) and in three approximately orthogonal derivations from ear to ear, chin to vertex, and inion to nasion.

side of the brain stem, and those in a right-ear derivation come from the right side of the brain stem. But aside from the initial portion of wave I, the generators of the BAEP are far from the surface and lie only a few centimeters apart—much closer to each other than to the scalp.[29] Passage through the skull and CSF distorts the electrical potential that appears at the scalp. As a consequence, it is appropriate to treat waves II–V as if they represented electrical vectors pointing outward from the center of a sphere.[28, 35, 39, 51] Even if multiple generators discharge at the same time, what we record at the scalp is a single net dipole vector, because the sources are so deep and so close together. The relative size of different peaks in different derivations is therefore not dependent on the relative location of the generators; instead, it is mostly a function of how well the recording electrodes "line up" with the direction of the electrical dipole.

Figure 2 shows a normal BAEP recorded with right-ear stimulation in four channels. The top channel is a conventional derivation from stimulated ear to vertex. Channels 2, 3, and 4 are from approximately orthogonal (right-angle) derivations along ear-to-ear, chin-to-vertex, and inion-nasion (posterior-anterior) axes, respectively. The individual waves of the BAEP have quite different appearances and latencies in each axis. Some of the posterior-anterior components in the bottom channel are not seen in conventional recording and do not appear to correspond to any of the classical "waves."

To illustrate the importance of three-dimensional (3-D) concepts in understanding the effects of different derivations, Figure 3 shows wave V plotted on a 3-D Cartesian system centered near the middle of the head. The three orthogonal axes point from right to left, bottom to top, and back to front. The direction of the dipole at any single moment is represented by a cone pointing outward from the center of the coordinate axes. The size of the potential is represented by the distance from the cone to the origin. To be consistent with conventional line graphs, the cones point toward positivity at the vertex, positivity at the left ear, and positivity at

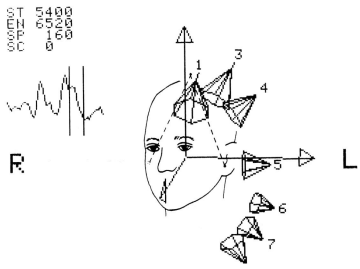

Figure 3. 3-D graph of wave V using left ear stimulation, showing vector orientations in relation to the head. Large cones with small lines at the tip come up out of the page; small cones without tips point into the page. Dashed lines represent the direction of ear-vertex derivations. STart, ENd, and SPacing between adjacent cones are noted in μsec at the upper left. The wave V vector loop rotates from the patient's right to left and from anterior to posterior. The vector parallel to A_1–C_z reaches its largest value sooner than the vector along A_2–C_z, so that the "peak" of the wave appears to come earlier in the ipsilateral derivation.

the nasion. The smaller line graph at the left in Figure 3 shows the portion of the BAEP between the two bars from which the 3-D graph is taken. In three dimensions, wave V forms a broad, open loop that reflects the complexity of its generator sources. The fact that BAEP vectors form loops in three dimensions is the reason that the latencies and amplitudes of individual waves commonly appear different in different derivations.

In normal subjects, wave V consistently turns toward the stimulated ear, and rotates clockwise with left-ear stimulation and counterclockwise with right-ear stimulation. For conventional BAEPs we measure the latency of a wave to its peak, but where is the "peak" in a 3-D loop? It depends on where we put the electrodes. For any recording derivation, the "peak" of a BAEP wave occurs when the loop attains its maximum amplitude in the direction of that derivation. Unless the loop forms a perfect circle around the origin, its apparent magnitude will be different in different recording derivations. Because the loop of wave V characteristically moves clockwise with left-ear stimulation, it will reach its "peak" along the line from left ear to vertex sooner than it will reach a peak along the line from right ear to vertex. Therefore, wave V will generally appear to peak later in the contralateral ear-vertex derivation. Wave IV usually rotates in the opposite direction from wave V, so that it seems to peak earlier in the contralateral ear-vertex derivation than in the ipsilateral one.

WAVEFORM IDENTIFICATION AND INTERPRETATION

With conventional recording techniques, wave I is most reliably identified by comparing responses from derivations connected separately to each ear, because the initial portion is present only on the stimulated side. Wave I is a major landmark for BAEP interpretation, but may be difficult to find in older subjects or in the presence of hearing loss. It may often be enhanced by increasing stimulus intensity, by using rarefaction clicks, by recording the ear-to-ear derivation, or by using a special electrode in the anterior portion of the external auditory canal.

Wave II may be difficult to identify in some normal subjects, especially if it is buried in the slope of the adjacent wave I or III; it is not considered as important a landmark. Wave II is often larger in the contralateral ear-vertex derivation. Wave III, in contrast, is usually larger (and later) in the ipsilateral ear-vertex derivation, and should be identifiable in almost all neurologically normal subjects who have normal or near-normal hearing and cooperation. Waves IV and V are generally fused together on a broad base. As noted above, these peaks usually appear to be separated more in the contralateral ear derivation, but in some patients they may be completely fused in any derivation with either click polarity. In attempting to distinguish the absence of IV or V from a completely fused IV/V, it is useful to remember that the "base" of either wave alone should be less than 1.5 msec wide, whereas the base of a combined IV/V is still greater than 1.5 msec. Wave V is further distinguished by a deep terminal downstroke carrying well below the baseline. When it is difficult to find, wave V may often be brought out more clearly by changing click polarity or by *decreasing* stimulus intensity. Waves VI and VII are so often absent, and so variable, that they can rarely be used for diagnostic purposes. Normal variants are common in BAEPs; unexpected results should not, therefore, be automatically assumed to represent abnormalities. Some possible variant patterns are discussed below.

Bifid Waves

Waves I and III are occasionally bifid in normal subjects (Fig. 4A); both may resume their conventional appearance with a change in click polarity (Fig. 4B). The earlier component of a bifid wave I appears at higher stimulus amplitudes. It is not good form to compare the earlier portion of a bifid wave I on one side with the later portion of a bifid wave I on the other.

Mega-I

Occasional subjects have a gigantic wave I on one side, with a very deep terminal downstroke as large as 1 μV (Fig. 5A). Relative to wave I, IV/V in these subjects can appear abnormally small. However, in this particular patient, comparison with Figure 5B shows that the IV/V complex is symmetrical and would not be considered abnormal on the other side. If we called the left side abnormal in this patient, we would be inferring the presence of a lesion in the brain stem on the basis of an unusually large signal from the distal acoustic nerve. Such an inference would not be very

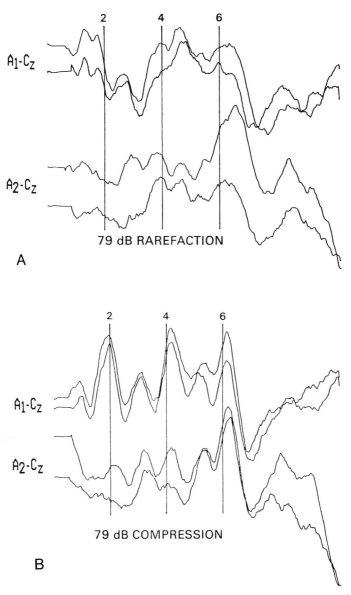

Figure 4. A, Bifid waves I and III. B, Same ear with nonbifid appearance of all waves using different click polarity. (*From* Epstein CM, Andriola MR: Introduction to EEG and Evoked Potentials. Philadelphia, JB Lippincott Co, 1983; with permission.)

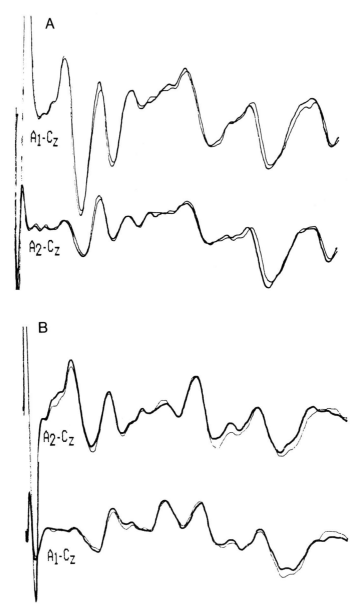

Figure 5. *A*, From A_1–C_z derivation, wave I is more than twice as large as IV/V, which constitutes an apparent amplitude ratio abnormality for IV/V. *B*, In the right ear, the IV/V amplitude is symmetrical, but wave I is smaller. Should an unusually large response from one acoustic nerve be interpreted as a lesion of the pons or midbrain?

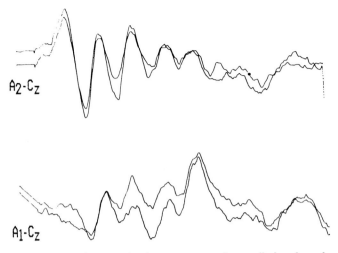

Figure 6. The amplitude ratio of IV/V to I is again abnormally low from the stimulated ear, but wave V is normal size from the opposite ear. Does this 3-D aberration of the wave V vector indicate disease?

logical, and is best avoided. A more subtle variant on this theme is shown in Figure 6. Here IV/V is abnormally small in the ipsilateral derivation, but wave V has a higher amplitude in the contralateral derivation. Recalling the 3-D vector analysis, we can infer that in this subject wave V is actually quite large, but is tilted at an unfavorable recording angle to the stimulated ear. A tilt in the 3-D vector may or may not represent brain-stem pathology, but until it is shown specifically that it does, interpreters should be cautious.

V Only

Especially when hearing loss or excess background noise is present, some studies show a characteristic reproducible wave V, with few earlier identifiable peaks. This is not necessarily the fault of the brain stem. Provided that the peak of wave V comes by 6.1 msec with regular earphones (or 7.0 msec with tubular insert phones), the study should be considered suboptimal but provisionally normal. If the absolute latency of wave V is delayed further than this, interpretation becomes quite difficult. Latency-intensity curves[18] have been advocated to resolve these cases but are not always satisfactory. When it is successful, the best approach is to find wave I by means of the techniques described above. Otherwise, such patients should have a formal audiogram.

VI-on-V

Wave VI may occur on the falling phase of the IV/V complex, leading the unwary interpreter to number these waves incorrectly (Fig. 7). *Decreasing* stimulus intensity helps to sort out this variant.

Effects of Click Polarity

Emerson and co-workers[15] noted that in 20 of 600 patients wave V could be seen with only one click polarity, and not the other. These studies

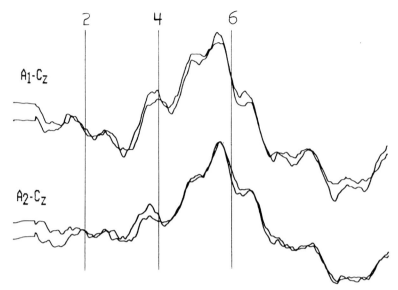

Figure 7. Wave VI merging into the shoulder of wave V.

used only a single derivation to ipsilateral ear, and the possibility of a rare normal variant could not be excluded. Yamada and colleagues[62] reported a patient with basilar migraine, in whom a reversibly delayed wave V was found only with rarefaction clicks. Unfortunately, the extraordinarily detailed studies on this patient can rarely be duplicated. Under ordinary circumstances, it may be prudent to accept as most valid the result that makes the BAEP appear most nearly normal.

In General

An abnormality is *not* necessarily present when wave I cannot be recorded in adults, when minor waves like II, IV, VI, and VII are not seen, when the IV/V complex is fused, or when the response "looks funny" to the observer. When funny-looking, noisy, or ambiguous waveforms appear, a competent technician should *automatically* try different stimulus parameters and recording strategies in an attempt to sort out noise, normal variants, and true abnormalities, and should *try to make the BAEP look normal*. It is not acceptable practice simply to quit after one or two runs, when interpretable waveforms may or may not have been recorded.

BAEP ABNORMALITIES

An abnormality of BAEPs may be defined when statistical limits of IPL or amplitude are reproducibly exceeded, or when the early peaks are recorded and later major waves are obliterated. Because they are most consistently present, waves I, III, and V are the major landmarks for BAEP interpretation. Interpeak latencies (IPL) rather than absolute latencies are

Table 1. *Normal Interpeak Latencies*

	IPSILATERAL		CONTRALATERAL	
I–V	< 4.59 msec	Inc–Vnc	< 5.15	
I–III	< 2.63 msec	Inc–Vc	< 4.12	
III–V	< 2.31 msec			

used whenever possible because they are much less sensitive to changes in stimulus intensity. Several large control series have now been published. One of the most comprehensive is that collected by Stockard, Stockard, and Sharbrough,[54] with the results seen in Table 1.

The values in Table 1 represent the "99 per cent one-sided tolerance limits" for rarefaction clicks at 60 dB SL or more in subjects older than 18 months. For compression or alternate polarity clicks they would be slightly conservative. The IPL for females separately are slightly shorter, and those for males slightly longer.

Clinical neurophysiologists establishing new laboratories are often advised to collect their own normative data for EPs. This may be essential for VEPs or long-latency EPs, where stimulus and recording characteristics vary widely; but with BAEPs most laboratories do things about the same way. The mean IPLs calculated separately by Stockard, Stockard, and Sharbrough[54] and by Chiappa, Gladstone, and Young[8] are identical, the standard deviations are similar, and the main difference is in the statistical choice of defining "normal." Large published series are generally reliable sources of control data, and can be used safely by other laboratories *provided that the hardware is similar and the stimulus and recording parameters are identical.* The real value to collecting one's own control series with BAEPs is in exposure to the broad range of normal variability.

A difference of 0.5 msec in I–V interpeak latency between the two ears may be considered abnormal, provided that peripheral auditory function and stimulus characteristics are identical on the two sides. With the electrode positions described above, a statistical abnormality exists when the amplitude from wave I to the following negative peak is more than twice as big as wave IV and wave V. (The IV/V amplitude is measured from the higher of these peaks to the base of the trough following wave V). As discussed in the section on normal variants, a mild amplitude decrease in the range of 2:1 should be considered pathologic only when a more benign interpretation cannot be found.

Hoth[26] has estimated that in the presence of typical background noise, latency estimates may be distorted by 0.05 to 0.10 msec, and amplitude estimates by a comparable amount. Trying to interpret IPL differences to within 0.01 msec or relative amplitudes to within 1 per cent may overstretch the intrinsic accuracy of the data; at times the word "borderline" is still applicable.

SPECIFIC ABNORMAL PATTERNS

Absence of All Waves

The most likely causes are severe peripheral hearing loss, excess noise, and technical error. When these possibilities can be excluded by formal

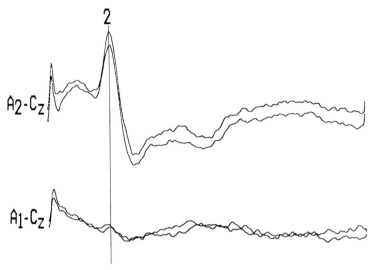

Figure 8. Wave I only recorded from patient with neonatal asphyxia.

audiometry, a well-trained operator, and ideally a clear response from the other side, a pathologic cause can be inferred. The differential diagnosis includes a very distal lesion of the eighth nerve (such as an acoustic neuroma within the temporal bone), Friedreich's ataxia,[49] and rare system atrophies.[42] Because hearing cannot be tested independently in comatose patients, and technical errors cannot be completely excluded in the absence of wave I, this pattern should never be used to diagnose brain death.

Wave I Only, Waves I and II Only, Increased I–III IPL (Fig. 8)

Lesions of the proximal acoustic nerve or pontomedullary junction near the root entry zone: The differential diagnosis includes peripheral demyelination or inflammation,[36, 50, 52] tumors of the cerebellopontine angle,[14] pontine glioma, multiple sclerosis (MS), leukodystrophies, neonatal anoxia or malformation, and brain-stem infarction. Some laboratories use a pattern of "wave I only" to confirm brain death. Because this pattern has a wide differential diagnosis, and is not automatically incompatible with survival, most interpreters do not.

Waves I–III Only, Increased III–V IPL, Decreased IV/V Amplitude (Figs. 9 and 10)

Lesions sparing the pontomedullary junction, but involving the upper pons to low midbrain: These patterns are fairly characteristic of MS, which is probably the most common etiology. However, they may be produced by any other disorder of the pontine tegmentum, and also by large extrinsic masses compressing the brain stem, especially tumors of the cerebellopontine angle opposite the stimulated ear.[40] The complexity of wave IV and V generators makes lateralization of lesions difficult at this level.

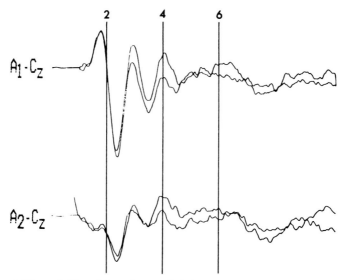

Figure 9. Waves I, II, and III only recorded from patient with multiple sclerosis. (*From* Epstein CM, Andriola MR: Introduction to EEG and Evoked Potentials. Philadelphia, JB Lippincott Co, 1983; with permission.)

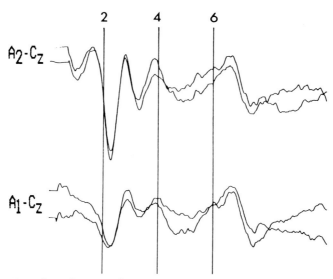

Figure 10. Prolonged III–V and I–V IPLs recorded from patient with multiple sclerosis. (*From* Epstein CM, Andriola MR: Introduction to EEG and Evoked Potentials. Philadelphia, JB Lippincott Co, 1983; with permission.)

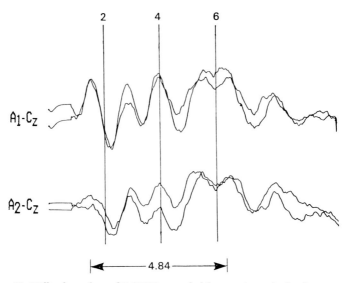

Figure 11. Diffusely prolonged I–V IPL recorded from patient who has brain-stem glioma. (*From* Epstein CM, Andriola MR: Introduction to EEG and Evoked Potentials. Philadelphia, JB Lippincott Co, 1983; with permission.)

Increased I–III IPL, III–V IPL, and I–V IPL (Fig. 11)

This pattern suggests diffuse or multifocal disease of the brain-stem auditory pathways, such as diffuse demyelination or glioma. It also occurs predictably with hypothermia.

Other Proposed Patterns of Abnormality

The patterns previously discussed constitute the great majority of currently recognized abnormalities in BAEPs. Other criteria of abnormality are theoretically possible, however, and some of these are described below.

Delayed wave I. The portion of the acoustic nerve producing wave I is invested with peripheral myelin, but some cases of MS have been said to show this finding (and rare cases of MS have peripheral demyelination). One obvious cause to be excluded is inadequate stimulus intensity. Even when intensity is adequate, high-frequency sensorineural or conductive hearing loss will still tend to delay wave I.

Abnormal wave shape. There is no *a priori* reason such a criterion could not be developed. Thus far, however, no published series has provided the data that would be required, including detailed analysis of many normal subjects and specific correlations with known anatomic and pathologic diseases. In the absence of such experience, "abnormal wave shape" seems to represent mostly a nonquantitative esthetic judgment.

Response variability. When a BAEP is difficult to reproduce despite careful efforts, it is reasonable to wonder if the problem might lie not in the test procedure or the external noise, but within the brain stem itself. Perhaps some damaged pathway is conducting only intermittently? Response variability within a single average certainly occurs in other EPs and is pathologic in some; but so far researchers skilled in signal analysis have found no evidence of this with BAEPs. As far as we can tell at present, response variability in BAEPs simply reflects external noise.[3, 61]

SPECIFIC INDICATIONS

Disorders of Myelin

BAEPs are exquisitely sensitive to white matter disease, including both inflammatory and degenerative disorders. According to many published series, more than 50 per cent of patients with definite multiple sclerosis have abnormalities of the BAEP; 30 per cent to 40 per cent of "probable" or "possible" cases have abnormalities as well.[2, 7, 9, 10, 20, 21, 31, 45, 46] Perhaps a third of patients have abnormalities in the absence of clinical brain-stem signs, which makes the BAEP diagnostically useful in many cases. This utility is dependent on the clinical situation, because an abnormal BAEP is helpful primarily in MS patients who lack other evidence of brain-stem lesions. BAEP abnormalities usually accompany internuclear opthalmoplegia but will not alter clinical localization in that setting.[59] Available data suggest that the BAEP has sensitivity equal to or better than MRI for demonstrating demyelination in the posterior fossa.[10, 20] However, serial EP studies in MS patients have shown poor correlation between appearance or remission of electrophysiological abnormalities and the overall clinical course, suggesting that EPs sample too small a fraction of the CNS white matter to be useful in routine follow-up or in clinical trials.[2]

BAEP abnormalities may be found in other disorders of myelin, especially leukodystrophies[5, 19, 43] but also including spinocerebellar degenerations,[42, 48, 49] and some cases of subacute combined degeneration.[32]

Posterior Fossa Tumors

In brain-stem glioma the incidence of BAEP abnormalities appears to be 100 per cent, except for a few cases with anatomic involvement that completely spares the pons.[11, 60] The earliest finding is prolongation of IPLs, with eventual obliteration of major waves as the tumor progresses. In our experience BAEPs are more sensitive than CT at detecting brain-stem glioma, although probably not more sensitive than MRI. BAEPs remain extremely useful and cost-effective at screening for acoustic neuroma, with a sensitivity that exceeds all other noninvasive procedures short of MRI. This application is discussed more extensively in article 9. Other tumors of the cerebellopontine angle have a lower but still significant yield of abnormalities. These are usually the result of anatomic compression and distortion of the brain stem, expressed as increased III–V IPL on stimulation of the opposite ear.[40]

Toxic/Metabolic Encephalopathies

BAEPs in adults are extraordinarily resistant to toxic and metabolic encephalopathies, and normal potentials can be recorded from patients in deep barbiturate coma with isoelectric EEGs.[41, 57] Hepatic[63] and renal[27] failure have no effect. Although inhalation anesthetics can mildly prolong the I–V IPL,[34] drug effects are mediated predominantly through hypothermia.[13,57] There is an exponential relationship between temperature and latencies as core body temperature falls below normal. The latencies of waves I, III, and V and the I–V IPL increase by roughly 7 per cent for a drop of one degree Centigrade.[37] Temperature effects are especially important in experiments with small animals, which can lose body heat very rapidly. Unfortunately, some reports of toxic or metabolic effects on the BAEP are difficult to evaluate because temperature was not carefully noted or controlled. Without discussion of possible hypothermia, increased IPLs or loss of waveforms have been reported with hypothyroidism[24] and phenytoin intoxication,[25] although previous studies of phenytoin found no major effect.[57]

The demonstration of normal BAEPs can be extremely valuable for comatose patients in whom toxic and structural factors are difficult to sort out. On the other hand, as discussed previously, many authorities do not consider the use of BAEPs helpful in the positive diagnosis of brain death.

Head Trauma

Abnormalities of the BAEP are correlated with a poor outcome in patients comatose after closed head trauma.[30, 47] Sensitivity is limited, with normal findings in some patients who have suffered extensive cerebral injury and fail to recover despite their robust BAEPs. Thus it should not be surprising that in the much milder postconcussion syndromes, individually definable abnormalities are rare. When present the BAEP abnormalities are usually minor and difficult to correlate with the nature or severity of symptoms.[53]

Brain-Stem Ischemia

Infarction of the auditory pathways within the pons or low midbrain produces appropriate BAEP abnormalities, although a competent neurologist should be able to define these classical syndromes without much difficulty. Most of the time he or she will not learn anything useful by adding EPs. Lateral medullary or even locked-in syndromes[4] may often spare the auditory pathways and produce no abnormalities. Authorities differ on the yield of BAEP abnormalities after vertebral-basilar TIAs, some considering them rare, although at least one report finds them common.[16] The latter is surprising but suggests a useful indication if corroborated.

Miscellaneous

Depending on the extent of anatomic involvement, BAEP abnormalities may be found in Friedreich's ataxia,[42, 49] Wilson's disease,[6, 17] subacute combined degeneration,[32] central pontine myelinolysis,[58] syringobulbia, and Arnold-Chiari malformation.[46] Overall, abnormalities appear to occur rarely in other spinocerebellar degenerations and multisystem atrophies that primarily involve gray matter.[42, 44, 48] We have seen prolonged IPLs in one case of atypical Jacob-Creutzfeldt disease that began with cerebellar symptoms, although in general, this rarely occurs. The utility of BAEPs in all these disorders depends on the clinical circumstance.

BAEPS IN INFANCY

Infants under 30 weeks conceptual age may have no recordable BAEPs or very long interpeak latencies. The I–V interpeak latency decreases at about 0.5 msec per week until term.[23] Compared with wave V, wave I is larger than it is in adults, and the same relative amplitude criteria should not be used. Wave III is more commonly bifid or forms a broad plateau. Infants weighing less than 1400 grams frequently have a delayed wave I suggestive of conductive hearing loss; these high-risk babies are often intubated or have other etiologies of middle ear dysfunction. The use of BAEPs to screen for infantile hearing loss is discussed more extensively in article 9.

BAEP abnormalities appear to be less specific and more reversible in neonates than in older subjects. Abnormal or absent potentials suggest significant auditory or neurologic impairment, but must be confirmed later during the first year of life before a diagnosis can be considered final. Abnormalities have been reported in many structural and metabolic disorders of infancy, with hypoxia and intracranial hemorrhage being the most common. Such abnormalities may later reverse, coinciding with improvement in clinical state. Specific localization is difficult, and in many instances abnormal BAEPs may reflect dysfunction at more than one site in the auditory pathway. A normal BAEP does not exclude long-term sequelae from neonatal anoxia.[22]

BAEPs are abnormal in symptomatic cases of infantile leukodystrophies,[5, 43] in Leigh's syndrome,[11] in nonketotic hyperglycinemia,[36] and in infantile Gaucher's disease.[33] Depending on anatomic involvement, abnormalities can be found in Möbius syndrome and other congenital brain-stem malformations. The latter tend to manifest as obliteration of waveforms rather than prolonged IPLs. Despite a few early reports, more recent data suggest that BAEPs have no predictive value for sudden infant death syndrome.[58]

REFERENCES

1. American Electroencephalographic Society: Guidelines for Clinical Evoked Potential Studies. J Clin Neurophysiol 1:3–53, 1984
2. Aminoff MJ, Davis SL, Panitch HS: Serial evoked potential studies in patients with definite multiple sclerosis. Arch Neurol 41:1197–1202, 1984
3. Boston JR: Noise cancellation for brainstem auditory evoked potentials. IEEE Trans Biomed Engr 32:1066–1070, 1985
4. Brown RH, Chiappa KH, Brooks EB: Brainstem auditory evoked responses in 22 patients with intrinsic brainstem lesions: Implications for clinical interpretations. Electroencephalogr Clin Neurophysiol 51:38, 1981
5. Chen YJ, Kurokawa T, Mitsudome A, et al: Brainstem auditory evoked potentials in children with neurodegenerative diseases. Eur J Pediatr 145:471–474, 1986
6. Chew N-S, Yang SS: Brain-stem auditory evoked potentials in different types of hepatic diseases. Electroencephalogr Clin Neurophysiol 67:337–339, 1987
7. Chiappa KH: Pattern shift visual, brainstem auditory, and short-latency somatosensory evoked potentials in multiple sclerosis. Neurology 30:110–123, 1980
8. Chiappa KH, Gladstone KJ, Young RR: Brainstem auditory evoked responses: Studies of waveform variations in 50 normal human subjects. Arch Neurol 36:81–87, 1979

9. Chiappa KH, Harrison JL, Brooks EB, et al: Brainstem auditory evoked responses in 200 patients with multiple sclerosis. Ann Neurol 7:135–143, 1980

10. Cutler JR, Aminoff MJ, Brant-Zawadzki M: Evaluation of patients with multiple sclerosis by evoked potentials and magnetic resonance imaging: A comparative study. Ann Neurol 20:645–648, 1986

11. Davis SL, Aminoff MJ, Berg BO: Brain-stem auditory evoked potentials in children with brain-stem or cerebellar dysfunction. Arch Neurol 42:156–160, 1985

12. Debruyne F: Influence of age and hearing loss on the latency shifts of the auditory brainstem response as a result of increased stimulus rate. Audiology 25:101–106, 1986

13. Döring WH, Daub D: Acoustically evoked responses under sedation with diazepam. Arch Otorhinolaryngol 227:522–525, 1980

14. Eggermont JJ, Don M: Mechanisms of central conduction time prolongation in brain stem auditory evoked potentials. Arch Neurol 43:116–120, 1986

15. Emerson RG, Brooks EB, Parker SW, et al: Effects of click polarity on brainstem auditory evoked potentials in normal subjects and patients: Unexpected sensitivity of wave V. Ann NY Acad Sci 388:710–721, 1982

16. Factor SA, Dentinger MP: Early brain-stem auditory evoked responses in vertebrobasilar transient ischemic attacks. Arch Neurol 44:544–547, 1987

17. Fujita M, Hosoki M, Miyazaki M: Brainstem auditory evoked responses in spinocerebellar degeneration and Wilson disease. Ann Neurol 9:42–47, 1981

18. Galambos R, Hecox KE: Clinical applications of the auditory brain stem response. Otolaryngol Clin N Am 11:709–722, 1978

19. Garg BP, Markand OM, DeMyer WE, et al: Evoked response studies in patients with adrenoleukodystrophy and heterozygous relatives. Arch Neurol 40:356–359, 1983

20. Giesser BS, Kurtzberg D, Vaughan HG: Trimodal evoked potentials compared with magnetic resonance imaging in the diagnosis of multiple sclerosis. Arch Neurol 44:281–284, 1987

21. Hammond KS, Yiannikas C: The relevance of contralateral recordings and patient disability to assessment of brain-stem auditory evoked potential abnormalities in multiple sclerosis. Arch Neurol 44:382–387, 1987

22. Hecox KE, Cone B: Prognostic importance of brainstem auditory evoked responses after asphyxia. Neurology 31:1429–1433, 1981

23. Hecox K, Cone B, Blaw M: Brainstem auditory evoked responses in the diagnosis of pediatric neurologic diseases. Neurology 31:832–840, 1981

24. Himelfarb MZ, Lakretz T, Gold S, et al. Auditory brain stem responses in thyroid dysfunction. J Laryngol Otol 95:679–686, 1981

25. Hirose G, Kitagawa Y, Chujo T: Acute effects of phenytoin on brainstem potentials: Clinical and experimental study. Neurology 36:1521–1524, 1986

26. Hoth S: Reliability of latency and amplitude values of auditory evoked potentials. Audiology 25:248–257, 1986

27. Hutchinson JC, Klodd DA: Electrophysiologic analysis of auditory, vestibular and brain stem function in chronic renal failure. Laryngoscope 92:833–843, 1982

28. Ino T, Mizoi K: Vector analysis of auditory brain stem responses (BSR) in human beings. Arch Otorhinolaryngol 226:55–62, 1980

29. Jewett DL, Williston JS: Auditory evoked far-fields averaged from the scalp of humans. Brain 94:681–696, 1971

30. Karnaze DS, Marshall LF, McCarthy CS, et al: Localizing and prognostic value of auditory evoked responses in coma after closed head injury. Neurology 32:299–302, 1982

31. Khoshbin S, Hallet M: Multimodality evoked potentials and blink reflex in multiple sclerosis. Neurology 31:138–144, 1981

32. Krumholz A, Weiss HD, Goldstein PJ, et al: Evoked responses in vitamin B12 deficiency. Ann Neurol 9:407–409, 1981

33. Lacey DJ, Terplan K: Correlating auditory evoked and brainstem histologic abnormalities in infantile Gaucher's disease. Neurology 34:539–541, 1984

34. Manninen PH, Lam AM, Nicholas JF: The effects of isoflurane and isoflurane-nitrous oxide anesthesia on brainstem auditory evoked potentials in humans. Anesth Analg 64:43–47, 1985

35. Marillaud A, Paquereau J, Ingrand P: Caracteristiques des représentations tridimensionnelles des potentiels évoqués auditifs du tronc cérébral. Rev EEG Neurophysiol Clin 16:411–422, 1986

36. Markand ON, Garg BP, Brandt IK: Nonketotic hyperglycinemia: Electrocephalographic and evoked potential abnormalities. Neurology 32:151–156, 1982
37. Markand ON, Lee BI, Warren C, et al: Effects of hypothermia on brainstem auditory evoked potentials in humans. Ann Neurol 22:507–513, 1987
38. Maurizzi M, Ottaviani F, Almadori G: Auditory brainstem and middle-latency responses in Bell's palsy. Audiology 26:111–116, 1987
39. Mizoi K, Ino T, Isogai Y: Vector analysis of evoked brain potentials—Theoretical background of a newly developed method by the stimulation. Nippon Jibiinkoka Gakkai Kaiho 81:131–140, 1978
40. Musiek FE, Kibbe K: Auditory brain stem response wave IV–V abnormalities from the ear opposite large cerebellopontine lesions. Am J Otology 7:253–260, 1986
41. Newlon PG, Greenberg RP, Enas GG, et al: Effects of therapeutic pentobarbital coma on multimodality evoked potentials recorded from severely head-injured patients. Neurosurgery 12:613–619, 1983
42. Nuwer MR, Perlman SL, Packwood JW, et al: Evoked potential abnormalities in the various inherited ataxias. Ann Neurol 13:20–27, 1983
43. Ochs R, Markand ON, DeMyer WE: Brainstem auditory evoked responses in leukodystrophies. Neurology 29:1089–1093, 1979
44. Prasher D, Bannister R: Brainstem auditory evoked potentials in patients with multiple system atrophy with progressive autonomic failure (Shy-Drager syndrome). J Neurol Neurosurg Psychiatry 49:278–289, 1986
45. Purves SJ, Low MD, Galloway J, et al: A comparison of visual, brainstem auditory, and somatosensory evoked potentials in multiple sclerosis. Can J Neurol Sci 8:15–19, 1981
46. Robinson K, Rudge P: The use of the auditory evoked potential in the diagnosis of multiple sclerosis. J Neurol Sci 45:235–244, 1980
47. Rosenberg C, Wogensen K, Starr A: Auditory brain-stem and middle- and long-latency evoked potentials in coma. Arch Neurol 41:835–838, 1984
48. Rossini PM, Cracco JB: Somatosensory and brainstem auditory evoked potentials in neurodegenerative system disorders. Eur Neurol 26:176–188, 1987
49. Satya-Murti S, Cacace AT, Hanson PA: Auditory dysfunction in Friedreich's ataxia: Result of spiral ganglion degeneration. Neurology 30:1047–1053, 1980
50. Satya-Murti S, Cacace AT, Hanson PA: Abnormal auditory evoked potentials in hereditary motor-sensory neuropathy. Ann Neurol 5:445–448, 1979
51. Scherg M, Von Cramon D: A new interpretation of the generators of BAEP waves I–V: Results of a spatio-temporal dipole model. Electroencephalogr Clin Neurophysiol 62:290–299, 1985
52. Schiff JA, Cracco RQ, Cracco JB: Brainstem auditory evoked potentials in Guillian-Barre syndrome. Neurology 35:771–773, 1985
53. Schoenhuber R, Gentilini M: Auditory brain stem responses in the prognosis of late postconcussional symptoms and neuropsychological dysfunction after minor head injury. Neurosurgery 19:532–534, 1986
54. Stockard JE, Stockard JJ, Sharbrough FW: Nonpathologic factors influencing brainstem auditory evoked potentials. Am J EEG Technol 18:177–209, 1978
55. Stockard JE, Stockard JJ, Westmoreland BF, et al: Brainstem auditory evoked responses: Normal variation as a function of stimulus and response characteristics. Arch Neurol 36:823–831, 1979
56. Stockard JJ: Brainstem auditory evoked potentials in adult and infant sleep apnea syndromes, including sudden infant death syndrome and near-miss for sudden infant death. Ann NY Acad Sci 388:443–465, 1982
57. Stockard JJ, Rossiter VS, Jones TA, et al: Effects of centrally acting drugs on brainstem auditory responses. Electroencephalogr Clin Neurophysiol 43:550–551, 1977
58. Stockard JJ, Rossiter VS, Wiederholt WC, et al: Brain stem auditory-evoked responses in suspected central pontine myelinolysis. Arch Neurol 33:726–728, 1976
59. Stockard JJ, Stockard JE, Sharbrough FW: Detection and localization of occult lesions with brainstem auditory evoked responses. Mayo Clin Proc 52:761–769, 1977
60. Weston PF, Manson JI, Abbott KJ: Auditory brainstem-evoked response in childhood brainstem glioma. Child Nerv Syst 2:301–305, 1986
61. Wong PKH, Bickford RG: Brainstem auditory evoked potentials: The use of noise estimate. Electroencephalogr Clin Neurophysiol 50:25–34, 1980

62. Yamada T, Dickins QS, Arensdorf K, et al: Basilar migraine: Polarity-dependent alteration of brainstem auditory evoked potential. Neurology 36:1256–1260, 1986
63. Yang S-S, Chu N-S, Liaw Y-F: Brainstem auditory evoked potentials in hepatic encephalopathy. Hepatology 6:1352–1355, 1986

Department of Neurology
Emory University School of Medicine
Atlanta, Georgia 30322

Evoked Potentials   0733 8619/88 $0.00 + .20

Auditory Evoked Potentials in the Assessment of Hearing

Terence W. Picton, MD, PhD, FRCP(C),*
and Andrée Durieux-Smith, PhD†

The clinician concerned with hearing impairment must bear in mind four basic principles. First, the hearing loss must be *detected* as quickly and as accurately as possible. Detection is usually done by the patient or the patient's family. However, hearing impairment in infancy can easily go undetected for many months or even years, unless it is actively sought out. Second, the hearing impairment must be fully *described*. The initial description of the hearing loss presents the hearing thresholds at different frequencies to air- and bone-conducted tones—the "audiogram." Third, the etiology of the hearing impairment must be *diagnosed*. Where in the auditory system is the primary defect and what is the cause of this defect? Fourth, the effects of the hearing loss must be *diminished*. The management of a hearing impairment will require removing the cause, if this is possible, or counteracting the effect of the impairment by amplification and training.

Audiometry

The auditory evoked potentials (AEPs) can play a role in all these procedures. It is important to realize, however, that the AEPs are only one part of the full audiometric evaluation. In *behavioral audiometry*, sounds are presented and the patient is asked to detect them, identify them, or discriminate them from other sounds. The behavioral response can require conscious processing—the pressing of a button—or it can be reflexive—the orienting of the eyes to the location of a sound. *Impedance audiometry* measures the impedance of the middle ear and describes how it changes during artificial variations of the pressure in the external auditory meatus or reflex contractions of the middle ear muscles. *Evoked potential audiometry* is the third part of the audiometric triangle.

*Professor of Medicine, University of Ottawa; Attending Physician, Ottawa General Hospital; and Consultant Physician, Children's Hospital of Eastern Ontario, Canada
†Associate Professor of Otolaryngology, University of Ottawa; and Director of Audiology, Children's Hospital of Eastern Ontario, Canada

Table 1. *Auditory Evoked Potentials*

LATENCY	TRANSIENT	STEADY STATE	SUSTAINED
First	Cochlear nerve action potential (N1, N2)	Cochlear Microphonic (CM)	Summating Potential (SP)
Fast	Auditory brain-stem response (I–VII)	Frequency-following response (FFR)	Pedestal of frequency following response
Middle	Middle-latency response (Na, Pa, Nb)	40 Hz potential	
Slow	Vertex potential (P1, N1, P2, N2)	Slow steady-state response	Cortical sustained potential
Late	Endogenous evoked potentials (e.g., P3 or P300)		Contingent negative variation (CNV)

Evoked potential audiometry has certain advantages over behavioral audiometry. The AEPs require less cooperation on the part of the patient and are therefore considered "objective." Furthermore, they measure specific parts of the auditory pathway rather than just the overall responsiveness of the auditory system. However, the performance of AEPs requires more time and may require sedation of the patient. AEPs are also less accurate and are more limited in scope than behavioral tests.

Auditory Evoked Potentials

Many different AEPs can be recorded from the human subject. These can be classified in different ways.[51, 61] The most common classification is based on the *latency* of the responses.[11] A second classification is in relation to the *temporal characteristics* of the stimulus. This classification determines whether the response is to an intermittent change in the stimulus (transient), to the continuation of a stimulus (sustained), or to the repetition of a stimulus (steady-state). Table 1 shows these systems of classification. Another possible means of classifying the evoked potentials is by the *nature of the stimulus*. Thus we may have evoked potentials to "clicks," "tones," "words," and so on. A final means of classification is based on the *origin* of the evoked potentials. Thus we can discuss "cochlear nerve action potentials," "auditory brain-stem responses," and "cortical evoked potentials," among others.

Although all AEPs may be useful in the evaluation of hearing, the auditory brain stem response (ABR) to a click is most commonly used for several reasons. First, the response is relatively easy to record. It does not require special electrodes or special stimuli. Second, the response does not vary with the state of the subject. Third, there are extensive normative data describing the threshold for the response and the amplitudes and latencies of its components. Despite these advantages, it is well to bear in mind that other AEPs—those elicited by a stimulus other than clicks, and those generated in regions other than the brain stem—may become essential to the full evaluation of certain patients.

Table 2. *Infants at Risk for Hearing Impairment*[35]

Family history of hearing loss
Craniofacial anomalies
Asphyxia (low Apgar score)
Bacterial meningitis
Congenital infection
Hyperbilirubinemia
Birth weight < 1500 g

IDENTIFICATION OF INFANTS WITH HEARING IMPAIRMENT

One in 750 children is born with a hearing impairment significant enough to impede the learning of speech and language.[23] Other children develop such a hearing loss in the first few years of life. Infants with hearing impairment should be identified as soon as possible so that management can be initiated at a time when the brain is sensitive to the development of speech and language—preferably by the age of 6 months. Over the past 20 years, there has been much research and debate about the most efficient means of identifying these infants.

Because of the low incidence of hearing impairment, it is probably not worthwhile to test all newborn babies. Table 2 shows the risk factors for hearing loss in infancy.[35] Babies "at risk" for hearing impairment should be evaluated. The high-risk register will include approximately two thirds of all babies who have a significant hearing impairment.[23] The other third must be referred to the clinician by parents and family physicians. Many of the high-risk factors are present in babies admitted to a neonatal intensive care unit. It is therefore worthwhile to assess the hearing of all babies who graduate from such a unit.

The various procedures for assessing the hearing of newborn infants can be evaluated by three main measurements. *Reliability* is how reproducible the results are from one testing session to another. *Sensitivity* is the percentage of impaired children correctly detected by the test. *Specificity* is the percentage of unimpaired children that show normal test results. The skeptical reviewer will look closely at the mistakes—the number of patients with a hearing impairment who are *missed* by the test and the number of normal patients who are considered impaired by the test (*false positives* or *false alarms*). The incidence of misses is 100 per cent less the sensitivity and the incidence of false alarms is 100 per cent less the specificity. A test is seldom perfect. The criterion level of a test is usually chosen to minimize the sum of the costs incurred by missing some impaired patients and the costs incurred by misidentifying normal patients as impaired.

When evaluating the various techniques for identifying infants with a hearing impairment, it is difficult to define what should be considered a *significant hearing loss*. A hearing loss in which the average threshold for the frequencies 500, 1000, and 2000 Hz is greater than 45 dB HL for both ears[30] will certainly require amplification. However, a bilateral sensorineural loss of more than 30 dB HL may also benefit from amplification. Bilateral mild conductive losses should also be identified because they may require active management.[18]

Behavioral Testing

In the 1970s, there was some enthusiasm for the behavioral screening of newborn infants—observing the startle reflex (eye blink, muscle movement, arousal from sleep) in response to loud sounds. This procedure was woefully insensitive. About one third of newborn infants with a severe bilateral hearing impairment were missed by the testing procedure.[25, 48] Behavioral testing also has very low specificity. About one half of normal newborn babies fail a behavioral screening test.[16] This is an even greater problem for sick babies—over 80 per cent of babies in a neonatal intensive care unit fail a behavioral screening test.[16]

Behavioral testing in the newborn suffers from three major problems. First, it is difficult to determine whether a baby's movement is spontaneous or in response to a sound. Second, the response depends as much on the motor system as on the auditory system. Babies who are sick tend not to respond to any stimulus. Third, the test requires relatively high intensities of sound and therefore misses mild or moderate hearing losses.

Automatic detection of behavioral responsiveness by means of a Crib-O-Gram removes the inaccuracy and bias of the human observer.[30] However, the results of Crib-O-Gram screening are still not very sensitive. The percentage of children with a bilateral hearing loss greater than 45 dB HL who are missed by the Crib-O-Gram has been reported as 21 per cent[30] and 23 per cent.[18] Also the Crib-O-Gram results are unreliable; many infants pass only one of two tests.

ABR Testing

A far better approach to identifying infants with a hearing impairment is to assess infants at risk with the auditory evoked potentials. The middle-latency and slow AEPs are not reliable because they vary significantly with both maturation and arousal. The ABR is, however, very effective.

The protocol for ABR testing in the first few months of life centers around demonstrating a wave V at click levels of 30 dB above normal adult thresholds (nHL). The test is most efficiently performed at rates of about 50/second because wave V is not significantly attenuated at these rates. The faster the stimulus is presented, the more responses can be averaged (and the more the background noise can be reduced) in a given amount of time.

Each ear is tested separately. If wave V is not present at 30 dB nHL, the intensity can be increased until a threshold is determined. Figure 1 shows some normal and abnormal results. It is probably also worthwhile to evaluate the response at a high intensity (70 dB nHL) and a slower rate (10 to 20/sec) to assess the amplitudes and latencies of the other components of the ABR. Abnormalities of these measurements can suggest some dysfunction in the auditory pathways of the brain stem.

Several provisos are important in evaluating hearing loss in the infant. First, babies should not be tested until they are well enough to go home. If possible, it is even better to wait until they are 2 to 4 months of age. Second, the final assessment of whether or not a hearing impairment is present should be based on two or more testing sessions separated by a month or more. Occasionally the threshold may improve significantly within

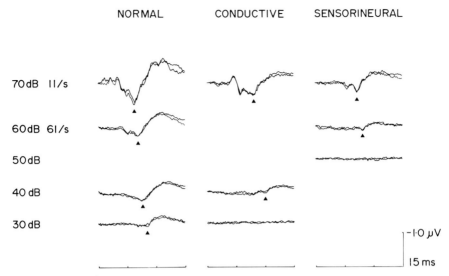

Figure 1. Auditory brain stem responses (ABRs) in infancy. On the *left* are the ABRs recorded from a normal infant; in the *middle* are the ABRs from an infant with a conductive hearing loss; and on the *right* are the ABRs from an infant with a sensorineural hearing loss. The recordings were obtained from the vertex using a mastoid reference. Negativity at the vertex is plotted upward. Wave V is indicated by the *triangles*. All intensities are expressed in dB nHL.

a short period of time. This is particularly true for mild conductive losses in the neonatal period. Third, the latencies of wave V decrease with maturation. Hence age-dependent normative data are necessary for interpretation.

The ABR has been extensively evaluated as a means for identifying babies with a hearing impairment. The result have shown that the incidence of a hearing loss requiring amplification in graduates of a neonatal intensive care unit is between 1 and 5 per cent.[24, 54, 57] Unfortunately, as yet there have been no published studies that have formally assessed the validity of the ABR procedures. Over the past several years, we have been able to follow up 600 babies that were evaluated by the ABR in the neonatal period or the first few months of life. Audiograms at the age of 2½ years or more have been obtained in 58 per cent of these babies. Two babies thought to have a unilateral sensorineural loss on the basis of ABR testing actually showed normal hearing on follow-up audiometry in at least one ear. These babies probably had transient conductive hearing losses that were not identified because of normal tympanometry and otoscopy. Six children who had been shown to have a bilateral sensorineural hearing loss by ABR testing had their losses confirmed on the follow-up audiogram. One child who had passed the initial ABR evaluation was determined by audiometry to have a bilateral sensorineural hearing loss. The audiogram of this child is shown in Figure 2. As can be seen, the behavioral threshold is within normal limits at 2000 and 4000 Hz. This explains the normal results on ABR testing. Because this child has some delay of speech and language, hearing aids are being tried.

If neonatal ABR testing is judged on its ability to identify infants with

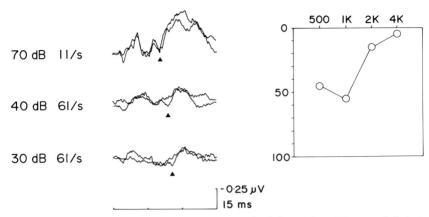

Figure 2. ABR and follow-up audiograms. On the *left* are the ABRs recorded during infancy. The recordings were obtained from the vertex using a mastoid reference. On the *right* is the audiogram showing a sensorineural hearing loss that was missed by ABR testing in infancy. Bone conduction thresholds were essentially the same as the air conduction thresholds. Both the audiogram and the ABRs are for stimulation of the child's right ear (the left ear showed a less severe sensorineural loss with a different audiometric pattern). Negativity at the vertex is plotted upward. Wave V is indicated by the *triangles*.

a bilateral sensorineural hearing loss of greater than 45 dB HL, the sensitivity is 100 per cent and the specificity 100 per cent. The child with a bilateral sensorineural hearing loss who was missed by ABR testing (see Fig. 2) did not fulfill the 45 dB criterion. However, we feel this judgment is overly enthusiastic. ABR testing can miss some children with a sensorineural hearing loss that may benefit from amplification. The reason for this is that the click ABR does not evaluate thresholds at specific frequencies.[32] Furthermore, it may at times be difficult to diagnose a conductive loss in infancy. Certain conductive losses can masquerade as a sensorineural loss until more definitive tests are available or until the transient otitis clears up.

Many mild to moderate conductive losses are picked up by the ABR testing in infancy. The final diagnosis of a conductive loss is made by a combination of features: the delayed latency of wave V, the normal ABR thresholds obtained with bone-conduction clicks, the abnormal tympanic membrane seen during otoscopy, the abnormal impedance results, and the absence of the stapedius reflex responses. Approximately 5 per cent of infants have a bilateral conductive hearing loss at some time during the first 2 years of life. Many of these are present at birth and return to normal; others develop after birth; some conductive losses persist or recur throughout the first 2 years. We do not feel these conductive losses should be considered "false-positive" results of ABR testing. For the most part, they represent clear diagnoses of hearing impairments that may, depending on their severity and persistence, require active treatment.

One problem with the ABR testing is that patients with neurologic disorders may have abnormalities of wave V that make it impossible to determine a clear threshold. In these patients, it is worthwhile to examine wave I of the response. If wave I is present at 40 dB nHL, one can probably

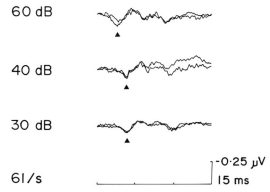

Figure 3. ABR of a patient with neurologic abnormalities affecting the brain stem. The infant has hydrocephalus. Wave I is more easily recognizable than wave V. Wave I is identified at intensities as low as 30 dB nHL. The recordings were obtained from the vertex using a mastoid reference. Negativity at the vertex was plotted upward. Wave I is indicated by the triangles.

state that there is no significant hearing loss. This is illustrated in Figure 3.

In recent years, several techniques have been developed to make the detection of ABR thresholds automatic.[22, 28, 50, 63] The continual calculation of the signal-to-noise ratio can support a decision either that a statistically reliable response is present or that the response is too small to be recognizable.

FREQUENCY-SPECIFIC AUDIOMETRY

One problem in evaluating a hearing loss with the click-evoked potential is the lack of frequency-specificity of the stimulus. A click has energy over a very broad band of frequencies. The region of the cochlea that contributes most prominently to the click ABR varies with the cochlear thresholds for different frequencies and with the degree of synchronization among the discharging fibers at each frequency region. The traveling wave spreads the different frequencies of a sound over the basilar membrane such that high frequencies cause maximal displacement in the region near the stapes and low frequencies in the region far from the stapes. The traveling wave slows down as it progresses along the basilar membrane, and the length of the membrane covered by a frequency band increases as the distance from the stapes increases. There is, therefore, little synchronization among fibers responding to frequencies below 1000 Hz. When the hearing is normal, the ABR derives mainly from the 2000 to 4000 Hz region of the cochlea.[15, 27] When there is a hearing loss at these frequencies, the click may evoke a response from the 1000 Hz region of the cochlea. Because this may have a normal threshold, a high-frequency hearing loss may go undetected.

An objective technique to assess the specific thresholds at different frequencies of sound would be very desirable: (1) It would help to detect hearing losses restricted to particular frequencies. (2) It would facilitate chosing the appropriate amplification for a hearing loss. (3) It would assist in determining the etiology of the hearing loss.

Tonal Stimuli

One approach to frequency-specific audiometry with evoked potentials is to use tonal stimuli. Unfortunately, very brief tones are necessary to obtain a synchronized response from the brain stem. Unlike a continuous pure tone, a brief tone contains energy dispersed over a range of frequencies. The amount of "frequency splatter" varies inversely with the duration and the rise-time of the tone. A patient with a hearing loss at the nominal frequency of a brief tone may still show a response to that tone. This response is evoked by the energy in the brief tone at a frequency different from its nominal frequency. This problem is similar to that with the click, although of a lesser degree because the brief tone does have more energy at its nominal frequency than at the other frequencies. Nevertheless, one may seriously underestimate a hearing loss at a particular frequency when using brief tones.

The longer the duration or the rise-time of a tone, the more frequency-specific is its energy content. Thus, a second approach to frequency-specific audiometry is to record AEPs to long-duration tones. Unfortunately, such tones do not elicit a response that is sufficiently synchronized to generate a measurable ABR. Even if the tone had an abrupt rise, the response is generated by the very beginning of the tone that contains "frequency splatter." One is therefore restricted to the middle-latency or slow AEPs that can be evoked by tones with longer rise-times. The slow evoked potentials can provide a good threshold estimation in waking children and adults. However, the potentials vary with attention and the state of arousal, and they are difficult to record in infants. The transient and steady-state middle latency responses can also be evoked with stimuli that are relatively frequency-specific. Brief tones lasting 15 msec are one approach. Pure tones that are sinusoidally modulated in amplitude can elicit steady-state middle-latency responses at the frequency of the modulation.[40, 53] However, the middle-latency responses are attenuated by sleep and may be difficult to record in young children and infants[39] unless very slow rates are used.[33]

The ABR has great advantages over the later auditory evoked potentials because it does not vary with sleep,[6] is easily recordable in infants, and is recognizable at rapid rates of stimulation. Masking techniques can provide frequency-specific thresholds with the ABR. One technique presents clicks in noise that has been high-pass filtered. The response to this stimulus comes from the region of the cochlea that is not masked by the high-pass noise. If the cutoff frequency of the high-pass noise is decreased, the extent of the masking will increase and the response will come from a smaller region of the cochlea. Subtraction of the second response from the first leaves a *derived response* equivalent to the response of the region of the cochlea between the two high-pass cutoff frequencies. This technique yields very specific thresholds.[14] However, the noise levels used to mask the click are quite high, and the subtraction procedure decreases the signal-to-noise ratio of the response. Another masking technique is to use brief tones and to mask the effect of the frequency splatter in these brief tones with *notched noise*, with the notch centered at the frequency of the tone.[5, 52, 60] This is illustrated in Figure 4.

Another technique is to reverse the masking procedure. The brain-

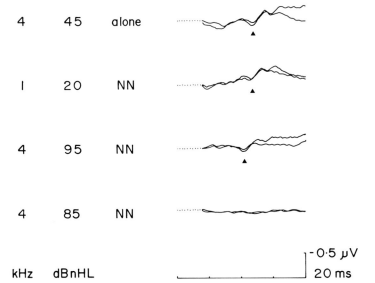

4	45	alone
1	20	NN
4	95	NN
4	85	NN

⌐−0·5 μV
20 ms

kHz   dBnHL

Figure 4. Notched noise masking. This figure shows the brain stem potentials evoked by tonepips with a duration of 4 msec. The initial part of the tracing has been blanked. These responses were obtained from a patient with a high frequency hearing loss. The audiometric thresholds were 15 dB nHL at 1 kHz, 70 dB at 2 kHz, and 95 dB at 4 kHz. The *top tracing* shows the response to a 4 kHz tonepip presented at an intensity of 45 dB nHL without any masking. There is a clearly recognizable wave V in the response *(triangle)*. This response is probably evoked by the spread of energy in the brief tone into the 1 kHz region. The second tracing shows the response to a 1 kHz tone presented at an intensity of 20 dB nHL. This response is similar to that recorded to the 4 kHz tone. When notched noise (NN) is used for the 4 kHz tonepips, the response is recognizable at 95 dB nHL but not at 85 dB nHL. The response now accurately reflects the patient's behavioral threshold.

stem evoked potentials are recorded to clicks. A *pure-tone masking* stimulus is then added to the clicks and the response recorded again. The difference between the two responses is the part of the click evoked brain-stem response that is also activated by the pure tone.[49] Because the pure tone is of long duration, the response derived in this manner is as frequency-specific as that obtained during behavioral pure tone audiometry.

All these techniques have difficulty when evaluating the low-frequency regions of the cochlea. In these regions, the response even to a click stimulus is very unsynchronized. This problem could be overcome by finding some way to bypass the traveling wave in the cochlea. Direct electrical stimulation of the nerve in experimental animals can provide a highly synchronized response from all the fibers in the cochlear nerve—both high-frequency fibers and low-frequency fibers. Pure-tone masking can then provide highly synchronized derived responses.[2] The problem is how to obtain a similarly synchronized response from the human subject. Magnetic stimulation may help in this regard.

The clinician therefore has several techniques to obtain frequency-specific auditory thresholds. These thresholds are most reliably obtained for frequencies between 1000 and 4000 Hz. The thresholds at 500 Hz or at lower frequencies are somewhat less reliable. Each of the techniques has its advantages and disadvantages.

THE ETIOLOGY OF A HEARING LOSS

As well as providing an estimate of the amount of hearing loss, the auditory evoked potentials can help in the differential diagnosis of the etiology. The components generated in the cochlea and the eighth nerve are particularly helpful. These potentials are not as well recorded using earlobe or mastoid electrodes as they are with electrodes placed in the external auditory meatus or inserted transtympanically to rest on the cochlear promontory. The "transtympanic" electrode has changed little since it was initially described.[56] There are several ways to place an "extratympanic" electrode in the external auditory meatus.[7, 43, 45, 62, 64, 65]

Conductive Hearing Loss

The clearest diagnosis of a conductive hearing loss is the demonstration that the thresholds for bone-conducted sounds are better than those for air-conducted sounds. Auditory evoked potentials can be recorded in response to bone-conducted sounds. The range of intensities is somewhat limited and the frequency content of a bone-conducted click differs from that of an air-conducted click. Nevertheless, useful thresholds can be obtained.[29, 44]

The auditory evoked potentials to bone-conducted sounds can be used to evaluate patients with a possible conductive hearing loss who are unable to respond to normal behavioral tests. Approximately 30 per cent of neonates in an ICU have middle-ear effusions most likely associated with a conductive hearing loss.[3] Others may develop a conductive hearing loss later. Children with craniofacial anomalies have a particularly high incidence of conductive hearing loss. The overall prevalence of otitis media with effusion in childhood is between 15 and 20 per cent.[31, 47] Approximately 4 per cent of children at age 5 years have a bilateral conductive loss that decreases their ability to perceive speech.[47] An accurate assessment of this hearing loss is important so that it can be differentiated from a sensorineural hearing loss and treated appropriately. Auditory evoked potentials to bone-conducted stimuli are also important in older children who may be unable to respond appropriately because of mental retardation or emotional disorders.

The auditory evoked potentials can help solve the masking dilemma that occurs in a patient with bilateral hearing losses, one of which (at least) is conductive. In such a patient, it is difficult to determine the extent of any sensorineural hearing loss because one ear cannot be masked without possibly masking the other. Because the electrocochleographic potentials are purely monaural, they can be used to assess each ear's response individually to air- or bone-conducted stimuli. Electrocochleographic recordings are not possible in patients with bilateral atresia. In these patients, it is possible that the asymmetry of the auditory brain-stem response may be helpful. Normal monaural stimulation in an infant causes a very asymmetric auditory brain-stem response.[19] The response recorded between the vertex and the mastoid contralateral to the stimulated ear is much smaller

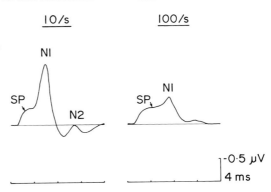

Figure 5. Electrocochleography. This figure is a diagrammatic representation of the potentials recorded using an extratympanic electrode. Clicks of alternating polarity were used to cancel the cochlear microphonic. At slow click rates (10 per sec), the summating potential (SP) is recognized as a shoulder on the beginning of the Nl wave of the cochlear nerve action potential. At more rapid rates (100 per sec), the Nl is attenuated and delayed, making the SP more prominent.

than the response recorded between the vertex and the ipsilateral responses. If the response to a bone-conducted click in a child with bilateral atresia is quite asymmetric between the vertex-to-left-mastoid and vertex-to-right-mastoid recordings, one internal ear is probably more responsive than the other.

Differential Diagnosis of Cochlear Hearing Loss

Basically there are two kinds of cochlear hearing loss: those associated with hair cell loss (for example, ototoxic drugs) and those that spare the hair cells (for example, Menière's disease). The auditory evoked potentials that directly reflect hair cell function are the "cochlear microphonic" and the "summating potential." The cochlear microphonic is very difficult to record because it is so easily contaminated by stimulus artifact. The summating potential, however, has become clinically important in the assessment of cochlear hearing loss.

The summating potential varies greatly with the location of the recording electrode. Transtympanic recordings may show a positive SP at high tonal frequencies and a negative SP at lower frequencies. Extratympanic recordings typically show negative SPs at all frequencies. The amplitude of the SP varies greatly from one individual to another. It is therefore usual to measure the ratio between the SP amplitude and the amplitude of the cochlear nerve action potential (Nl component). This measurement is the SP/AP ratio.

In the click-evoked response the SP is usually seen as a shoulder on the way up to the Nl peak of the cochlear nerve action potential. It can be dissociated from the Nl peak by increasing the rate of stimulation.[8] High rates of stimulation attenuate the Nl, but leave the SP unaffected. The SP is distinguished from the cochlear microphonic by using stimuli of alternating polarity. The extratympanic SP/AP ratio in patients with Menière's disease is usually greater than 0.4, the upper limits of normal.[45] The AP and SP measurements are shown in Figure 5.

Another approach to the diagnosis of Menière's disease is to evaluate the change in the summating potential with changes in the fluid-electrolyte balance of the cochlea. The SP recorded in patients with Menière's disease decreases significantly after glycerol dehydration.[9, 10]

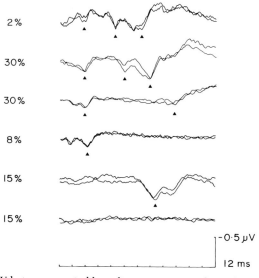

2%

30%

30%

8%

15%

15%

-0.5 µV

12 ms

Figure 6. Cerebellopontine angle (CPA) tumors. This figure shows the different kinds of ABR waveforms that can be recorded in patients with CPA tumors. On the *left* are shown the approximate incidences of the different patterns. These incidences are based upon our own experience and that of several other laboratories. The *triangles* show waves I, III, and V where they are recognizable. The first pattern shows an ABR with normal latencies. In this patient, both the I–III and the I–V latencies are at the upper limits of normal. The second pattern shows a delayed wave I–III interval. The third pattern shows a delayed I–V interval with no recognizable wave III. In the fourth pattern, only wave I is recognizable. In the fifth pattern, there is a delayed wave V but no recognizable earlier components. The sixth pattern shows no recognizable response.

The Diagnosis of Retrocochlear Hearing Loss

The auditory brain-stem response is almost always abnormal in patients with tumors of the eighth nerve. The ABR is therefore one of the most sensitive tests in detecting an acoustic neuroma.[1, 4, 13, 20, 21, 59] Between 98 and 100 per cent of patients with tumors of the eighth nerve show an abnormal ABR.[1, 4] As such, the test is far more sensitive than behavioral audiometry and better than many types of imaging.

However, abnormalities of the ABR are very nonspecific. Many different patterns of ABR abnormality can be seen (Fig. 6) and all of these patterns can be associated with disorders other than an acoustic neuroma. Perhaps the "classic" ABR abnormality is an abnormally delayed interval between wave I generated in the cochlear nerve and wave III generated in the pons. However, in many patients, wave III is often difficult to recognize and one measures an abnormally long I–V interval. Both the I–III and I–V abnormalities may, however, be caused by lesions involving the brain stem rather than the eighth nerve. The presence of the first wave of the response with no recognizable later components is another pattern of abnormality that can be seen in patients with tumors of the eighth nerve. However, this may also be seen in patients with multiple sclerosis. Approximately one third of patients with acoustic neuroma have no recordable ABR.[21] This pattern can of course be seen in any patient with a severe to profound hearing loss.

One problem with the recording of the ABR in patients with tumors of the eighth nerve is that it is often difficult to recognize wave I. One is left with a very nonspecific delay in wave V. A conductive hearing loss can delay wave V. This can be diagnosed by otoscopy, impedance audiometry,

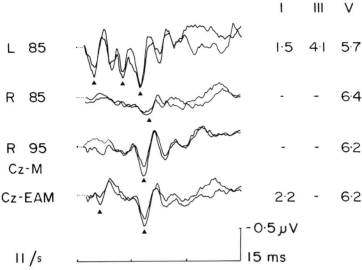

Figure 7. High-frequency hearing loss. This figure shows the ABRs recorded from a patient with a high-frequency hearing loss in the right ear. The right ear audiometric thresholds at 1000, 2000, and 4000 Hz were 15 dB, 85 dB, and 110 dB. The left ear thresholds were 10 dB, 15 dB, and 45 dB, respectively. The clicks were presented at a rate of 11 per sec. At 85 dB nHL, the ABR to right ear stimulation shows a delayed wave V and no earlier components. At 95 dB, there is a questionable wave I on the vertex-mastoid recording. Wave I is much more easily recognized using a needle electrode in the external auditory meatus (EAM). As the wave I–V interval is within normal limits, there is no evidence for any retrocochlear hearing impairment.

or bone conduction. A delayed wave V can also be caused by a cochlear hearing loss. Damage to the high-frequency region of the cochlea can attenuate wave I and delay wave V. In these patients, it is impossible to determine whether the delayed wave V is related to the high-frequency cochlear hearing loss or to a retrocochlear lesion. This is a particular problem because many patients with tumors of the eighth nerve present with a high-frequency hearing loss.[34] Various techniques can be used to enhance wave I: the rate can be slowed, the intensity can be increased, and the recording electrode changed from the mastoid (or earlobe) to one in the external auditory meatus or to a transtympanic electrode. Figure 7 shows the ABR of a patient with a unilateral high-frequency hearing loss.

Central Auditory Dysfunction

The ABR is very helpful in demonstrating lesions of the brain-stem auditory pathways. The middle- and long-latency potentials have been less successful. One of the problems is that several different generators may contribute to the scalp-recorded potentials during the middle and slow responses.[46] The changes in the scalp-recorded field that follow lesions to one of the generators may be difficult to measure. Nevertheless, there have been some recent demonstrations of cortical lesions using evoked potentials.[38] Furthermore, new techniques to derive the generators of the scalp-recorded potentials may be important in evaluating lesions of the auditory system beyond the brain stem.[58]

Patients with disorders of auditory perception have been loosely grouped under the diagnostic category of "central auditory dysfunction."[36, 55] These disorders involve the central auditory system rather than the cochlea or eighth nerve. They manifest themselves as difficulties with auditory perception. The cause of these problems is unknown. The diagnosis of these disorders is difficult because most tests have very wide limits of normality. Several auditory processes are specifically tested because they are mainly central in origin. Speech perception involves the integration of auditory information over both time and frequency. Binaural functions like localization involve the integration of auditory information between the two ears. In the next few years, it is possible that one may record evoked potentials to stimuli that are specifically processed in the central auditory system. These may become helpful in diagnosing patients with central auditory dysfunction.

Recently we have been recording the potentials evoked by changes in the lateralization of a sound. In the past, the potentials related to binaural interaction have been measured by comparing monaural with binaural stimuli.[12, 41] Our stimulus is specifically binaural in nature. A continuous noise is generated by running a sequence of random numbers through a digital-analog converter and connecting the analog output through an amplifier and filter to a speaker. Two channels of a digital-analog converter can be programmed to generate identical noise stimuli with one channel delayed relative to the other. If these two channels are presented separately to the two ears through earphones, the subject hears a noise that is lateralized to the side receiving the leading stimulus. Changes in the relative timing of the two channels cause the sound to shift its lateralization. These shifts have a very rapid onset (less than 1 msec). Furthermore, they occur independently of any detectable change in the ongoing monaural stimulus. The potentials evoked by these shifts in lateralization can therefore be used as a specific measurement of binaural interaction in the brain. Figure 8 shows the stimulus and the late cortical evoked potentials to such a stimulus.

Nonorganic Hearing Losses

In patients who have a nonorganic hearing loss, the auditory evoked potentials may demonstrate normal responsiveness or may describe an underlying hearing loss that is being exaggerated. The ABR is the most reliable technique in determining thresholds. However, later components of the auditory evoked potential may be useful in obtaining more frequency-specific information and in demonstrating that the auditory information is reaching the cortex.

MONITORING THERAPY

Once a significant hearing loss has been identified, it is important that management be initiated either medically or audiologically. For a sensorineural hearing loss, amplification is recommended to attempt to compensate for the loss. Many new techniques have been developed for electroacoust-

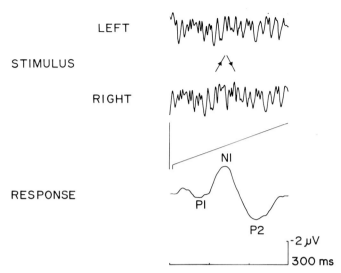

Figure 8. Evoked potentials to binaural interaction. The dichotic white noise stimulus is shown in the *top two tracings.* At the beginning of the 10 msec time interval, the right ear leads. Halfway through the tracing, the stimulus changes so that the left ear leads. The subject heard this stimulus as a noise switching in lateralization from right to left. The *bottom tracing* is the auditory evoked potential recorded at the vertex during the perception of this shift in lateralization. The tracing is the grand mean waveform from eight subjects. Negativity at the vertex is recorded as an upward deflection.

ically fitting a hearing aid to a patient's loss. However, the ultimate test of a hearing aid is the patient's ability to use the amplified auditory information. The most important use of this information is in the understanding of speech. An adult or an older child can show the benefit of amplification by his or her ability to discriminate speech sounds. However, when fitting a young child or infant, such testing is not reliable. Continual evaluation during the habilitation program is necessary to evaluate the hearing status and to determine the auditory needs of the child. The family is as important in this evaluation as the audiologist.

Several papers have suggested that the ABR may be useful in fitting a hearing aid.[37, 42] However, there are problems with this approach because the hearing aid may amplify transient sounds such as a click or brief tone differently from more continuous sounds such as speech.[26] Steady-state potentials like the middle-latency response to frequency- or amplitude-modulated tones may prove helpful in this regard.[53]

CONCLUSION

The human auditory evoked potentials are an essential part of the audiometric test battery. They are by far the best means of detecting a hearing loss in infants before the age of 1 year. They are important in the evaluation of the type of hearing loss, particularly in dissociating retrocochlear from cochlear disorders. In the near future, the auditory evoked potentials will probably become important in the diagnosis of central auditory dysfunction and in the fitting and monitoring of hearing aids.

REFERENCES

1. Antonelli AR, Bellotto R, Grandori F: Audiologic diagnosis of central versus eighth nerve and cochlear auditory impairment. Audiology 26:209, 1987
2. Aran J-M, Erre J-P, Charlet de Sauvage R: Derived evoked potentials for continuous tones using a hybrid electrical-acoustical stimulation. Hear Res 20:289, 1985
3. Balkany TJ, Berman SA, Simmons MA, et al: Middle ear effusions in neonates. Laryngoscope 88:398, 1978
4. Barrs DM, Brackmann DE, Olson JE, et al: Changing concepts of acoustic neuroma diagnosis. Arch Otolaryngol 111:17, 1985
5. Beattie RC, Boyd RL: Early/middle evoked potentials to tone bursts in quiet, white noise and notched noise. Audiology 24:406, 1985
6. Campbell KB, Bartoli EA: Human auditory evoked potentials during natural sleep: The early components. Electroencephalogr Clin Neurophysiol 65:142, 1986
7. Chiappa KH: Evoked potentials in clinical medicine. New York, Raven Press, 1983
8. Coats AC: The summating potential and Menière's disease. I. Summating potential amplitude in Menière's and non-Menière's ears. Arch Otolaryngol 107:199, 1981
9. Coats AC, Alford BR: Menière's disease and the summating potential. III. Effect of glycerol administration. Arch Otolaryngol 107:469, 1981
10. Dauman R, Aran J-M, Portmann M: Summating potential and water balance in Menière's disease. Ann Otol Rhinol Laryngol 95:389, 1986
11. Davis H: Principles of electric response audiometry. Ann Otol Rhinol Laryngol 85(suppl) 28:1, 1976
12. Dobie RA, Berlin CI: Binaural interaction in brainstem-evoked responses. Arch Otolaryngol 105:391, 1979
13. Don M: ABR in acoustic tumor diagnosis. In Moller AR (ed): Brainstem Auditory Evoked Potentials Paper Presented at the International Congress on Auditory Evoked Potentials, New York, October 21, 1986
14. Don M, Eggermont JJ, Brackmann DE: Reconstruction of the audiogram using brain stem responses and high-pass noise masking. Ann Otol Rhinol Laryngol 88(suppl) 57:1, 1979
15. van der Drift JFC, Brocaar MP, van Zanten GA: The relation between the pure-tone audiogram and the click auditory brainstem response threshold in cochlear hearing loss. Audiology 26:1, 1987
16. Durieux-Smith A, Jacobson JT: Comparison of auditory brainstem response and behavioral screening in neonates. J Otolaryngol 14:47, 1985
17. Durieux-Smith A, Picton TW, Edwards CG, et al: Brainstem electric-response audiometry in infants of a neonatal intensive care unit. Audiology 26:284, 1987
18. Durieux-Smith A, Picton T, Edwards C, et al: The Crib-O-Gram in the NICU: An evaluation based on brainstem electric response audiometry. Ear Hear 6:20, 1985
19. Edwards CG, Durieux-Smith A, Picton TW: Neonatal auditory brain stem responses from ipsilateral and contralateral recording montages. Ear Hear 6:175, 1985
20. Eggermont JJ, Don M: Mechanisms of central conduction time prolongation in brainstem auditory evoked potentials. Arch Neurol 43:116, 1986
21. Eggermont JJ, Don M, Brackmann DE: Electrocochleography and auditory brainstem electric responses in patients with pontine angle tumors. Ann Otol Rhinol Laryngol 89 (suppl)75:1, 1980
22. Elberling C, Don M: Threshold characteristics of the human auditory brain stem response. J Acoust Soc Am 81:115, 1987
23. Feinmesser M, Tell L, Levi H: Follow-up of 40,000 infants screened for hearing defect. Audiology 21:197, 1982
24. Galambos R, Hicks G, Wilson MJ: The auditory brainstem response reliably predicts hearing loss in graduates of a tertiary intensive care nursery. Ear Hear 5:254, 1984
25. Gerber SE: Newborn screening and diagnostic tests. In Jaffe BF (ed): Hearing Loss in Children. Maryland, University Park Press, 1977, p 78

26. Gorga MP, Beauchaine KA, Reiland JK: Comparison of onset and steady-state responses of hearing aids: Implications for use of the auditory brainstem response in the selection of hearing aids. J Speech Hear Res 30:130, 1987
27. Gorga MP, Worthington DW, Reiland JK, et al: Some comparisons between auditory brain stem response thresholds, latencies, and the pure-tone audiogram. Ear Hear 6:105, 1985
28. Greenblatt E, Zappulla RA, Kaye S, et al: Response threshold determination of the brain stem auditory evoked response: A comparison of the phase versus magnitude derived from the fast Fourier transform. Audiology 24:288, 1985
29. Hooks RG, Weber BA: Auditory brainstem responses of premature infants to bone-conducted stimuli: A feasibility study. Ear Hear 5:42, 1984
30. Hosford-Dunn H, Johnson S, Simmons FB, et al: Infant hearing screening: Program implementation and validation. Ear Hear 8:12, 1987
31. Howie VM: Acute and recurrent acute otitis media. In Jaffe BF (ed): Hearing Loss in Children. Baltimore, University Park Press, 1977, p 421
32. Hyde ML: Frequency-specific BERA in infants. J Otolaryngol 14:19, 1985
33. Jerger J, Chmiel R, Glaze D, et al: Rate and filter dependence of the middle-latency response in infants. Audiology 26:269, 1987
34. Johnson EW: Auditory test results in 500 cases of acoustic neuroma surgically confirmed. Arch Otolaryngol 103:152, 1977
35. Joint Committee on Infant Hearing: Position statement. Pediatrics 70:496, 1982
36. Keith RW: Central Auditory and Language Disorders in Children. San Diego, College-Hill Press, 1981
37. Kileny P: Auditory brainstem responses as indicators of hearing aid performance. Ann Otol 91:61, 1982
38. Kraus N, Ozdamar O, Hier D, et al: Auditory middle latency responses (MLRs) in patients with cortical lesions. Electroencephalogr Clin Neurophysiol 54:275, 1982
39. Kraus N, Reed N, Smith D, et al: Auditory middle latency responses in children: Effects of age and diagnostic category. Electroencephalogr Clin Neurophysiol 62:343, 1985
40. Kuwada S, Batra R, Maher VL: Scalp potentials of normal and hearing-impaired subjects in response to sinusoidally amplitude-modulated tones. Hear Res 21:179, 1986
41. Levine RA: Binaural interaction in brainstem potentials of human subjects. Ann Neurol 9:384, 1981
42. Mahoney TM: Auditory brainstem response hearing aid applications. In Jacobson JT (ed): The Auditory Brainstem Response. San Diego, College-Hill Press, 1985, p 349
43. Mason SM, Singh CB, Brown PM: Assessment of non-invasive electrocochleography. J Laryngol Otol 94:707, 1980
44. Maudlin L, Jerger S: Auditory brainstem evoked responses to bone conducted signals. Arch Otolaryngol 105:656, 1979
45. Mori N, Asai H, Doi K, et al: Diagnostic value of extratympanic electrocochleography in Menière's disease. Audiology 26:103, 1987
46. Näätänen R, Picton TW: The N1 wave of the human electric and magnetic response to sound: A review and an analysis of the component structure. Psychophysiology 24:375, 1987
47. Northern JL, Downs MP: Hearing in Children. Ed 2. Baltimore, Williams & Wilkins, 1978, p 2
48. Northern JL, Downs MP: Hearing in Children. Ed 2. Baltimore, Williams & Wilkins, 1974, p 108
49. Pantev C, Lagidze S, Pantev M, et al: Frequency-specific contributions to the auditory brain stem response derived by means of pure-tone masking. Audiology 24:275, 1985
50. Peters JG: An automated infant screener using advanced evoked response technology. Hear J 39(9):25, 1986
51. Picton TW, Fitzgerald PG: A general description of the human auditory evoked potentials. In Moore EJ (ed): Bases of Auditory Brain-Stem Evoked Responses. New York, Grune and Stratton, 1983, p 141
52. Picton TW, Ouellette J, Hamel G, et al: Brainstem evoked potentials to tonepips in notched noise. J Otolaryngol 8:289, 1979
53. Picton TW, Skinner CR, Champagne SC, et al: Potentials evoked by the sinusoidal modulation of the amplitude or frequency of a tone. J Acoust Soc Am 82:165, 1987
54. Picton TW, Taylor MJ, Durieux-Smith A, et al: Brainstem auditory evoked potentials in

pediatrics. *In* Aminoff MJ (ed): Electrodiagnosis in Clinical Neurology, 2nd ed. New York, Churchill Livingstone, 1986, p 505

55. Pinheiro M, Musiek F (eds): Assessment of Central Auditory Dysfunction: Foundation and Correlates. Baltimore, Williams & Wilkins, 1985
56. Portmann M, Lebert G, Aran JM: Potentiels cochléaires obtenues chez l'homme en dehors de toute intervention chirurgicale. Note préliminaire. Rev Laryngol Otol Rhinol 88:157, 1967
57. Sanders R, Durieux-Smith A, Hyde ML, et al: Incidence of hearing loss in high-risk and intensive care nursery infants. J Otolaryngol 14:28, 1985
58. Scherg M, von Cramon D: Evoked dipole source potentials of the human auditory cortex. Electroencephalogr Clin Neurophysiol 65:344, 1986
59. Selters WA, Brackmann DE: Acoustic tumor detection with brain stem electric response audiometry. Arch Otolaryngol 103:181, 1977
60. Stapells D, Picton T, Perez-Abalo M, et al: Frequency specificity in evoked potential audiometry. *In* Jacobson JT (ed): The Auditory Brainstem Response. San Diego, College-Hill Press, 1985, p 147
61. Starr A, Don M: Brain potentials evoked by acoustic stimuli. *In* Picton TW (ed): Human Event-Related Potentials. New York, Elsevier, 1988, p 97
62. Stypulkowski PH, Staller SJ: Clinical evaluation of a new ECoG recording electrode. Ear Hear 8:304, 1987
63. Valdes-Sosa MJ, Bobes MA, Perez-Abalo MC, et al: Comparison of auditory-evoked potential detection methods using signal detection theory. Audiology 26:166, 1987
64. Yanz JL, Dodds HJ: An ear-canal electrode for the measurement of the human auditory brain stem response. Ear Hear 6:98, 1985
65. Yoshie N, Ohashi T, Suzuki T: Non-surgical recording of auditory nerve action potentials in man. Laryngoscope 77:76, 1967

Ottawa General Hospital
501 Smyth Road
Ottawa, Canada K1H 8L6

The Use of Somatosensory Evoked Potentials in the Evaluation of the Central Nervous System

*Michael J. Aminoff, MD, FRCP**

SEPs have been used increasingly over the last few years to evaluate the function of the central and peripheral somatosensory pathways. They can be obtained by a variety of different sensory stimuli, but for clinical purposes are most easily elicited electrically. Either a mixed or cutaneous nerve can be stimulated, or stimuli can be applied to the skin in the territory of an individual nerve or nerve root, depending on the reason that the SEPs were requested. For studies performed to evaluate central somatosensory function, nerve stimulation is appropriate. Electrical stimulation of peripheral nerve activates particularly the large-diameter, fast-conducting group Ia and group II afferent fibers, giving rise to a relatively synchronous volley. The electrical stimuli are usually of an intensity that is just above motor threshold (thereby producing a small muscle twitch when a mixed nerve is stimulated), or about two or three times above sensory threshold. The stimuli are of short duration (for example, 200 μsec), are repeated at 3 or 5 Hz, and are delivered with the stimulating cathode placed proximally to the anode. The nerves most commonly stimulated to elicit SEPs are the median or ulnar nerve at the wrist, the peroneal nerve at the knee, and the posterior tibial nerve at the ankle.

The responses can be recorded using either surface or needle electrodes. Needle electrodes are quick and easy to apply but may be a little more uncomfortable, carry a small risk of infection, and may be more difficult to position accurately. The author therefore prefers surface disk or cup electrodes. Unfortunately, there is no general agreement concerning the optimal recording montage, although the American Electroencephalographic Society has published guidelines in this regard.[2] These guidelines recommend that for recording cerebral responses over the scalp to stimulation of a nerve in the upper limb, both a cephalic bipolar and a noncephalic

*Professor of Neurology, Department of Neurology, University of California School of Medicine, San Francisco, California

referential recording derivation should be used. Responses are also generally recorded over the spine, as well as peripherally in the stimulated limb,
to confirm the adequacy of the stimulus and to ensure there is no
postganglionic lesion of afferent pathways. The montage recommended by
the American Electroencephalographic Society, for use with a four-channel
recording system, is to record from the contralateral C3'/C4' electrode
placement with reference to FZ and also referenced to contralateral Erb's
point (channels 1 and 2), from over the second cervical spine referenced to
FZ (channel 3), and from ipsilateral to contralateral Erb's point (channel
4).[2] When SEPs are elicited by stimulation of a nerve in the lower limbs,
one channel is commonly used to record between L3 and L1 over the
spine, and another to record between CZ' and FpZ' or FZ; other channels
can be used to record between different levels of the spine (for example,
between T12 and T10, and T6 and T4), although in our laboratory we have
preferred to record from other cephalic bipolar derivations.

A relatively broad filter bandpass, such as 10–3000 Hz, is employed
for recording purposes. The number of trials that needs to be averaged
depends on the quality of the recording and the amount of background
noise, but often between 500 and 2000 trials are necessary to obtain
satisfactory responses when a nerve in the arms is stimulated, and between
1000 and 4000 trials for a nerve in the lower limbs. An analysis time of 50
msec from stimulus onset is appropriate with upper-limb stimulation, and
of 100 msec with lower-limb stimulation. As with all evoked potential work,
at least two averages should always be obtained to ensure the replicability
of the findings.

Before SEPs are used to evaluate patients with neurologic disorders,
it is important to gain experience in recording them in normal subjects,
and also to gather normal data that can be compared with the data obtained
from individual patients. Responses are evaluated with regard to the
absolute latency of the various components and the latency between specific
components. Latency depends on limb length and height, and also on age.
Conduction velocity along the entire somatosensory pathway may not reach
the adult range of values until patients are about 8 years of age, and latency
values increase again in the elderly.[15] Latency or interpeak latency values
should not be regarded as abnormal unless they exceed the normal mean
by 3 standard deviations. In addition to the evaluation of latency and
interpeak latency, SEPs are also examined for the presence or absence of
individual components and for the amplitude of the responses. In many
laboratories, an interside difference in amplitude of more than 50 per cent
is regarded as abnormal, but at least in this author's experience, such
variation is found occasionally in normal subjects and caution should
therefore be exercised in regarding SEPs as abnormal on this criterion
alone. There is certainly considerable variation in amplitude of responses
among individuals. Furthermore, the absence of a spinal potential should
not be regarded as abnormal when normal scalp responses are obtained
following stimulation of a nerve in the lower limbs. Responses are sometimes
judged to have an abnormal configuration, but this parameter is much
harder to quantify without using more sophisticated methods of analysis
than are currently available in most clinical laboratories.

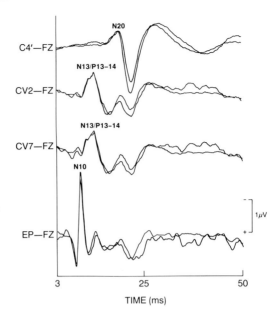

Figure 1. Normal somatosensory evoked potentials recorded over Erb's point (EP), the cervical spine over the 7th and 2nd cervical vertebrae (CV7 and CV2), and the "hand" area of the contralateral scalp (C4') using a midfrontal (FZ) reference, in response to stimulation of the left median nerve at the wrist. Two trials, each of 1024 responses, have been superimposed to demonstrate the replicability of the findings. The various components of the response have been labeled.

In median- or ulnar-derived SEPs, it is normally possible to recognize an Erb's point potential, an N13/P13–14 in the neck-FZ derivation, and the P13–14 and N20 in the C3'/C4'–FZ derivation (Fig. 1). When a scalp-noncephalic reference derivation is also used, it is usually possible to recognize P9, P13–14, and N20. The N20 is probably generated in the somatosensory cortex. It is followed by a P25–N35–P40 complex when recorded postcentrally, whereas precentrally there is a P22–N30 complex. Distinct cortical generators are probably responsible for these different components.

Following stimulation of a nerve in the lower extremity, potentials can generally be recorded over the cauda equina and spine; over the scalp, conspicuous P27 and N35 peaks can be identified with stimulation of the common peroneal nerve at the knee (Fig. 2), and P37 (sometimes designated P40) and N45 components are found after stimulation of the posterior tibial nerve at the ankle. Immediately preceding the positive peaks (P27 or P37), there is sometimes a smaller negativity that may also be cortically generated,[14] but it is usually easier to measure the latency of the positive wave because it is so prominent.

CLINICAL APPLICATIONS

The SEP findings are never pathognomonic of specific diseases. The role of SEPs in the clinical evaluation of the central nervous system can be considered under several different headings.

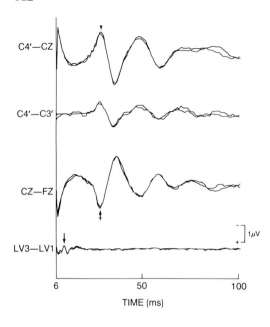

Figure 2. Responses recorded between the 3rd and 1st lumbar vertebrae (LV3–LV1) and over the scalp in response to left peroneal nerve stimulation at the knee in a normal subject. Two trials, each of 1024 responses, have been superimposed. There is a well-marked cauda equina potential (*arrow*) recorded between LV3 and LV1. A reproducible positive wave is recorded at CZ with reference to FZ (⬍), and a corresponding negativity is recorded between C4′ and either CZ or C3′ (*arrowhead*).

Detection of Lesions in Central Somatosensory Pathways

Multiple Sclerosis. Somatosensory evoked potentials are requested most often to evaluate patients in whom a diagnosis of multiple sclerosis is suspected. In this context, the presence of SEP abnormalities may be helpful in detecting subclinical lesions involving the central somatosensory pathways, and thus in establishing the presence of multiple lesions in patients who present with clinical evidence of only one lesion that does not involve these pathways. An abnormality of the SEPs may also be important in indicating that vague sensory complaints have an organic basis when this is otherwise uncertain. In patients with multiple sclerosis, the likelihood of finding an SEP abnormality increases as the diagnostic certainty increases, if there is clinical evidence of a lesion in the sensory pathway being tested, or if pyramidal signs are present in the stimulated limb[12] or in the legs.[45] In patients with suspected multiple sclerosis, SEPs generally have a higher diagnostic yield in revealing abnormalities in clinically unaffected pathways than do either visual or brain-stem auditory evoked potentials.[23, 28, 40] Moreover, SEPs elicited by stimulation of a nerve in the legs are more likely to show an abnormality than median- or ulnar-elicited SEPs,[16] although technically satisfactory responses may be harder to elicit from a nerve in the lower limbs, especially in patients with spasticity. A variety of abnormalities have been described in patients with multiple sclerosis, including loss of components of the response or a prolongation in absolute or interpeak latency (Figs. 3 and 4). A frequently encountered abnormality is loss of the response recorded over the cervical spine, with preservation of the cortically generated responses, following stimulation of a nerve in the upper limb. There may also be an alteration in morphology or a marked asymmetry in amplitude of the response on the two sides, but it is difficult

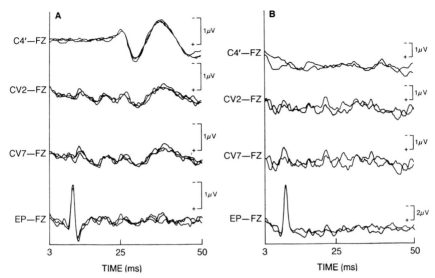

Figure 3. Somatosensory evoked potentials elicited by stimulation of the right median nerve at the wrist in two subjects with multiple sclerosis. *A*, There is a well-marked Erb's point potential, but the cervical responses are poorly formed or absent, and the N20 component over the scalp is delayed, having a latency of 26 msec. *B*, There is a well-marked Erb's point potential, but there is no recognizable response over the cervical spine or scalp.

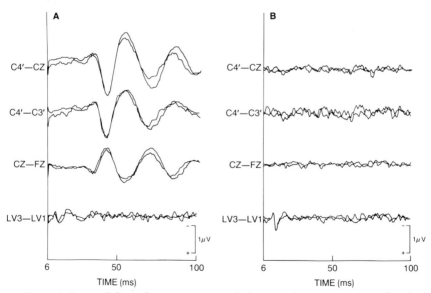

Figure 4. Peroneal-derived somatosensory evoked potentials in two patients with multiple sclerosis. *A*, There is a prolongation in the latency of the response recorded over the scalp, and the interval between the cauda equina potential and the scalp positivity is also prolonged by 5 msec above the upper limit of normal for subjects of the same height. *B*, There is a reproducible cauda equina potential, but no response can be recorded over the scalp.

to provide precise quantitative measures of these parameters and to define the limits of normality.

Evoked potential abnormalities never provide a diagnosis in themselves. They must be interpreted in the clinical context of the case and with regard to the other laboratory investigations to provide support for a clinical diagnosis. With regard to the diagnosis of multiple sclerosis, a variety of other neurologic disorders that can simulate it clinically may also lead to subclinical SEP abnormalities or to multimodality evoked potential abnormalities. Such disorders include the hereditary spinocerebellar degenerations, vitamin B12 or vitamin E deficiency, and hereditary spastic paraplegia.[19, 37, 38, 47]

With recent developments in neurologic imaging procedures, and in particular with the advent of magnetic resonance imaging (MRI), it is necessary to reevaluate the utility of SEP and other electrophysiological studies in the investigation of patients with suspected multiple sclerosis. In this regard, several important points can be made. First, in this author's experience, electrophysiologic techniques and MRI appear to be equally sensitive in detecting lesions in patients with definite multiple sclerosis, but MRI is somewhat more sensitive in patients in whom the diagnosis is less certain.[11] However, a number of patients without multiple sclerosis clinically may have MRI abnormalities of a sort that previously have been taken as pathognomonic of multiple sclerosis—the MRI findings do not therefore establish in themselves a diagnosis of multiple sclerosis. Second, there is some evidence that electrophysiologic techniques may be a little more sensitive than MRI in detecting lesions in the posterior fossa.[11] Third, evoked potential studies, particularly if selected with regard to the individual clinical context, are generally considerably cheaper than MRI, and this is important to consider at a time of escalating medical costs.[11] Fourth, the electrophysiologic findings may be helpful in defining the underlying pathophysiology. Eisen and associates[16] recently pointed out that in many patients with abnormal tibial-derived SEPs, the early cortically generated P40 and N45 components are absent, and the first measurable component is a positive wave having a mean latency of 51 msec. Because this closely approximates the latency of the next normal positive peak, that is, the P50, they took their findings to suggest that conduction block rather than delay of P40/N45 had occurred.

Serial evoked potential studies have been used to follow the course of multiple sclerosis or its response to therapy,[36] but its role in this context is unclear. Thus, when Matthews and Small[31] recorded median-derived SEPs in seven patients at intervals over an average period of 18 months, they found in three patients with frequent relapses that responses fluctuated between normality and abnormality without any obvious relationship to clinical status. Aminoff and associates[3] could find no consistent relationship between clinical deterioration and electrophysiologic change in patients with SEPs that were already abnormal. They studied changes in multimodality evoked potentials over time in patients with definite multiple sclerosis, and concluded that the evoked potentials could sometimes change without any accompanying clinical disturbance, or vice versa, that electrophysiologic abnormalities could revert to normal despite persisting or

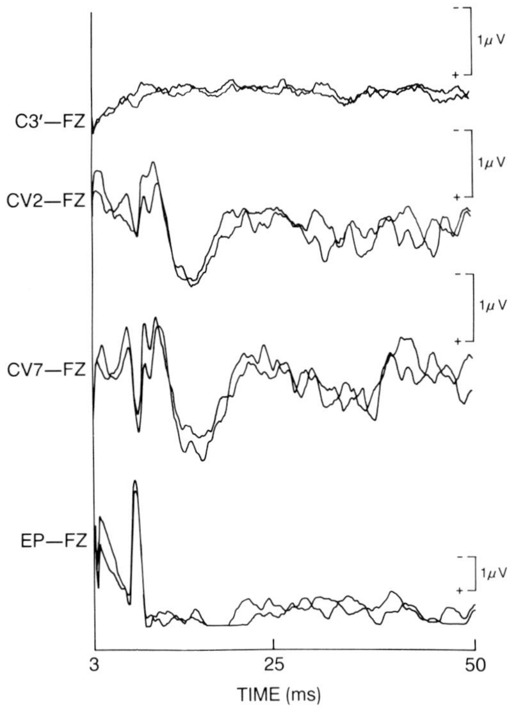

Figure 5. Somatosensory evoked potential following stimulation of the right median nerve at the wrist in a 15-year-old boy with a structural lesion at the level of the foramen magnum. There is a reproducible Erb's point potential, and responses can also be recorded over the cervical spine, but there is no response over the scalp.

worsening clinical deficits, and that any further change in an already abnormal response had little localizing significance. A lack of clear correlation between clinical and electrophysiologic abnormalities has also been found by others.[25]

Other Neurologic Disorders. SEPs may be abnormal in a variety of other disorders affecting the central nervous system, depending on the site of the lesion. For example, they may be abnormal in patients with tumors of the spinal cord (Fig. 5) or brain stem when these lesions are so placed that they involve the afferent pathways being stimulated. SEPs are normal in patients with Wallenberg syndrome,[34] but are often abnormal in patients with lesions involving the medial lemniscus. They may also be abnormal in patients with locked-in syndrome owing to pontine infarction.[34]

In patients with vascular or neoplastic thalamic lesions, the SEPs tend to be abnormal in patients with significant clinical deficits.

Chu[10] has recently examined the effect on short- and long-latency components of the median- and tibial-derived SEP of lesions in the thalamus and the thalamocortical radiation. When lesions were located primarily in the ventroposterior thalamus, the SEP changes consisted of loss or attenuation of overall response amplitude, an increase in peak latency, and attenuation of the median N20–P25 or tibial P40, in some combination. Laterally situated lesions tended to preferentially affect the tibial SEP, and more medially situated lesions the median-derived SEP. These SEP findings correlated with clinical observations that patients with lateral lesions tended to have more severe involvement of the lower extremity than the upper, whereas the opposite was true for patients with medial lesions. Infarcts involving the corona radiata produced SEP changes similar to those with ventroposterior thalamic lesions, except that evoked potentials were never entirely lost. With subcortical infarcts there was relative preservation of the short-latency SEP compared with the mid- and long-latency components. Tumors affecting the thalamus influence the SEP differently depending on whether the lesion is extrinsic or intrinsic. The SEPs may be relatively preserved with slowly growing noninfiltrating extrinsic tumors compressing the thalamus, whereas extrinsic mass lesions compressing the thalamus acutely may markedly influence the SEPs. Thus, Chu[10] found that many patients with basal ganglia hemorrhage had lost both median- and tibial-derived SEPs; when responses were present, the tibial SEPs were almost always the more severely affected. The SEPs are often markedly abnormal in patients with intrinsic thalamic tumors and a clinical sensory deficit.

With parietal lesions secondary to vascular pathology, Alajouanine and colleagues[1] found that the SEP to median nerve stimulation is often abolished over the affected hemisphere. The findings depend in part on the clinical status of the patient, in that SEPs are often normal in patients without sensory deficit and abolished in those with severe cortical sensory disturbances.[21] In 22 selected patients with a single circumscribed hemispheric lesion, Mauguiere and associates[32] found that a complete parietal lesion produced contralateral hemianesthesia without pyramidal signs, and eliminated the parietal complex that they designated N20–P27–P45 without affecting the prerolandic P22–N30, indicating that the N20 and P22 components have distinct neural generators. There was enhancement of the P22–N30 after chronic parietal lesions. Small postcentral lesions produced astereognosis (with preserved sensation otherwise), and they led to attenuation or loss of N20 and P27 without affecting P22–N30.

SEPs as a Guide to Prognosis

The SEP findings may help in providing a guide to the prognosis of patients who have had a hemispheric stroke. Thus, La Joie and associates[29] found that among patients with a right hemiplegia due to a stroke, 3 of the 8 who had a normal median-derived SEP showed some functional improvement by the time of discharge from hospital, whereas only 1 of 42 patients who had no cortical SEPs showed any functional improvement.

SEPs have been used to provide a guide to prognosis following head injury that was severe enough to cause coma. The most comprehensive study is that of Hume and Cant,[24] who correctly predicted the outcome by the SEP findings in 38 of 49 patients studied within 3½ days of onset of coma. The loss of median-derived SEPs over both hemispheres was regarded as indicative of a fatal outcome, whereas responses that were consistently reduced or absent over one side, or of prolonged latency on that side, were held to imply the probable development of a severe residual neurologic deficit such as a hemiplegia. However, SEPs were obtained on a number of different occasions for each patient and the outcome in individual patients did not always correlate well with the SEP findings.

The SEP findings showed some variation among different tests in the same patient, and the outcome in individual patients did not show a good correlation with the results obtained in every SEP. For example, 44 patients ultimately fared poorly, either dying or being left with a severe residual deficit; among these, the SEP findings were normal on at least some occasions in 10 patients, and 3 patients had normal SEPs on every occasion. Conversely, among 31 patients who did well, 15 had abnormal SEPs on some occasions. Such findings suggest that although SEPs may provide important prognostic information for groups of patients, they are not sufficiently reliable to provide a useful guide to prognosis in individual cases.

SEPs have been used to evaluate patients following anoxic-ischemic coma. In one recent study, none of 30 such patients with no cortical SEPs recovered cognition. By contrast, prognosis was more varied in patients in whom cortical responses were present. Thus, the presence of normal short-latency cortical SEPs several hours after cardiac arrest was associated with recovery of cognition in some patients and persistence of coma or development of a vegetative state in others.[8] As might have been anticipated, however, the presence or absence of cortical SEPs also corresponded with the clinical signs. One or several brain-stem reflexes (which are known to be of prognostic importance) were absent on initial examination in 60 per cent of patients with no cortical SEPs but in only 20 per cent of those with preserved SEPs. The different susceptibility of frontal and parietal cortex to anoxia was reflected by a dissociated loss of parietal or frontal potentials in six patients.

In both post-traumatic and postanoxic coma, however, reliable prognostic information can be obtained easily and at an early stage by clinical examination, without the necessity of more expensive, time-consuming procedures such as the recording of SEPs.

The role of SEPs in evaluating patients with suspected brain death is also controversial. For example, Anziska and Cracco[4] studied 11 patients who were clinically brain-dead, and in 1 of these patients, in whom brain death was confirmed by arteriography, it was possible to record an SEP component thought to be cortically generated. Whether in fact the response represented a subcortically generated N17 component rather than the cortically generated N20 peak cannot now be determined. Other authors have found that the recording of SEPs to median nerve stimulation has been more helpful in the evaluation of brain death suspects than the recording of BAEPs. Thus, Goldie and colleagues[22] found that among 35 patients with clinical brain death, 69 per cent had N13–N14 components recorded over the neck, but none had any later components. Similar data were reported by Belsh and Chokroverty,[5] who also noted that P13–P14 was clearly identifiable bilaterally in three patients using a scalp-noncephalic montage but was absent with a scalp-scalp montage, unlike the findings in normal subjects. Their findings were taken to imply two generators of P13–P14: a caudal P13 (for example, high cervical cord or dorsal column nuclei) and a rostral P14 (medial lemniscal pathways). With death of both generators, P13–P14 is lost, whereas with destruction of only the more rostral generator, the intact P13 will be recorded with the noncephalic reference but not with the active scalp reference (because of a cancellation effect).

SEPs have been used to evaluate patients following spinal injury. Following such injury, the responses recorded over the scalp to stimulation of a nerve below the level of the lesion may be normal or abnormal, depending in part on the extent and severity of the lesion and on the timing of the examination. However, early hopes that the presence or absence of a response over the scalp could provide a guide concerning the completeness of the cord lesion have not been substantiated. Thus, it is often not possible to record any cortical response in the acute stage after a spinal injury regardless of whether or not the lesion is complete. Nevertheless, preserved responses or the early return of responses after a spinal injury would indicate an incomplete lesion, and therefore a better prognosis than otherwise.[15]

Use of SEPs to Prevent or Minimize Neurologic Problems

SEPs have been used to monitor spinal cord function during surgery. Unfortunately, their role in this regard is not clear at the present time, and the overall utility of the technique remains to be clarified. The procedure has been used most often to monitor patients undergoing corrective surgery for spinal scoliosis. Such a procedure carries a definite risk of postoperative neurologic deficit in the legs, and it was hoped that by monitoring SEPs it would be possible to detect evidence of cord damage at an early stage during the operative procedure, when it might still be reversible. A number of studies have been published in this regard,[18, 26, 42, 48] but because of the very low surgical morbidity, it has not been possible to determine whether or not such electrophysiologic monitoring has prevented the incidence of major neurologic sequelae. In a recent study, a marked change in the intraoperative SEP findings was found to indicate a high probability of developing a neurologic deficit (43 per cent of cases, or three of seven patients),[13] but the crucial clinical question not addressed by this study was whether a change in surgical technique at the time of a detected SEP change alters the outlook.

Postoperative neurologic deficits may occur despite preservation of the SEPs during intraoperative monitoring.[30] There are several reasons why such "false-negative" results may occur. First, the SEP may remain normal if the operative procedure leads to a lesion that does not involve the somatosensory pathways being monitored. Second, if the pathways being monitored are already abnormal and have led to a preexisting electrophysiologic and neurologic deficit, it may not be possible to use SEPs to monitor them further. Third, a perioperative complication may occur after the monitoring procedure has been discontinued, so that a neurologic deficit occurs despite an SEP that was normal at the time of surgery. Fourth, certain technical factors, such as suboptimal "noisy" recordings or the effect of hypotension or general anesthetics on the response, may confound the use of SEPs in monitoring operative procedures. Technical refinements, such as the stimulation of motor pathways, either electrically or magnetically, in conjunction with the recording of SEPs, may enhance the value of electrophysiologic monitoring procedures in the operating room.

Central conduction time (that is, the N14–N20 interpeak latency) of the median SEP may be prolonged in patients with cerebral ischemic complications of subarachnoid hemorrhage or of surgery undertaken for ruptured intracranial aneurysm, and it has therefore been suggested that SEPs be used to monitor for the development of ischemia during such surgery.[46]

In patients with cervical spondylosis, SEPs do not help in distinguishing spondylosis from other lesions, and the findings obtained by stimulation of nerves in the upper limbs do not provide a guide to either the severity of the neurologic disorder or its prognosis. In patients with symptoms but no neurologic signs, the SEPs from upper-limb nerves are usually normal, whereas in patients with spondylotic radiculopathy associated with objective neurologic signs, the SEPs may be abnormal irrespective of whether or not there is any cord involvement.[17, 20] Noel and Desmedt[33] reported that with cervical cord compression the SEP elicited by sural nerve stimulation was often more abnormal than that elicited by stimulation of a digit in the upper limb. This suggests that the recording of sural-derived SEPs in patients with no clinical evidence of cord involvement may indicate which patients with cervical spondylosis are likely to develop a significant cord deficit, so that surgical treatment can be considered at an early stage. In this regard, Perlik and Fisher[39] recently studied 13 patients with cervical spondylotic myelopathy and found that posterior tibial SEPs were absent or delayed in all, including 1 patient with a pure motor syndrome. Scalp responses were bilaterally absent in six patients and bilaterally delayed in six others. In the remaining patient, a Brown-Sequard syndrome was associated with loss of scalp potentials with stimulation of the tibial nerve on one side, and prolonged response latency with stimulation of the other. These patients all had chronic symptoms and a definite clinical and radiologic diagnosis of cervical spondylotic myelopathy. Yu and Jones[49] found that tibial-derived SEP abnormalities were strongly correlated with ipsilateral posterior column signs but not with anterolateral column sensory signs, and that in patients with spondylotic myelopathy the SEP findings seemed more sensitive to sensory pathway involvement than clinical examination. The role of SEPs in patients with less definite cord involvement awaits delineation, although Yu and Jones[49] did find abnormal SEPs consistent with subclinical posterior column involvement in three patients with cervical spondylosis, of whom two had neck pain alone and one had radiculopathy.

Defining the Extent of Neuropathologic Involvement

As was referred to earlier, the SEP findings may be abnormal but are of no diagnostic help in the hereditary spinocerebellar degenerations, hereditary spastic paraplegia, and vitamin B12 or vitamin E deficiency states. The SEP findings are often more severely abnormal in Friedreich's ataxia than in the other inherited ataxias.[37] The SEP findings are of interest in defining the extent of pathology in these disorders, but are of little immediate clinical relevance. Nevertheless, because these disorders are sometimes confused clinically with multiple sclerosis, it is important to bear in mind the possibility that evoked potential studies may be abnormal in both contexts. In the hereditary ataxias, however, there tends to be greater symmetry of abnormality on the two sides than in disorders such as multiple sclerosis, in which pathology is more scattered.[37]

In Friedreich's ataxia, the peripheral Erb's point potential and the responses recorded over the cervical spine are often small or absent, but when present show little or no delay.[27, 37] Nevertheless, the response recorded over the scalp is often dispersed and delayed, implying that conduction is slowed in central pathways.

In patients with amyotrophic lateral sclerosis or motor neuron disease, SEP abnormalities have been found following upper- or lower-limb stimulation,[41] confirming previous clinical and pathologic reports of sensory involvement in this disorder. In another recent electrophysiologic study, abnormalities were found not only of the N20 of the median SEP, but also of certain longer-latency negative peaks.[7]

In Wilson's disease, multimodality evoked potential studies may show abnormalities, with subclinical dysfunction occurring in each of the major sensory pathways,[9] as might have been expected from the neuropathologic and neuroradiologic findings of widespread degeneration of the brain in that disease. In Huntington's disease, central somatosensory conduction time is normal, but there may be a reduction in amplitude of the early cortical components, with little or no change in latency.[6, 35] Such findings are of no clinical relevance at the present time.

Marked enhancement of the SEP occurs in certain types of myoclonus and epilepsy, but the significance of this is unclear.[44]

Determination of Whether Sensory Symptoms Have an Organic Basis

It is sometimes difficult to determine whether sensory symptoms have an organic basis when there are no consistent objective findings on examination. In this regard, an abnormal SEP would imply an organic cause for such symptoms. A normal SEP, together with normal peripheral sensory nerve conduction studies, would support clinical suspicions that symptoms are not organic in origin, but such electrophysiologic findings do not in themselves establish this with certainty. Indeed, it is not uncommon for SEPs to be normal in patients with pure sensory stroke owing, for example, to lacunar infarcts.[43]

SUMMARY

SEPs may be recorded over the spine and scalp to stimulation of any accessible mixed or sensory nerve in the extremities. SEP abnormalities are useful in detecting lesions in central somatosensory pathways. They do not establish a specific diagnosis, but they may suggest or support a diagnosis made on clinical grounds. They have been used particularly to detect subclinical lesions in multiple sclerosis, but their role in following the course of this disorder is unclear. SEPs have been used as a prognostic guide in patients with hemispheric stroke and in patients who are comatose following head injury or severe cerebral anoxia; in such instances, however, the SEP often adds little to what can be determined by clinical examination. Their role in the evaluation of patients with brain death is controversial. Preserved SEPs or their early return after a spinal injury suggests an incomplete lesion, and therefore a better prognosis than otherwise. SEPs have been used to minimize or prevent intraoperative neurologic complications by monitoring spinal cord function, but their role in this regard awaits adequate validation. In patients with cervical spondylosis, SEPs elicited by stimulation of a nerve in the lower extremities may be helpful in indicating which patients are liable to develop a significant cord deficit, so that surgical treatment can be considered at an early stage. SEP abnormalities have been described in a number of other neurologic contexts, but the findings may be of more academic than clinical relevance in that they help to define the extent of neuropathologic involvement without altering the management of individual patients.

REFERENCES

1. Alajouanine T, Scherrer J, Barbizet J, et al: Potentiels évoqués corticaux chez des sujets atteints de troubles somesthésiques. Rev Neurol 98:757, 1958
2. American Electroencephalographic Society: Guidelines for clinical evoked potential studies. J Clin Neurophysiol 1:3, 1984
3. Aminoff MJ, Davis SL, Panitch HS: Serial evoked potential studies in patients with definite multiple sclerosis: Clinical relevance. Arch Neurol 41:1197, 1984
4. Anziska BJ, Cracco RQ: Short latency somatosensory evoked potentials in brain dead patients. Arch Neurol 37:222, 1980
5. Belsh JM, Chokroverty S: Short-latency somatosensory evoked potentials in brain-dead patients. Electroencephalogr Clin Neurophysiol 68:75, 1987
6. Bollen EL, Arts RJ, Roos RA, et al: Somatosensory evoked potentials in Huntington's chorea. Electroencephalogr Clin Neurophysiol 62:235, 1985
7. Bosch EP, Yamada T, Kimura J: Somatosensory evoked potentials in motor neuron disease. Muscle Nerve 8:556, 1985
8. Brunko E, Zegers de Beyl D: Prognostic value of early cortical somatosensory evoked potentials after resuscitation from cardiac arrest. Electroencephalogr Clin Neurophysiol 66:15, 1987
9. Chu N-S: Sensory evoked potentials in Wilson's disease. Brain 109:491, 1986
10. Chu N-S: Median and tibial somatosensory evoked potentials. Changes in short- and long-latency components in patients with lesions of the thalamus and thalamo-cortical radiations. J Neurol Sci 76:199, 1986
11. Cutler JR, Aminoff MJ, Brant-Zawadzki M: Evaluation of patients with multiple sclerosis by evoked potentials and magnetic resonance imaging: A comparative study. Ann Neurol 20:645, 1986
12. Davis SL, Aminoff MJ, Panitch HS: Clinical correlations of serial somatosensory evoked potentials in multiple sclerosis. Neurology 35:359, 1985
13. Dinner DS, Luders H, Lesser RP, et al: Intraoperative spinal somatosensory evoked potential monitoring. J Neurosurg 65:807, 1986
14. Eisen A: The somatosensory evoked potential. Can J Neurol Sci 9:65, 1982
15. Eisen A, Aminoff MJ: Somatosensory evoked potentials. In Aminoff MJ (ed): Electrodiagnosis in Clinical Neurology, 2nd ed. New York, Churchill Livingstone, 1986, p 535
16. Eisen A, Odusote K, Li D, et al: Comparison of magnetic resonance imaging with somatosensory testing in MS subjects. Muscle Nerve 10:385, 1987
17. El Negamy E, Sedgwick EM: Delayed cervical somatosensory evoked potentials in cervical spondylosis. J Neurol Neurosurg Psychiatry 42:238, 1979
18. Engler GL, Spielholz NI, Bernhard WN, et al: Somatosensory evoked potentials during Harrington instrumentation for scoliosis. J Bone Joint Surg 60–A:528, 1978
19. Fine EJ, Hallett M: Neurophysiological study of subacute combined degeneration. J Neurol Sci 45:331, 1980
20. Ganes T: Somatosensory conduction times and peripheral, cervical and cortical evoked potentials in patients with cervical spondylosis. J Neurol Neurosurg Psychiatry 43:683, 1980

21. Giblin DR: The effect of lesions of the nervous system on cerebral responses to peripheral nerve stimulation. Electroencephalogr Clin Neurophysiol 12:262, 1960
22. Goldie WD, Chiappa KH, Young RR, et al: Brainstem auditory and short-latency somatosensory evoked responses in brain death. Neurology 31:248, 1981
23. Green JB, Price R, Woodbury SG: Short-latency somatosensory evoked potentials in multiple sclerosis: Comparison with auditory and visual evoked potentials. Arch Neurol 37:630, 1980
24. Hume AL, Cant BR: Central somatosensory conduction after head injury. Ann Neurol 10:411, 1981
25. Iragui VI, Wiederholt WC, Romine JS: Serial recordings of multimodality evoked potentials in multiple sclerosis: A four year follow-up study. Can J Neurol Sci 13:320, 1986
26. Jones SJ: Clinical applications of short-latency somatosensory evoked potentials. Ann NY Acad Sci 388:369, 1982
27. Jones SJ, Baraitser M, Halliday AM: Peripheral and central somatosensory nerve conduction defects in Friedreich's ataxia. J Neurol Neurosurg Psychiatry 43:495, 1980
28. Khoshbin S, Hallett M: Multimodality evoked potentials and blink reflex in multiple sclerosis. Neurology 31:138, 1981
29. La Joie WJ, Reddy NM, Melvin JL: Somatosensory evoked potentials: Their predictive value in right hemiplegia. Arch Phys Med Rehabil 63:223, 1982
30. Lesser RP, Raudzens P, Luders H, et al: Postoperative neurological deficits may occur despite unchanged intraoperative somatosensory evoked potentials. Ann Neurol 19:22, 1986
31. Matthews WB, Small DG: Serial recording of visual and somatosensory evoked potentials in normal man and patients with multiple sclerosis. J Neurol Sci 40:11, 1979
32. Mauguiere F, Desmedt JE, Courjon J: Astereognosis and dissociated loss of frontal or parietal components of somatosensory evoked potentials in hemispheric lesions. Brain 106:271, 1983
33. Noel P, Desmedt JE: Cerebral and far-field somatosensory evoked potentials in neurological disorders involving the cervical spinal cord, brainstem, thalamus and cortex. In Desmedt JE (ed): Clinical Uses of Cerebral, Brainstem and Spinal Somatosensory Evoked Potentials: Progress in Clinical Neurophysiology. Vol. 7. Basel, Karger, 1980, p 205
34. Noel P, Desmedt JE: Somatosensory cerebral evoked potentials after vascular lesions of the brain-stem and diencephalon. Brain 98:113, 1975
35. Noth J, Engel L, Friedemann H-H, et al: Evoked potentials in patients with Huntington's disease and their offspring. I. Somatosensory evoked potentials. Electroencephalogr Clin Neurophysiol 59:134, 1984
36. Nuwer MR, Packwood JW, Myers LW, et al: Evoked potentials predict the clinical changes in a multiple sclerosis drug study. Neurology 37:1754, 1987
37. Nuwer MR, Perlman SL, Packwood JW, et al: Evoked potential abnormalities in the various inherited ataxias. Ann Neurol 13:20, 1983
38. Pedersen L, Trojaborg W: Visual, auditory and somatosensory pathway involvement in hereditary cerebellar ataxia, Friedreich's ataxia and familial spastic paraplegia. Electroencephalogr Clin Neurophysiol 52:283, 1981
39. Perlik SJ, Fisher MA: Somatosensory evoked response evaluation of cervical spondylotic myelopathy. Muscle Nerve 10:481, 1987
40. Purves SJ, Low MD, Galloway J, et al: A comparison of visual, brainstem auditory, and somatosensory evoked potentials in multiple sclerosis. Can J Neurol Sci 8:15, 1981
41. Radtke RA, Erwin A, Erwin CW: Abnormal sensory evoked potentials in amyotrophic lateral sclerosis. Neurology 36:796, 1986
42. Raudzens PA: Intraoperative monitoring of evoked potentials. Ann NY Acad Sci 388:308, 1982
43. Robinson RK, Richey ET, Kase CS, et al: Somatosensory evoked potentials in pure sensory stroke and related conditions. Stroke 16:818, 1985
44. Rothwell JC, Obeso JA, Marsden CD: On the significance of giant somatosensory evoked potentials in cortical myoclonus. J Neurol Neurosurg Psychiatry 47:33, 1984
45. Small DG, Matthews WB, Small M: The cervical somatosensory evoked potential (SEP) in the diagnosis of multiple sclerosis. J Neurol Sci 35:211, 1978

46. Symon L, Hargadine J, Zawirski M, et al: Central conduction time as an index of ischaemia in subarachnoid haemorrhage. J Neurol Sci 44:95, 1979
47. Thomas PK, Jefferys JGR, Smith IS, et al: Spinal somatosensory evoked potentials in hereditary spastic paraplegia. J Neurol Neurosurg Psychiatry 44:243, 1981
48. Worth RM, Markand ON, DeRosa GP, et al: Intraoperative somatosensory evoked potential monitoring during spinal cord surgery. In Courjon J, Mauguiere F, Revol M (eds): Clinical Applications of Evoked Potentials in Neurology. New York, Raven Press, 1982, p 367
49. Yu YL, Jones SJ: Somatosensory evoked potentials in cervical spondylosis. Correlation of median, ulnar and posterior tibial nerve responses with clinical and radiological findings. Brain 108:273, 1985

Department of Neurology
Box 0114, Room 794-M
University of California
School of Medicine
San Francisco, California 94143

Evoked Potentials   0733–8619/88 $0.00 + .20

The Use of Somatosensory Evoked Potentials for the Evaluation of the Peripheral Nervous System

Andrew Eisen, MD, FRCP(C)*

The somatosensory evoked potential (SEP) is mediated peripherally by group Ia muscle and group II cutaneous afferents.[6, 15] These sensory nerves are the largest-diameter nerve fibers and are those routinely and most easily accessible to conventional study. The SEP can be used indirectly to assess peripheral nerve disease, and there are several indications for using SEPs to evaluate peripheral nerve disease: (1) to measure conduction along a normal or diseased nerve that by reason of anatomic location is not easily accessible to stimulation or recording using standard electromyographic methods; (2) to document axonal continuity when a sensory nerve action potential cannot be recorded; (3) to evaluate radiculopathies, especially when sensory signs or symptoms predominate; and (4) to evaluate plexopathies. These different applications of the SEP are the subject of this article.

Although the SEP has been shown to play a useful role in assessing the peripheral nervous system, routine and more direct techniques should first be shown to have been of no or limited value. Furthermore, when the SEP is used to evaluate the peripheral nervous system, it is assumed that the central nervous system is normal. This conclusion, which is usually based on clinical judgment, can be misleading because several conditions may be associated with clinically occult involvement of the central nervous system. Diabetes,[9, 31] collagen vascular diseases, complications of cancer, Guillain-Barré syndrome,[41] and Charcot-Marie-Tooth disease[32] are examples. In these and other diseases where one might suspect additional involvement of the central nervous system, central conduction times should be measured. This can be achieved by recording the cervical and lumbar spinal potentials at the same time as the SEP and subtracting their latencies

*Professor, Division of Neurology; Acting Head, Department of Medicine, University of British Columbia; Director, Department of Diagnostic Neurophysiology, Neuromuscular Diseases Unit (EMG), Vancouver General Hospital, Vancouver, British Columbia, Canada

from N20 (arm SEP) or P40 (leg SEP). These central conduction times should not exceed 7.5 msec (N20–N13) and 22.5 msec (P40–N1).[15]

PERIPHERAL NERVE DISEASE

Assessment of Some Specific Nerves

Although it is possible to measure conduction along the lateral femoral cutaneous nerve, employing either orthodromic or antidromic stimulation,[7, 44, 48] the potentials elicited are frequently small and not recordable in all normal, especially obese, subjects. Entrapment or infarction of this nerve is common in association with diabetes, producing meralgia paresthetica.[34] The nerve can be stimulated four finger breadths inferior and two finger breadths lateral to the anterior superior iliac spine. Either trans- or percutaneous stimulation can be employed. A correct stimulation site is confirmed by the subject's feeling sensory radiation in a correct anatomic distribution. In a severely diseased nerve, this may not be possible. A SEP is usually easily elicited and best recorded using a conventional bipolar cephalic montage (Cz–Fz, Cz–C3, or C4 contralateral to the side of stimulation). The normal mean latency measured to "P_{40}" is 31.8 ± 1.8 msec ($n = 25$). It is useful to compare SEPs elicited by stimulation of the normal with the diseased nerve (Fig. 1). SEPs may be used in a similar way to assess several other cutaneous nerves where difficulty is encountered in conventionally recording sensory action potentials. The lateral and medial antebrachial nerves, the saphenous nerve, the dorsal cutaneous branch of the ulnar nerve, the intercostal nerves, and dorsal primary cutaneous rami are other examples (Fig. 2).

Nerve Injury

Following nerve trauma, nerve action potentials may become small, dispersed, or unrecordable for many months, depending on the degree of axonal degeneration that has occurred.[5] Despite the absence of peripherally recorded potentials, it is often possible to elicit a SEP. The ability to do so indicates that some axons have regenerated and are in continuity (Fig. 3). This has important prognostic implications, especially when reconstructive surgery is contemplated. The ability to record a SEP in the apparent absence of a sizable peripheral volley suggests the intervention of a central nervous system amplifying mechanism. Such would indeed seem to be the case and an amplifying capability has been demonstrated in normal subjects.[19] When the amplitude of a sensory nerve action potential (SNAP) and SEP are reduced by progressively reducing current intensity, the amplitude of the SNAP is reduced more rapidly than the SEP (Fig. 4). In engineering terms, the gain of the central nervous system is about 2, being greatest at stimulus intensities of between 30 to 60 per cent of maximum, where maximum is defined as 2½ times sensory threshold.[19] How and at what level(s) of the nervous system amplification occurs are not known, but probably very few intact axons are needed to initiate a volley capable of eliciting a recordable SEP. During the regenerative process, SEPs are

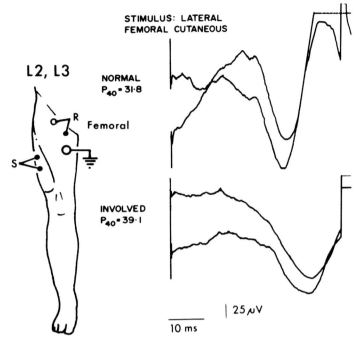

Figure 1. Meralgia paresthetica. SEPs evoked by stimulation of the lateral femoral cutaneous nerve. The stimulation site, S, is indicated. Near nerve recording, R is used to monitor any peripheral response. The top traces are normal and were elicited by stimulation of the uninvolved side. The lower traces are prolonged and reduced in amplitude, indicating conduction block in a patient with diabetes.

recordable much earlier than the SNAP or mixed nerve action potential. Absence of peripheral potentials should be regarded as positive proof of failed nerve regeneration only if the SEP is also unrecordable.

Peripheral Neuropathies

The central nervous system amplification principle can be equally applied to generalized neuropathies in which it may also be impossible to record sensory action potentials. This is frequently the case in Charcot-Marie-Tooth disease and other chronic hereditary neuropathies, chronic diabetic neuropathy, and Friedreich's ataxia. The ability to indirectly measure sensory conduction by recording SEPs is diagnostically helpful. Demonstration of conduction slowing of greater than 60 per cent of normal is good evidence of a demyelinating as opposed to an axonal degenerating neuropathy.[27] Recording the SEP also allows one to detect peripheral sensory nerve slowing proximally, which can be difficult using conventional methods. This has particular relevance in the Guillain-Barré syndrome, in which distal conduction is often normal but in which the SEP is prolonged, of reduced amplitude, or dispersed.[18, 41]

RADICULOPATHIES

There is no electrophysiologic test that is specific for the investigation and assessment of radiculopathies. Nevertheless, there is an important role

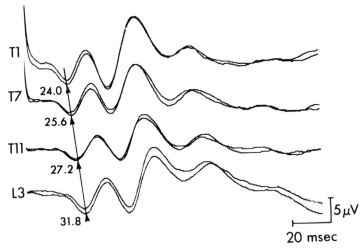

Figure 2. Paraspinal stimulation. The paraspinal region is stimulated bilaterally and simultaneously at given spinal levels. The cutaneous branches of the dorsal root rami are among the structures activated. The method can be used to study segmental sensory radiculopathies such as occurs in diabetes. (*From* Goodridge A, Eisen A, Hoirch M: Paraspinal stimulation to elicit somatosensory evoked potentials: An approach to physiological localization of spinal lesions. Electroencphalogr Clin Neurophysiol 68:268–276, 1987; with permission.)

of electrophysiology in the evaluation of radiculopathies.[13] Computed tomography (CT) scan and, more recently, magnetic resonance imaging (MRI) allow for excellent anatomic localization of a root lesion, but they give little or no information regarding the severity of the lesion or its possible prognosis. Additionally there are situations where despite extensive electrophysiologic evidence of a root lesion, imaging may be inconsequential. On the other hand, minor or moderate defects without clinical counterpart are fairly frequently seen on CT scan or MRI. This is particularly true in those over the age of 50 years, after which time asymptomatic degenerative disk disease is common.[13] Finally, even when a clinically suspected root lesion is confirmed radiologically, caution is required before concluding a causal relationship, because the same electrophysiologic abnormalities occur in amyotrophic lateral sclerosis, syringomyelia, and other diseases that are much rarer than radiculopathy due to a degenerative disk, but that can coexist.

Of the several available electrophysiologic tests, each has advantages and disadvantages. Using SEPs to evaluate radiculopathies should therefore be considered in the context of being part of a battery of available physiologic tests.[13, 14, 53] Needle electromyography, particularly of the paraspinal muscles, confirms the presence of a lesion at least as proximal as the dorsal root ganglion cell and is still the best means of delineating which specific myotome(s) is/are involved.[29, 35] It is the only definitive means of documenting the presence of axonal degeneration indicated by the presence of fibrillation or positive sharp waves. Development of these, however, takes days to weeks to develop, depending on how proximal is the particular muscle tested. Fibrillation and positive sharp waves do not develop in

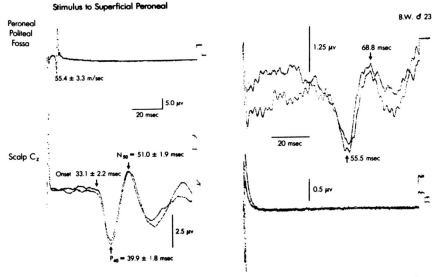

Figure 3. SEPs following nerve trauma. The left panel is a normal near nerve recording of a superficial peroneal sensory nerve action potential (*top*). Lower trace shows the SEP, also normal, that was recorded simultaneously on another channel. Right panel represents corresponding recordings from the contralateral side. No sensory nerve action potential was recorded but a SEP was recordable. It is small, dispersed, and prolonged. The patient had sustained an injury to the superficial peroneal nerve. Ability to record a SEP even in the absence of a SNAP confirms the presence of nerve continuity.

neurapraxic lesions,[13, 14] and then one has to rely on abnormal recruitment patterns that are harder to interpret. Hence the continual search for a useful conduction test in radiculopathies.

Thus far, all conduction tests, including SEPs, designed to evaluate root lesions have fallen short of their initial promise. This is not too surprising when one considers that they all attempt to detect conduction slowing over a small (few millimeters) segment of diseased nerve diluted in a long length of normally conducting nerve distal to the root. Prolonged F wave latencies may be helpful in confirming a root lesion.[20, 21, 24] F waves are, however, recordable only from a select group of muscles with limited segmental representation, and they give no information about disease involving the sensory roots.[38, 40, 42] Similarly the H reflex is usually recordable only from the gastrocnemius-soleus muscle complex, limiting its use to assessment of the S1 sensory root.[2, 3, 46] H reflexes can be unmasked from other muscles by voluntary contraction of the muscle from which the response is being elicited. This may widen the scope of the H reflex in radiculopathies[17] (Fig. 5).

Sensory symptoms or signs often predominate or occur in isolation in root disease, especially if due to compression when the type Ia afferents and type II cutaneous sensory fibers, the largest-diameter ones, are most likely to be compromised. In this situation, both needle electromyography and F-wave studies are likely to be normal, which prompted consideration of using SEPs to study sensory root lesions. There are several possible approaches to using SEPs for evaluating radiculopathies.

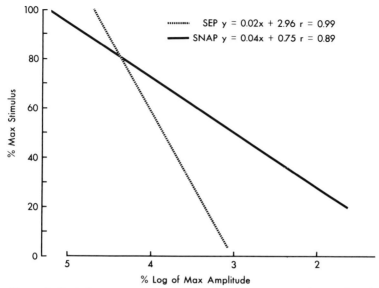

Figure 4. Central nervous system amplification. The regression lines reflect the normal decline in amplitude of the SEP and SNAP in relation to reduction of stimulus intensity. Between about 30 per cent and 60 per cent of maximum stimulus, defined as the stimulus that elicits a near maximal response, the SNAP amplitude declines proportionally at about twice the rate of the SEP.

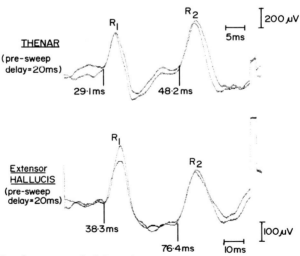

Figure 5. H reflexes unmasked by voluntary muscle contraction. R1 (H reflex) was recorded from the thenar and extensor hallucis muscles. The median and common peroneal nerves, respectively, were stimulated at 1 Hz whereas the muscles were voluntarily contracted at about 30 per cent of their maximum force. 200 sweeps were averaged. R2 is a long latency response in all probability synapsing in the motor cortex.[29]

Mixed Nerve Stimulation

The most convenient method of eliciting a sizable and therefore easily measurable SEP is by stimulating a mixed nerve trunk that generates a large, synchronous volley in the type Ia afferents. However, this invariably entails multisegmental activation, precluding detection of abnormality in a single root lesion. For the same reason, F-wave latencies are often normal. Use of mixed nerve stimulation to evoke SEPs has proven of some value in the diagnosis of cervical disk disease, but only in the context of myelopathic cervical spondylosis.[22, 25, 47] Eliciting potentials over Erb's point and over the cervical spine is easily achieved by mixed nerve stimulation. The conduction difference between these points includes transmission through the roots. It normally measures less than 7.0 msec and, if prolonged, would be supportive evidence of a proximal peripheral nerve lesion.

Spinal SEPs

In suspected lumbosacral radiculopathies, it would seem appropriate to study spinal evoked potentials elicited by tibial or peroneal nerve stimulation.[10, 11] Unfortunately, these potentials are not universally record-able in all normal subjects, making interpretation of small or unrecordable responses in disease difficult. In infants and children, they are much more easily recorded and have a role in assessing root lesions.[10, 11] In adults, latency is the only consistently measurable characteristic of spinal evoked potentials, and this is unlikely to be significantly affected because of the distal nerve dilution factor referred to previously. Spinal recording is greatly facilitated by epidural or intradural recording, which enables measurement of amplitude as well as latency.[8] Although these invasive techniques are unacceptable for routine use, they may prove helpful intraoperatively, and can be modified into a "semi near-nerve" recording technique by percuta-neous introduction of a monopolar needle to the level of the lamina.[39] This is safe and not overly uncomfortable, being essentially the same technique as used for recording paraspinal EMG.[13, 14]

Segmental Cutaneous Nerve Stimulation

In an attempt to increase segmental and modality specificity of SEPs when trying to isolate a radiculopathy, several groups have turned to cutaneous nerve stimulation.[12, 16, 37, 45] Three different techniques are worthy of consideration. They are cutaneous nerve trunk stimulation, dermatomal stimulation, and motor point stimulation. Of these, cutaneous nerve trunk stimulation excites the largest peripheral volley and elicits the most easily measurable SEPs[16] (see Fig. 3). However, it is not possible to stimulate a single dermatomal representation this way, because most peripheral cuta-neous nerves contain fibers from two or more roots.

Relevant data are summarized in Table 1. The cutaneous nerve is stimulated at 2 to 2½ times sensory threshold at a rate of 3 to 5 Hz; in other respects, recording and data acquisition are comparable to that employed when stimulating a mixed nerve. The latencies of the different SEP components are, however, slightly longer than those of a corresponding SEP evoked by mixed nerve stimulation at a site that is equidistant from

Table 1. *Nerves and Stimulating Sites Used to Elicit SEPs*

CUTANEOUS NERVE	STIMULATING SITE	SEGMENT	LATENCY (N20/P40)
Musculocutaneous	Forearm	C5	17.4 + 1.2
Median	Thumb	C6	22.5 + 1.1
Median	Adjacent surfaces Fingers 2 and 3	C7	21.2 + 1.2
Ulnar	Finger 5	C8	22.5 + 1.1
Lateral femoral cutaneous	Thigh	L2	31.8 + 1.8
Saphenous	Knee	L3	37.6 + 2.0
Saphenous	Ankle	L4	43.4 + 2.2
Superficial peroneal	Ankle	L5	39.9 + 1.8
Sural	Ankle	S1	42.1 + 1.4

the cortex.[15] Correctness of the stimulation site is confirmed by recording a sensory nerve action potential along the course of the appropriate nerve (see Fig. 3) and by subjective sensation in the expected distribution of the cutaneous nerve. By definition, a root lesion is proximal to the dorsal root ganglion cell, and therefore in radiculopathies, the sensory nerve action potential will be normal, whereas the SEP may be abnormal in one or more respects. If both are abnormal, it indicates additional or isolated pathology distal to the dorsal root. The exception to this occurs in ganglion-opathies associated with marked cell loss within the dorsal root ganglion. When this happens, both the sensory nerve action potential and SEP are small, dispersed, or more usually unrecordable. Examples of ganglionopa-thies are acute diabetic radicular infarction,[4] herpes zoster,[52] Friedreich's ataxia,[12] as well as a spontaneous variety.

Dermatomal stimulation is more selective in terms of dermatomal input, but is technically more difficult. A representative area of skin is stimulated preferably employing a large cathode against a small anode, again at 2 to 2½ times sensory threshold.[1, 30] The nerve terminals are of small diameter, relatively few, and of variable conduction. Because of this, the volley that is initiated is desynchronized and the resulting SEP is usually small and dispersed. This makes it difficult to measure latencies and virtually impossible to measure other SEP characteristics.

A more synchronous volley and larger SEP can be elicited using motor point stimulation. This can be achieved by surface stimulation, but for large muscles a monopolar needle-stimulating electrode is more satisfactory. A long duration stimulus (1.0 msec) of small intensity preferentially activates the type Ia muscle afferents that exist in association with the motor fibers at the motor point. If the needle electrode is in close proximity to the motor point, a stimulus intensity of fewer than 3 mA is sufficient to obtain a maximum response. Motor point stimulation has the advantage of being applicable to most muscles and is easier than dermatomal stimulation (Fig. 6). Its drawback lies in reduced specificity, because usually more than a single dorsal root is activated.

All the methods previously mentioned in eliciting SEPs using segmen-tal sensory stimulation have thus far had a disappointing diagnostic yield in

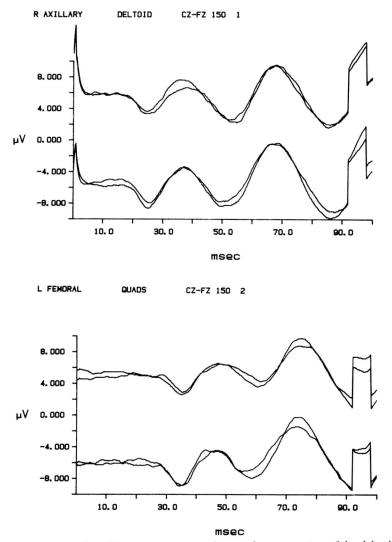

Figure 6. SEPs elicited by motor point stimulation. The motor points of the deltoid (*top* tracings) and quadriceps (*bottom* tracings) muscles were stimulated through a monopolar needle electrode. The normal SEPs elicited are an average of 250 sweeps.

radiculopathies, some reports being more encouraging than others.[13, 14] The main reason for this, undoubtedly, lies in dilution of the short segment of diseased nerve by the long length of normal nerve distally.

This should not deter one from use of SEPs in radiculopathies, because characteristics of the SEP other than latency require consideration and are likely to be more relevant. In most radiculopathies, conduction block usually underlies the neurologic deficit that would be reflected by amplitude reduction of the SEP (Fig. 7). Absolute values are too variable to be meaningful, but side-to-side or rostral caudal comparisons may be useful. Dispersion or poor morphology is another characteristic that might become

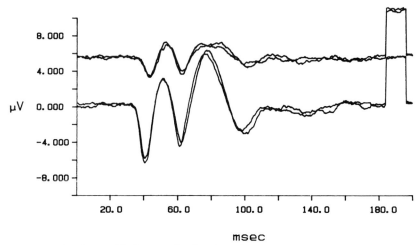

Figure 7. Conduction block in a radiculopathy. The SEPs were evoked by stimulation of the right (*top*) and left (*lower*) sural nerves (S1 root). The patient had a myelographically confirmed right S1 disk herniation. Paraspinal needle EMG did not show fibrillation or positive sharp waves. The SEP latencies are normal and comparable, but the amplitude on the involved side is reduced by more than 60 per cent. This type of abnormality, which reflects conduction block, is more likely than latency prolongation.

a helpful measure. Presently this is not easy to measure and requires computer-assisted techniques not yet sufficiently standardized for routine clinical use.[15] It is to be anticipated that future efforts directed to careful standardization of both morphology and amplitude of the SEP will yield much better results in root lesions.

PLEXOPATHIES

The need for accurate anatomic localization in traumatic plexopathies lies in the growing potential of microneurosurgical intervention using grafts. This is feasible only if root avulsion has not occurred. Avulsion may not always be evident as a meningocele on myelography, which is otherwise the most definitive means of its verification. Sometimes pseudomeningoceles may falsely indicate root avulsion when there is none. Root avulsion can also be confirmed electrophysiologically by the presence of a normal sensory nerve action potential in the absence of an elicitable motor action potential and SEP, paraspinal muscle denervation (fibrillation or positive sharp waves), and persistence of a histamine flare in response to an injection of intradermal histamine (Fig. 8).

Recording the SEP is useful in a traumatic plexopathy, enabling documentation of continuity between the peripheral and central nervous systems.[36, 50, 51, 57, 58] Ability to elicit a SEP, even when a sensory nerve action potential cannot be recorded and when there is significant motor weakness with fibrillation or positive sharp waves recorded on needle EMG, can be regarded as indicating a more favorable prognosis than if the

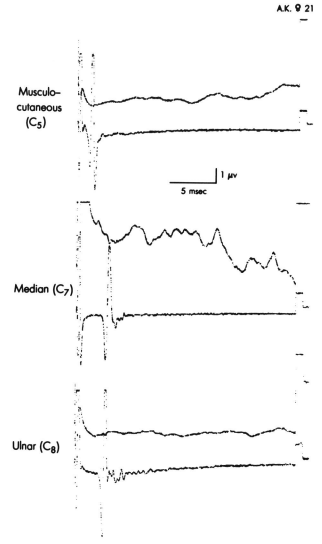

A.K. ♀ 21

Musculo-
cutaneous
(C₅)

1 µv

5 msec

Median (C₇)

Ulnar (C₈)

Figure 8. Brachial plexus avulsion. The patient had sustained a total brachial plexus avulsion involving upper, middle and lower trunks. Normal SNAPs were evoked by stimulation of the musculocutaneous (C5, upper trunk), the median (C6, middle trunk) and the ulnar (C8, T1, lower trunk). Attempts to elicit SEPs at the same time failed indicating interruption of peripheral and central nervous system structures.

SEP was not recordable. It is possible to roughly distinguish different trunks or cords of the brachial plexus by selecting particular nerves to stimulate, and these are listed in Table 2. This is helpful when it is not possible to delineate the lesion anatomically by needle EMG, as happens shortly after trauma before there has been time for fibrillation or positive sharp waves to develop. Specificity is achieved with more difficulty in

Table 2. *Nerves Employed to Elicit SEPs in the Evaluation of*
Brachial Plexopathies

NERVE	TRUNKS	CORDS
Musculocutaneous	Upper	Lateral
Radial	Middle	Posterior
Median	Upper	Medial
	Lower	Lateral
Ulnar	Lower	Medial

traumatic lumbosacral plexopathies because overlapping involvement frequently occurs.

Experience with SEPs in nontraumatic plexopathies is limited, but several situations lend themselves logically to their use. In the rare, neurogenic thoracic outlet syndrome,[26, 28, 55, 56] SEPs elicited by ulnar nerve stimulation might be expected to be abnormal, complementing other electrophysiologic tests of proven value in this disease. In contrast, in nonneurogenic outlet syndrome, in particular the "droopy shoulder syndrome," the SEP, as are other electrophysiologic tests, is normal.[49, 54] Another uncommon plexopathy in which SEPs are proving useful is that developing in association with open-heart surgery.[33] Here it has been shown through SEPs that patients may have a pure plexopathy, a pure ulnar neuropathy, or most often a mixture of the two.[43] Its pathogenesis is unclear, but simple mechanical pressure plays a small or irrelevant role. In paralytic brachial neuritis, lesion(s) is/are patchy, reflecting damage to nerve branching points as they arise from the plexus.[23] The SEP can help here by defining more accurately which nerve or nerves are predominantly involved.

REFERENCES

1. Aminoff MJ, Goodin DS, Barbaro NM, et al: Dermatomal somatosensory evoked potentials in unilateral lumbosacral radiculopathy. Ann Neurol 17:171–176, 1985
2. Braddom RL, Johnson EW: H reflex: Review and classification with suggested clinical uses. Arch Phys Med Rehabil 55:412–417, 1974
3. Braddom RL, Johnson EW: Standardization of H reflex and diagnostic use in S1 radiculopathy. Arch Phys Med Rehabil 55:161–166, 1966
4. Brown MJ, Asbury AK: Diabetic neuropathy. Ann Neurol 15:2–12, 1974
5. Buchthal F, Kuhl V: Nerve conduction, tactile sensibility and the electromyogram after suture or compression of peripheral nerve: A longitudinal study in man. J Neurol Neurosurg Psychiatry 42:436–451, 1979
6. Burke D, Skuse NF, Lethlean AK: Cutaneous and muscle afferent components of the cerebral potential evoked by electrical stimulation of human peripheral nerve. Electroencephalogr Clin Neurophysiol 51:579–588, 1981
7. Butler ET, Johnson EW, Kaye ZA: Normal conduction velocity in the lateral femoral cutaneous nerve. Arch Phys Med Rehabil 55:31–32, 1974
8. Caccia MR, Ubiali E, Andreusse L: Spinal evoked responses recorded from the epidural space in normal and diseased humans. J Neurol Neurosurg Psychiatry 39:962–972, 1976
9. Cracco J, Castells S, Mark E: Spinal somatosensory evoked potentials in juvenile diabetics. Ann Neurol 15:55–58, 1984
10. Cracco RQ: Spinal evoked response: Peripheral nerve stimulation in man. Electroencephalogr Clin Neurophysiol 35:379–386, 1973

11. Cracco RQ, Cracco JB: Spinal evoked potentials. *In* Buser PA, Cobb WA, Okuma T (eds): Kyoto Symposia (EEG suppl no 36). Amsterdam, Elsevier, 1982, pp 358–364

12. Desmedt JE, Noel P: Average cerebral evoked potentials in the evaluation of lesions of the sensory nerves and the central somatosensory pathways. *In* Desmedt JE (ed): New Developments in Electromyography and Clinical Neurophysiology. Vol. 2. Basel, Switzerland, Karger, 1973, p 352–371

13. Eisen A: Radiculopathies and plexopathies. *In* Brown WF, Bolton CF (eds): Clinical Electrodiagnosis. New York, Butterworths, 1987, pp 52–73

14. Eisen A: Electrodiagnosis of radiculopathies. Neurol Clin 3:495–510, 1985

15. Eisen A, Aminoff MJ: Somatosensory evoked potentials. *In* Aminoff MJ (ed): Electrodiagnosis in Clinical Neurology, 2nd ed. New York, Churchill Livingstone, 1986, pp 532–573

16. Eisen A, Elleker G: Sensory nerve stimulation and evoked cerebral potentials. Neurology 30:1097–1105, 1980

17. Eisen A, Hoirch M, White J, et al: Sensory group Ia proximal conduction velocity. Muscle Nerve 7:636–641, 1984

18. Eisen A, Humphreys P: The Guillain-Barre syndrome: A clinical and electrophysiological study of 25 cases. Arch Neurol 30:438–443, 1974

19. Eisen A, Purves S, Hoirch M: Central nervous system amplification: Its potential in the diagnosis of early multiple sclerosis. Neurology 32:359–364, 1982

20. Eisen A, Shomer D, Melmed C: An electrophysiological method for examining lumbosacral root compression. Can J Neurol Sci 4:117–123, 1977

21. Eisen A, Shomer D, Melmed C: The application of F-wave measurements in the differentiation of proximal and distal upper limb entrapments. Neurology 27:662–668, 1977

22. El Negamy E, Sedgwick EM: Delayed cervical somatosensory potentials in cervical spondylosis. J Neurol Neurosurg Psychiatry 42:238–241, 1979

23. England JD, Sumner AJ: Neuralgic amyotrophy: An increasingly diverse entity. Muscle Nerve 10:60–68, 1987

24. Fisher MA, Shivde AJ, Teixera C, et al: Clinical and electrophysiological appraisal of the significance of radicular injury in back pain. J Neurol Neurosurg Psychiatry 41:303–306, 1978

25. Ganes T: Somatosensory conduction times and peripheral cervical and cortical evoked potentials in patients with cervical spondylosis. J Neurol Neurosurg Psychiatry 43:683–689, 1980

26. Gilliatt RW: The clinical neurological syndrome associated with a cervical rib and band. *In* Greep JM, Lemmens HA, Roos DB, et al (eds): Pain in Shoulder and Arm. The Hague, Martinus Nijhoff, 1979, pp 173–183

27. Gilliat RW: Nerve conduction in human and experimental neuropathies. Proc Roy Soc Med 59:989–993, 1966

28. Gilliatt RW, LeQuesne PM, Logue V, et al: Wasting of the hand associated with cervical rib or band. J Neurol Neurosurg Psychiatry 33:615–624, 1970

29. Gough JC, Koepke GH: Electromyographic determination of motor root levels in erector spinae muscles. Arch Phys Med Rehabil 47:9–11, 1966

30. Green J, Gildemeister R, Hazelwood C: Dermatomally stimulated somatosensory cerebral evoked potentials in the clinical diagnosis of lumbar disc disease. Clin Electromyogr 14:152–160, 1983

31. Gupta PR, Dorfman LJ: Spinal somatosensory conduction in diabetes. Neurology 31:841–845, 1981

32. Halliday AM, Carrol WM, Jones SJ: Visual and somatosensory evoked potential studies in Charcot-Marie-Tooth disease. Electroencephalogr Clin Neurophysiol 52:584, 1981

33. Hanson MR, Breuer AC, Furlan AJ, et al: Brachial plexus lesions following open-heart surgery: A prospective analysis and possible new mechanism of injury. Neurology 30:441, 1980

34. Jefferson D, Eames RM: Subclinical entrapment of the lateral femoral cutaneous nerve: An autopsy study. Muscle Nerve 2:145–154, 1979

35. Johnson EW, Melvin JL: Value of electromyography in lumbar radiculopathy. Arch Phys Med Rehabil 52:239–243, 1971

36. Jones SI, Wynn Parry CB, Landi A: Diagnosis of brachial plexus traction by sensory nerve action potentials and somatosensory evoked potentials. Injury 12:376–382, 1981

37. Jorg J, Dullberg W, Koeppen S: Diagnostic value of segmental somatosensory evoked potentials in cases with chronic progressive para- or tetraspastic syndromes. *In* Courjon J, Mauguiere F, Revol M (eds): Clinical Applications of Evoked Potentials in Neurology. New York, Raven Press, 1982, pp 347–358

38. Kimura J: F-wave velocity in the central segment of the median and ulnar nerves. A study in normal subjects and in patients with Charcot-Marie-Tooth disease. Neurology 24:539–546, 1974

39. Lueders H: Surgical monitoring of spinal cord function: Cauda equina stimulation technique. Neurosurgery 11:482–485, 1982

40. Mayer RF, Feldman RG: Observations on the nature of the F-wave in man. Neurology 17:147–156, 1967

41. McLeod JG: Electrophysiological studies in the Guillain-Barre syndrome. Ann Neurol 9(Suppl 1):20–27, 1981

42. Miglietta OE: The F response after transverse myelotomy. *In* Desmedt JE (ed): New Developments in Electromyography and Clinical Neurophysiology, Vol. 3. Basel, Switzerland, Karger, 1973, pp 323–327

43. Morin JE, Long R, Elleker MG, et al: Upper extremity neuropathies following median sternotomy. Ann Thorac Surg 34:181–185, 1982

44. Sarala PK, Nishihara T, Oh SJ: Meralgia paresthetica: Electrophysiologic study. Arch Phys Med Rehabil 60:30–31, 1979

45. Schramm J, Oettle GJ, Pichert T: Clinical application of segmental somatosensory evoked potentials (SEP)—Experience in patients with non-space occupying lesions. *In* Barber C (ed): Evoked Potentials. Lancaster, MTP Press, 1980, pp 455–464

46. Schuchmann JA: H reflex latency in radiculopathy. Arch Phys Med Rehabil 59:185–187, 1978

47. Siivola J, Salg I, Heiskari M: Somatosensory evoked potentials in diagnostics of cervical spondylosis and herniated disc. Electroencephalogr Clin Neurophysiol 52:276–282, 1981

48. Stevens A, Rosselle N: The sensory conduction velocity in the cutaneous femoris lateralis nerve. *In* Desmedt JE (ed): New Developments in Electromyography and Clinical Neurophysiology, Vol. 2. Basel, Switzerland, Karger, 1973, pp 64–66

49. Swift TR, Nichols FT: The droopy shoulder syndrome. Neurology 34:212–215, 1984

50. Synek VM: Somatosensory evoked potentials from musculocutaneous nerve in the diagnosis of brachial plexus injury. J Neurol Sci 61:443–452, 1983

51. Synek VM, Cowan JC: Somatosensory evoked potentials in patients with supraclavicular brachial plexus injuries. Neurology 32:1347–1352, 1982

52. Thomas JE, Howard FM Jr: Segmental zoster paresis—A disease profile. Neurology 22:459–466, 1974

53. Tonzola RF, Ackil AA, Shahani BT, et al: Usefulness of electrophysiological studies in the diagnosis of lumbosacral root disease. Ann Neurol 9:305–308, 1981

54. Wilbourn AJ: Thoracic outlet syndrome surgery causing severe brachial plexopathy. Muscle Nerve 11:66–74, 1988

55. Wilbourn AJ: True neurogenic thoracic outlet syndrome. AAEE Case Report No 7. Rochester, Minnesota, Custom Printing, 1982

56. Wulff CH, Gilliatt RW: F waves in patients with hand wasting caused by a cervical rib and band. Muscle Nerve 2:452–457, 1979

57. Yiannikas C, Shahani BT, Young RR: The investigation of traumatic lesions of the brachial plexus by electromyography and short latency somatosensory potentials evoked by stimulation of multiple nerves. J Neurol Neurosurg Psychiatry 46:1014–1022, 1983

58. Zverina E, Kredba J: Somatosensory cerebral evoked potentials in diagnosing brachial plexus injuries. Scand J Rehabil Med 9:47–54, 1977

Neuromuscular Diseases Unit
Vancouver General Hospital
855 West 12th Avenue
Vancouver, British Columbia
Canada V5Z 1M9

Use of Somatosensory Evoked Potentials in Infants and Children

Robin Gilmore, MD*

Somatosensory evoked potentials (SEPs) provide the means to noninvasively study the somatosensory system of the peripheral and central nervous systems. The physical examination of the young child, especially that of the sensory system, is frequently difficult. In infants and preverbal children, SEPs can provide information about the functioning of these systems currently not assessed by other means. Hence, SEPs may be a valuable diagnostic aid to the clinician. In this article, we review short-latency SEPs after median nerve (MN-SEP) and posterior tibial nerve (PTN-SEP) stimulation: techniques, limitations, and some clinical applications.

As in the adult, the MN-SEP[2, 6, 12, 14, 42] has been more thoroughly investigated in children than the PTN-SEP.[25, 28] Some early work in SEPs from the lower extremity in infants and children involved peroneal nerve.[10] Neural generators of MN-SEPs and PTN-SEPs in adults have been delineated and are reviewed in articles 4 and 5, respectively. Current evidence[1, 15, 19, 46] is summarized in Tables 1 (MN-SEP) and 2 (PTN-SEP).

METHODOLOGIES

Several methods have been suggested for recording MN-SEPs in infants[11, 37, 68] and children,[8, 32] and three are reviewed in Table 3. Filter bandpass is generally 30 to 3000 Hz. Polarity conventions are indicated in the table.

Cracco has modified her method for recording Erb's point potential (EP pot), component of MN-SEPs in infants to record 1 cm above the axilla rather than at EP. In infants, and especially in newborns, this allows more reliable recording of the EP pot.[11] Methods for PTN-SEPs have been less frequently reported in children (than MN-SEP), but are similar to those

---

*Director, Clinical Neurophysiology Program, and Associate Professor, Department of Neurology, University of Kentucky Medical Center, Lexington, Kentucky

Dr. Gilmore is a recipient of CIDA 1 K08 NS1005

Table 1. *Presumed Generators of MN-SEPs*

COMPONENT	ORIGIN
P9 (EP pot)	Brachial plexus
P11	Cervical cord dorsal columns
P13–P14	Brain-stem lemniscal pathways
N20	Subcortical region and sensory cortex
P23	Sensory cortex

Table 2. *Presumed Generators of PTN-SEPs*

COMPONENT	ORIGIN
N8	Tibial nerve action potential
N19(PV)*	Cauda equina
N22	Lumbar cord gray matter
N29(N27)	Gracile nucleus
P38(P37)	Mesial sensory cortex

*PV = propagated volley.

Table 3. *Summary of Three Methods of MN-SEP Recording in Infants and Children*

CHANNELS	RECORDING SITE	COMPONENTS RECORDED
Cracco Method [11]		
1	C'c–NC (may be EPc or Shc)	P9, P11, P13–14, N20, P23
2	C'c–Ac	P13–14, N20, P23
3	spC2–Cz or spC5–Fz	N9, N11, N13, N14
4	EPi–EPc or Shc	EP pot
Negativity in grid 1 plotted as "up"		
Goldie Method [37]		
1	EPc–C'c	P9, P11, P13–14, N20, P23
2	Fpz–C'c	N20
3	Fpz–spC7	B complex, 2nd negative peak
4	Fpz–EPi	EP pot
Negativity in grid 1 plotted as "down"		
Willis Method [68]		
1	C'c–Fz	N1, P1, N2
2	spC2–Fz	CII
3	EPi–Fz	EP
Negativity in grid 1 plotted as "up"		

Abbreviations: C'c is either C3'c or C4'c, and is contralateral (c) to side of stimulation. C3' or C4' is 2 cm behind the standard placement of C3 or C4 of the International 10–20 system. EP is Erb's point. EPi is ipsilateral to stimulation. EPc is contralateral to stimulation. EP pot. is EP potential. Ai and Ac are ears ipsilateral and contralateral to stimulation. Notations of spC2, spC5, and spC7 refer to cervical spine at the C2, C5, and C7 levels, respectively. NC is noncephalic reference. It may be the dorsum of the contralateral hand, EPc, or contralateral shoulder, Shc.

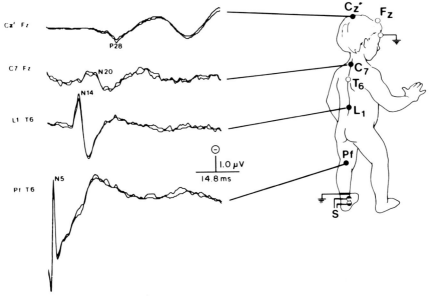

Figure 1. SEP after tibial nerve stimulation at the ankle recorded at various sites simultaneously. Label was based on surface polarity and mean peak latency observed in 32 normal young subjects (age = 1 to 8 years, height = 82 to 130 cm). Electrodes were placed at the popliteal fossa (Pf), first lumbar (spL₁) and sixth thoracic (spT₆) and seventh cervical (C7) spinous processes (sp) of vertebrae, Cz' (2 cm behind Cz) and Fz (10–20 electrode system). Fz was the reference for Cz' and spC₇ and spT₆ was the reference for spL₁ and Pf. Current pulses of 200 sec duration were delivered at 5/sec. Two independent averages of 1000 to 2000 responses were superimposed to show intertrial replicability. Original data were directly photographed to make illustration. (*From* Gilmore R, Bass NH, Wright EA, et al: Development assessment of spinal cord and cortical evoked potentials after tibial nerve stimulation: Effects of age and stature on normative data during childhood. Electroencephalogr Clin Neurophysiol 62:241–251, 1985; with permission.)

for adults[28] (Fig. 1). One may use height-, and as necessary, age-corrected normative data for the latencies of peaks, or one may calculate conduction ("propagation") velocities over the peripheral nerves and central fibers.[10] American EEG Society Guidelines recommend the use of velocity calculations.[3] However, there are legitimate objections to this method because there is a potential for error in the measurement of distance as a requisite for the calculation.[45, 62, 71] We have preferred using height-based normative data.[28, 29]

EFFECTS OF MATURATION

Postnatal development of the somatosensory system is exceedingly complex because of coincident nonparallel changes in parameters of maturation like (1) the length of the pathway; (2) varying rates of myelination of portions of the pathway; and (3) increasing numbers of synapses in the pathway. These developmental sequences are relatively simple compared with the maturation of brain, which includes the process of synaptogenesis as well as lengthening and myelination of complex polysynaptic pathways of the thalamocortical system.

Peripheral Nerve Maturation

In the developing human infant, the diameter of the peripheral nerve increases[53] in close association with increasing myelination. There is close correlation between fiber size and functional properties in developing peripheral nerve.[40] The length of the nerve increases as well, probably parallel to increasing leg length.[51] In newborns, the conduction velocity of posterior tibial nerve has been shown to directly increase linearly with postconceptional age (PCA) from approximately 20 m/sec at 33 weeks PCA to 33 m/sec at 44 weeks PCA.[18, 61] The conduction velocity of peripheral nerve has been shown to increase with age,[66] reaching maximal values at 18 to 27 postnatal months for sural nerve.[5]

Spinal Cord Maturation

During fetal and early postnatal growth and development, the spinal cord elongates and myelinates rapidly, but complete maturation occurs later than that of peripheral nerve. Elongation is such that at 26 weeks PCA, the most caudal portion of the spinal canal terminates at the fourth lumbar vertebra. At the 38th to 40th week, the terminal spinal cord is midway between the second and third lumbar vertebra.[4]

Myelinogenesis of the spinal cord has its onset during early prenatal life (Fig. 2). Sensory roots undergo myelination at 24 weeks gestational age (GA) and are fully myelinated by 6 months postterm.[69] The fasciculus cuneatus and fasciculus gracilis first appear at 8 weeks GA.[43] Myelin first appears in the fasciculus cuneatus at 14 weeks GA and in the fasciculus gracilis at 22 to 24 weeks GA in the human being. In contrast, in the developing cat the fasciculus gracilis has an increasing fiber diameter that approaches that of the adult cat by 3 postnatal months. This is associated with a parallel increase in central conduction velocity.[40] Presumably, in humans the increase in spinal cord conduction velocity exceeds spinal cord elongation in early infancy.[29]

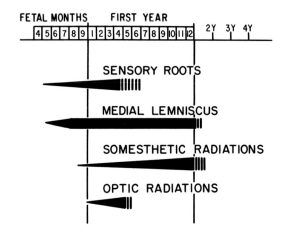

Figure 2. Myelogenetic cycles of selected somatosensory pathways. Optic radiations data provided for comparison. Point at left indicates when myelin starts to appear and point at right indicates when myelination is believed complete. (*Adapted from* Yakovlev P, Lecours A: The myelogenetic cycles of regional maturation of the brain. *In* Minkowski A (ed): Regional Development of the Brain in Early Life. Philadelphia, FA Davis, 1967, pp 3–69.)

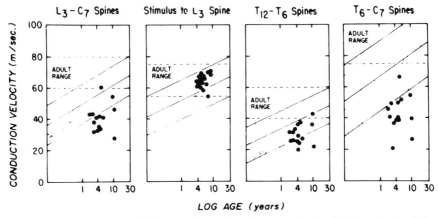

Figure 3. Distribution of the overall spinal conduction velocities (L_3-C_7 spines) and the segmental conduction velocities over peroneal nerve and cauda equina (stimulus to L_3 spine), caudal spinal cord (T_{12}-T_6 spines) and rostral spinal cord (T_6-C_7 spines) in the patients with degenerative disease. The shaded area represents the regression line with 95 per cent confidence limits for these conduction velocities in 95 normal subjects. The range of conduction velocities in normal adults is indicated by the dotted lines. (*From* Cracco JB, Bosch VV, Cracco RQ: Cerebral and spinal somatosensory evoked potentials in children with CNS degenerative disease. Electroencephalogr Clin Neurophysiol 49:437–445, 1980; with permission.)

Cracco and co-workers partitioned the spinal cord into several segments and calculated conduction velocities over these segments using surface distance measurements. They found that conduction velocity along the spinal cord progressively increased with age[10] (Fig. 3). It is likely that in children the increase in conduction velocity parallels the increase in spinal cord length.[28]

Brain Stem and Cerebrum Maturation

The most complex part of the lemniscal system is the intracranial portion: the brain stem, the thalamus, the somesthetic radiations, and the cerebral cortex. In the first 2 years of human postnatal life there is a fivefold increase in the amount of myelin.[17] The medial lemniscus starts to myelinate at approximately 23 to 25 weeks PCA, proceeds in a caudal-rostral order, and probably concludes myelination approximately 12 months post-term.[69] The functional development of transmission capacities and neuronal responsiveness requires, at the level of the nucleus cuneatus, a period of 2 to 3 months postnatally within the central pathways of the kitten[21] approximately equivalent to 24 human months post-term. At higher levels than the nucleus cuneatus, in the kitten, the acquisition of mature signaling capacities probably occurs even later.[57] Similar developmental data are not readily available for the nucleus gracilis.

Because of the complex maturational changes in infancy affecting pathways and generators of SEPs, not all components are recorded at term. The time when various components can be reliably recorded is important. It is possible that a component is absent not because of a pathologic process, but because from a maturational standpoint, the necessary central nervous system (CNS) substrate is not yet developed to the point of transmitting or generating the potential.

In humans there is almost certainly a period of time (probably months) during which the appearance of the scalp-recorded component of the MN-SEP will develop. Cracco and colleagues reported that the N20 was consistently recorded after 6 weeks[11]; Willis and co-workers has reported it after 8 weeks[68]; and Goldie and Spydell, after 12 weeks.[37] These times are postterm. The period of time during which the scalp-recorded component of the PTN-SEP develops is unknown, but is probably later than that for MN-SEP. Approximately 50 per cent will have the scalp-recorded component close to term[29] (see below for further details).

Because the thalamus is a critical element in cerebral transmission of peripheral signals, one might anticipate that the development of cortical EPs would be closely related to thalamic maturation and myelination. In preterm newborns, approximately 32 weeks PCA, the thalamus has no myelin; in newborns approximately 34 weeks PCA, myelin in the thalamus is seen in fewer than 20 per cent; by 36 weeks PCA, some thalamic myelin is seen in approximately 70 per cent of brains. By term, 87 per cent of brains contain myelin in the thalamus.[55] However, there is considerable interinfant or interfetus variability in the sequencing of myelination, not only in the thalamus but in other myelinative sites.[21] The somesthetic radiations start to myelinate at approximately 40 weeks PCA and are thought to be completely myelinated by approximately 12 to 18 months post-term.[69] The wide ranges of time over which the thalamus and subcortical radiations are myelinated may well be reflected in time variability of the appearance of scalp-recorded potentials in preterm newborns.[29] Gilmore and co-workers have reported that although the P37 was not seen in infants whose PCA was more than 31 weeks, it was not invariably present in infants > 31 weeks.

Variability in the presence or absence and the distribution and latency of cortical PTN-SEP components has been found in older infants as well.[25] Georgesco and associates reported PTN-SEPs in 26 presumably full-term infants aged 1 day to 3 months. In six infants, no scalp-recorded SEP was observed. In the other 20 infants, an electropositive scalp-recorded SEP was seen approximately 36 msec (probably P37) after stimulation. No factor, whether it be the baby's size, physiologic state of arousal, or intensity of stimulation, correlated with distribution or latency of the component. Even age failed to correlate. In fact, the oldest infant, approximately 3 months post-term, did not have a P37.[25] The appearance or absence of cortical EP as well as the wide range of cortical EP latency may parallel electrophysiologically the wide time range over which myelin appears at specific sites within the immature spinal cord and brain compared with the mature, fully myelinated somatosensory pathway of the adult.

Age and Height Effects on Latencies

The latencies of the various components, of course, change with age. One reason is because of functional changes in maturation of the nervous system as reviewed above. Another is because of changes in the length of the pathways over which SEPs are transmitted. This latter point is of more importance with PTN-SEPs, but it should be noted with MN-SEPs as well. In general, the latency of the N20 component decreases from early infancy (Fig. 4) to 2 to 3 years and then starts to increase.[10] The increase in latency is correlated with body length and arm length.[39] The latencies of the EP pot. and N13 are similar in newborns and older infants,[11] probably remaining stable until 2 to 3 years, at which age their latencies start to prolong, reaching adult values by approximately ages 14 to 18 years.[10] This is

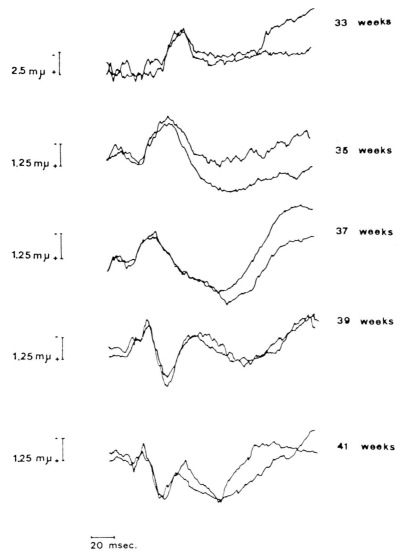

Figure 4. Examples of cortical components of MN-SEPs at different postconceptional ages. (*From* Gallai V: Maturation of the CNS and Evoked Potentials. Amsterdam, Elsevier, 1986; with permission.)

probably true for the central conduction time (CCT) also. Goldie and Spydell used the CCT for MN-SEP calculated as latency of N20 minus latency of the B-wave (CCT = N20 − B). After log transformation of CCT, they found a high inverse correlation ($r = -.85$) between age and CCT; that is, as the infant grew, CCT decreased.[37]

The latencies of the N8, N22, and N27 (referred to as N5, N14, and N20 in Figs. 5, 6, and 7, respectively) components of the PTN-SEP increase with increasing age or increasing height in children 1 to 8 years old.[28] The latency of the scalp-recorded potential P37 (P28 in children) is much more variable in children than adults and correlates only modestly with height (Fig. 8).

The latencies of the N22 (N16 in Fig. 9) and N27 (Fig. 10) of the PTN-SEP components in preterm infants decrease with increasing PCA.[29] These latencies decrease probably because conduction velocities (or propagation velocities) are increasing less rapidly than length of the conducting pathway.[29] Because the latency of N8 is constant in preterm newborns, it does not vary with PCA. The latency of N8 is approximately leg length divided by conduction velocity. Because that leg length is increasing,[51] and conduction velocity is increasing,[66] both must be increasing at parallel rates. The latency of the P37 (P55 in Fig. 11) is widely variable.

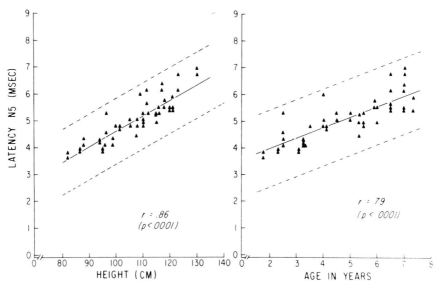

Figure 5. *Left:* Relationship between stature and absolute latency of N5 (N8 in adult) in children with height ranging 82 to 130 cm: $\hat{x} = -1.021 + 0.056$ (height). *Right:* Relationship between age and absolute latency of N5 in children aged 1 to 8 years: $\hat{x} = 3.23 + 0.38$ (age). In this and Figures 6 through 8, solid line is line of regression; dotted lines ± 3 S.D. (*From* Gilmore R, Bass NH, Wright EA, et al: Development assessment of spinal cord and cortical evoked potentials after tibial nerve stimulation: Effects of age and stature on normative data during childhood. Electroencephalogr Clin Neurophysiol 62:241–251, 1985; with permission.)

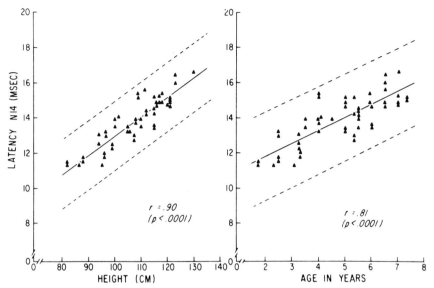

Figure 6. *Left:* Relationship between stature and absolute latency of N14 (N22 in adult) in children with height ranging 82 to 130 cm: $\hat{x} = 1.84 + 0.11$ (height). *Right:* Relationship between age and absolute latency of N14 in children aged 1 to 8 years: $\hat{x} = 10.26 + 0.74$ (age). (*From* Gilmore R, Bass NH, Wright EA, et al: Development assessment of spinal cord and cortical evoked potentials after tibial nerve stimulation: Effects of age and stature on normative data during childhood. Electroencephalogr Clin Neurophysiol 62:241–251, 1985; with permission.)

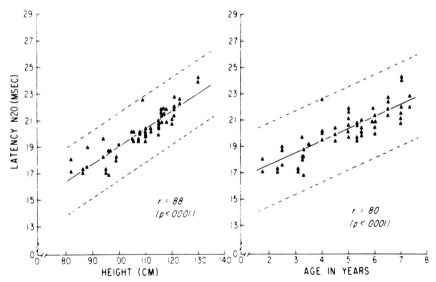

Figure 7. *Left:* Relationship between stature and absolute latency of N20 (N27 in adult) in children with height ranging 82 to 130 cm: $\hat{x} = 4.60 + 0.14$ (height). *Right:* Relationship between age and absolute latency of N20 in children aged 1 to 8 years: $\hat{x} = 15.51 + 0.95$ (age). (*From* Gilmore R, Bass NH, Wright EA, et al: Development assessment of spinal cord and cortical evoked potentials after tibial nerve stimulation: Effects of age and stature on normative data during childhood. Electroencephalogr Clin Neurophysiol 62:241–251, 1985; with permission.)

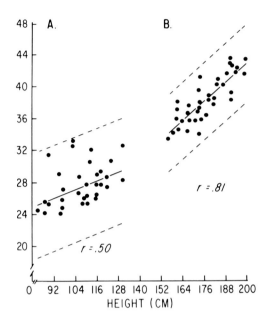

Figure 8. Effect on height on the cortical evoked potential (P28 in children and P37 in adults). A, during growth and development (1 to 8 years old). B, during adulthood (18 to 40 years old). (*From* Gilmore R, Bass NH, Wright EA, et al: Development assessment of spinal cord and cortical evoked potentials after tibial nerve stimulation: Effects of age and stature on normative data during childhood. Electroencephalogr Clin Neurophysiol 62:241–251, 1985; with permission.)

Figure 9. Relationship between PCA and absolute latency of N16 (N22 in adult) in preterm newborns with PCA ranging from 26 to 38.2 weeks. *Inset:* Relationship between age and absolute latency of N14 (N22 in adult terminology) in children aged 1 to 8 years. (*From* Gilmore RL, Brock J, Hermansen MC, et al: Development of lumbar spinal cord and cortical evoked potentials after tibial nerve stimulation: Effects of gestational age and other factors. Electroencephalogr Clin Neurophysiol 68:28–39, 1987; with permission.)

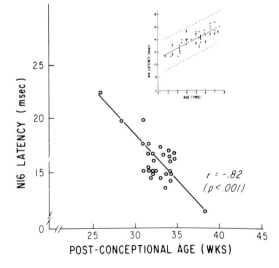

Figure 10. Relationship between PCA and absolute latency of N27 in preterm newborns with PCA ranging from 26 to 38 weeks. *Inset:* Relationship between age and absolute latency of N20 (N27 in adult terminology) in children aged 1 to 8 years. (*From* Cracco JB, Bosch VV, Cracco RQ: Cerebral and spinal somatosensory evoked potentials in children with CNS degenerative disease. Electroencephalogr Clin Neurophysiol 49:437–445, 1980; with permission.)

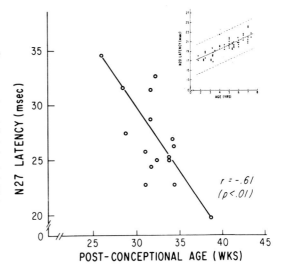

Figure 11. SEP after bilateral simultaneous tibial nerve stimulation at the ankles recorded at various sites simultaneously from a 35-week-old (PCA). Label was based on surface polarity and mean peak latency observed in 29 preterm newborns (GA, 26 to 38 weeks; length, 22.5 to 44 cm). Electrodes were placed at the popliteal fossa (PF), first lumbar (spL1), sixth thoracic (spT6), and seventh cervical (C7) spinous processes (sp) of vertebrae. Cz' (1 cm behind Cz) and Fpz (10–20 electrode system). Cz' and spC7 were referred to Fpz. The reference for spL1 and PF was spT6. Constant current pulses of 130 to 150 sec duration were delivered at 5/sec. Two independent averages of 1000 to 2000 responses were superimposed to show intertrial replicability. Original data were directly photographed to make illustration. (*From* Gilmore RL, Brock J, Hermansen MC, et al: Development of lumbar spinal cord and cortical evoked potentials after tibial nerve stimulation in the pre-term newborns: Effects of gestational age and other factors. Electroencephalogr Clin Neurophysiol 68:28–39, 1987; with permission.)

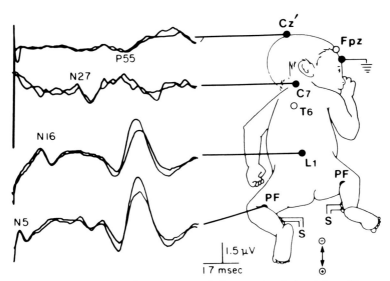

EFFECTS OF SLEEP

The effect of sleep on the short-latency MN-SEPs is poorly understood in infants and children. Desmedt and Manil reported the effects of quiet or slow-wave sleep and REM sleep on the longer-latency MN-SEPs in infants[16] (Fig. 12). Wakefulness and REM sleep appeared to have similar effects. The effects of sedating drugs are even less well understood. The only systematic report of sedative effects in children has been by Hashimoto and colleagues.[39] They examined MN-SEPs in 83 children and 7 adults. Patients less than 5 years of age received tricloryl syrup (50 to 100 mg/kg) to induce sleep. EEG monitoring was done simultaneously with SEP recording. Components comparable to N20 remained stable during sleep, whereas P22 demonstrated an increase in peak latency during deep sleep but not during REM sleep. The effect of sleep on the P37 of the PTN-SEP is even more marked and complicated in infants[29] and children.[27] In some preterm infants natural sleep will actually enhance the appearance of the P37 (Fig. 13). We have preferred not to sedate infants under 3 months old.[30] We sedate older infants as necessary, recognizing that this will

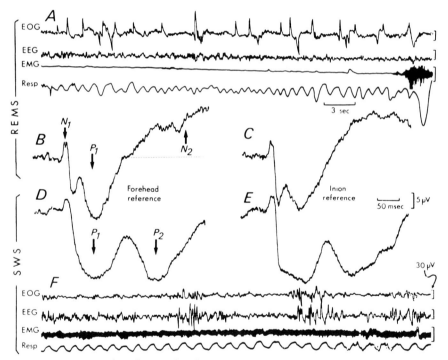

Figure 12. Female infant aged 3 days. Polygraph and evoked potential data recorded either in an REM stage (A,B,C) or in a SWS state (D,E,F) during the same session. A and F from above downwards; the electro-oculogram (EOG), the bipolar EEG between frontal and parietal leads, the EMG of the submentalis muscle and the respirogram. B and D, Evoked potentials recorded from the contralateral parietal focus against a forehead reference. C and E, Evoked potentials recorded between the same active electrode and an inion reference. (*From* Desmedt JE, Manil J: Somatosensory evoked potentials of the normal human neonate in REM sleep, in slow wave sleep and in waking. Electroencephalogr Clin Neurophysiol 29:113–126, 1970; with permission.)

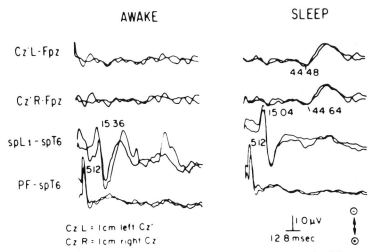

Figure 13. Short-latency PTN-SEP in the awake (*left*) and sleep (*right*) states in the infant. Note the appearance of the scalp recorded component during sleep. (*From* Gilmore RL, Brock J, Hermansen MC, et al: Development of lumbar spinal cord and cortical evoked potentials after tibial nerve stimulation in the pre-term newborns: Effects of gestational age and other factors. Electroencephalogr Clin Neurophysiol 68:28–39, 1987; with permission.)

attenuate the N20 of the MN-SEP and the P37 of the PTN-SEP. Sedation may also change the latencies of potentials, especially of the P37. We have used oral chloral hydrate (50 mg/kg), recognizing, as have others, that barbituates have an even more marked effect on cortical potentials than chloral hydrate.[58] If the study is abnormal, we will repeat it in the waking state. This can be a problem in a busy lab but must be done to avoid the possibility of false-positive results.

CLINICAL APPLICATIONS

Coma and Progressive Encephalopathies

SEPs may be useful in several clinical situations. The prognostic value of MN-SEPs has been examined in comatose infants and children.[22, 48, 67] It appears that SEPs, especially when combined with brain-stem auditory evoked potentials (BAEPs), provide useful information concerning prognosis. In one group of comatose children with hypoxic insults, BAEP and MN-SEP were better predictors of chronic vegetative state than the EEG and clinical assessment.[67] In cases of children with brain-stem pathology, the combined recordings of BAEP and MN-SEP together have provided more information than either test alone.[31, 35] De Meirleir and Taylor reported SEPs in comatose children with a variety of etiologies. Patients with bilaterally absent cortical SEPs either died or developed severe spastic quadriplegia.[13] Unilaterally abnormal cortical SEPs predicted a residual hemiparesis. Patients with normal outcomes had normal or only mildly abnormal SEPs that normalized within a few days.

An investigation of SEP in children with Reye's syndrome has indicated that serial studies were more helpful in prognostication than the EEG.[34] In this group, the cortical components were abnormal in the initial recordings. Patient survival correlated with early progressive recovery of short latency (N20–P30) components. Clinical recovery without neurologic sequelae was associated with recovery of later (more than 100 msec) components.

Neurologic dysfunction is described frequently in pediatric AIDS. Udani and colleagues investigated the clinical and developmental assessment, BAEPs, SEPs, and magnetic resonance images (MRI) in 18 HIV-positive children with AIDS or AIDS-related complex.[65] Thirty-three per cent had microcephaly; 56 per cent had motor impairment; 18 per cent had abnormal BAEP CCT; and 25 per cent had peripheral BAEP abnormalities. Seventy-nine per cent had abnormal MN-SEPs. Fewer than 20 per cent of the MRIs were specifically abnormal, although all had varying degrees of cerebral atrophy. These authors concluded that SEP abnormalities are common, are seen early in the course of the disease, and may be useful in follow-up.

Assessment of High-Risk Newborns

The assessment and prognosis of high-risk newborns (HRNs) can be quite difficult.[59] Assessment via evoked potentials is attractive because it is noninvasive, can be done at the bedside, and can give quantitative information that can be acquired longitudinally. An increasing number of studies evaluate the SEP in this setting. Hrbek and colleagues reported abnormal cortical components in 65 per cent of asphyxiated newborns.[41] All patients with persistent abnormalities had clinical evidence of brain injury. Laget and associates studied infants and children from 14 days to 13 years with motor deficits.[44] They reported that the SEP was more accurate than the EEG in localizing/lateralizing the lesion. Lutschg and co-workers combined SEPs and BAEPs to study 10 asphyxiated babies at 3 months of age, all with abnormal tone and severe leukomalacia on CT. Although BAEPs were normal or only slightly abnormal, there were no cortical components recorded at 3 months.[47] Gorke evaluated the prognostic value of the SEP in infants with cerebral palsy and neurodegenerative and CNS metabolic diseases.[38] Many infants had prolonged or absent cortical potentials, all of whom demonstrated handicaps after the first year of life. He concluded that the SEP was a valuable early indicator of severe motor impairment. He pointed out, though, a rather high false-negative rate and related this to the exclusive testing of the afferent pathway. Majnemer and associates assessed healthy and HRNs.[49] They found that approximately one third of newborns at risk for neurologic and/or developmental sequelae had abnormal SEPs consisting of prolongation of absolute cortical latency or CCT, or absence of potential. Patients were retested at 2 to 3 months of age and demonstrated the following: prolonged latencies at birth; later normal latencies—mild neurologic deficits; absent potentials initially and absent 3 months later—spastic quadriparesis.

Neurodegenerative Disorders

Several investigators have reported abnormalities in SEPs in a variety of neurodegenerative disorders[7, 10, 24, 36, 50, 56, 63, 64] (see Figs. 3 and 14). Severe

1024 Averaged Responses

Normal Infant

CNS Degenerative Disease with Myoclonus

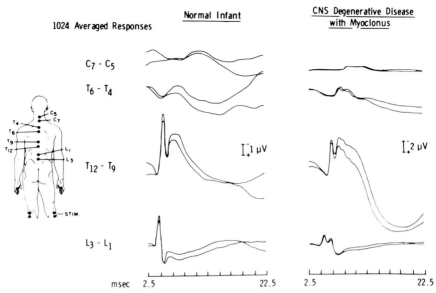

Figure 14. Comparison of spinal evoked potentials in a normal infant and a child with degenerative disease and myoclonus who had enhancement of longer-latency scalp-recorded SEPs. The positive potential that follows the large complex negative potential recorded over the caudal spinal cord (T_{12}-T_9 spines) is much larger in the patient. (Note the calibration difference.) (*From* Cracco JB, Bosch VV, Cracco RQ: Cerebral and spinal somatosensory evoked potentials in children with CNS degenerative disease. Electroencephalogr Clin Neurophysiol 49:437–445, 1980; with permission.)

abnormalities have been described in children with polioencephalopathies (affecting primarily gray matter) and leukodystrophies. In most of these disorders, the peripheral components are normal except for metachromatic leukodystrophy (MLD). More rostral components have been delayed or absent.[7, 50] Tobimatsu and co-workers have demonstrated that MN-SEP are valuable in differentiating adrenomyeloneuropathy (AMN) from adrenoleukodystrophy (ALD).[64] In both conditions CCT is prolonged, but in AMN the EP pot. is prolonged also. Garg and colleagues suggested that the SEP may be more sensitive than the BAEP in demonstrating abnormalities associated with the ALD gene.[24]

Rossini and associates have examined SEPs in patients with other neurodegenerative disorders[56]: Friedreich's ataxia (FA), hereditary motor sensory neuropathy (HMSN), familial spastic paraplegia (FSP), olivopontocerebellar atrophy (OPCA), and ataxia telangiectasia (AT). The MN-SEPs of patients with FA, OPCA, HMSN-II, and AT had impaired central conduction and normal or slightly prolonged peripheral potential latencies. In patients with FA and HMSN-II peripheral nerve potentials were of low amplitude. Lower-extremity SEPs in FA patients also indicate nearly normal peripheral potential latencies with impairment of transmission within spinal cord afferent pathways. This has been verified by others.[63] Patients with OPCA usually had normal MN-SEPs, but all SEPs from the lower extremities were abnormal. The patients with HMSN-II and AT usually had normal MN-SEPs with increased CCT of SEP after lower-extremity testing.

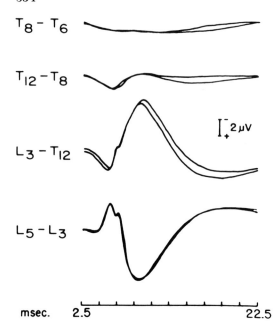

$T_8 - T_6$

$T_{12} - T_8$

$L_3 - T_{12}$

$L_5 - L_3$

$\left[\begin{smallmatrix} - \\ + \end{smallmatrix}\right. 2\mu V$

msec.   2.5   22.5

Figure 15. Spinal responses in a 3-year-old child with thoracolumbar myelomeningecele. The large complex response that is recorded over T_{12}-T_9 spines in normal children is present over L_3 spine in this child, suggesting caudal displacement of the spinal cord. (*From* Cracco JB, Cracco RQ: Spinal somatosensory evoked potentials: Maturational and clinical studies. Ann NY Acad Sci 388:526–537, 1982; with permission.)

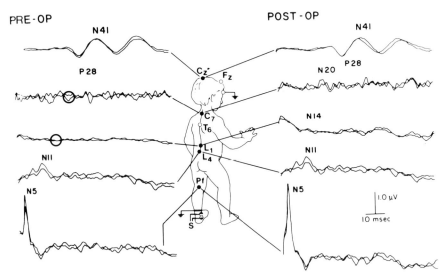

PRE-OP   POST-OP

N41   N41

P28   N20   P28

Cz* Fz

C7

T6

N14

L1
L4

NII   NII

N5   N5

1.0 μV

10 msec

Figure 16. Preoperative and postoperative PTN-SEP in a child who at surgery was found to have extensive tethering and rotation of the sacral spinal cord. Both N14 and N20 (lumbar and cervical spinal cord evoked potentials, respectively) were absent prior to operation (*circles*) and appeared postoperatively. (*From* Roy MW, Gilmore R, Walsh JW: Somatosensory evoked potentials in tethered cord syndrome. Encephalogr Clin Neurophysiol 64:42P, 1986; with permission.)

Patients with HMSN-I had prolonged latency of EP pot. and absence of more rostral potentials. In this study, patients with FSP had normal SEPs.

Metabolic disorders such as aminoacidopathies, neuronal storage diseases, or organic acidemias demonstrate mild prolongations of CCT. The most profound CCT delays have been seen in Leigh's disease and Krabbe's disease.[37]

Structural and Compressive Lesions

Structural and compressive lesions may also give rise to abnormal SEPs, depending on their site. Compressive cervical spine lesions such as foramen magnum stenosis are frequently associated with abnormal SEPs. The degree of abnormality correlates well with motor delay, hypotonia, and the propensity toward apnea.[37] Intrinsic cervical spine lesions, such as those seen in spinal cord gliomas and Arnold Chiari malformations, are associated with SEP abnormalities that correlate with the severity of clinical involvement.

Structural brain-stem lesions are frequently associated with abnormalities in both MN-SEPs[36] and PTN-SEPs.[54] They are probably most useful when used in conjunction with BAEPs. Infants with Moebius syndrome may have abnormal MN-SEPs.[37]

Structural noncervical spinal cord lesions are, of course, frequently associated with abnormalities in PTN-SEPs.[54] Cracco and colleagues were among the first to demonstrate the utility of recording the spinal components of SEPs in the evaluation of patients with myelodysplasia and occult spinal dysraphism.[9] The large spinal potential normally recorded over lower thoracic spine is caudally displaced and recorded over the lumbar spine in these children (Fig. 15). Others have recorded PTN-SEPs in patients with tethered spinal cord syndrome (TSCS)[58] (Fig. 16). To determine the diagnostic usefulness of the PTN-SEP in TSCS, Roy and co-workers studied 22 consecutive patients with symptoms of tethered spinal cord (aged 18 months to 22 years) who underwent recording of PTN-SEP. Results were correlated with clinical, myelographic, and operative findings. In patients with clinical symptoms but no myelographically demonstrable lesions, PTN-SEPs were within normal limits, suggesting normal physiologic function. In patients with myelographically and operatively confirmed tethering dysraphic lesions, PTN-SEPs were predictive of the level of laterality of the lesion. Similarly, ranking the severity of neurologic impairment and extent of dysraphism at operation, as well as the extent of abnormality of PTN-SEPs, revealed a significant ($r = 0.81$, $P < 0.001$) correlation.[58] It has been suggested that TSCS produces signs of neurologic impairment by producing subacute hypoxia superimposed on chronic hypoxia of the lumbosacral spinal cord.[70] The effect of hypoxia manifests itself by altered spinal and cortical SEPs (Fig. 17). If the traction is relieved the PTN-SEP may change (see Fig. 16).

Peripheral Lesions

Peripheral nerve plexus and root lesions can also be assessed with SEPs. Several have reported the findings in patients with Erb's palsy.[8, 20, 37] If there is a root avulsion, the dorsal root ganglion is intact, an EP pot. is

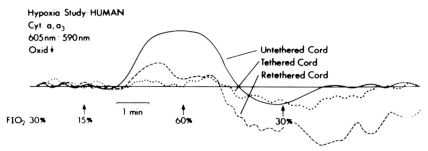

Figure 17. Redox changes during hypoxia in one group of the human tethered cords (type 1). No redox change is seen before untethering (*dotted line*), but reduction similar to that in normal cat cords is noted after untethering (*solid line*). No reduction occurs while the cord is temporarily retethered (*interrupted line*). FIO2 = fraction of oxygen in the respired gas mixture. (*From* Yamada S, Zinke DE, Sanders D, et al: Pathophysiology of "tethered cord syndrome." J Neurosurg 54:494–503, 1981; with permission.)

recorded, and more rostral components are abnormal.[8] If there is a plexus lesion, the EP pot. and more rostral components are absent.

Spine-to-scalp "propagation velocities" may be useful for evaluation of proximal peripheral nerve. Schiff and associates reported slowed propagation velocities in Guillain-Barré syndrome.[60] Combinations of prolongation or absence of peripheral potentials, and more rostral potentials of MN-SEP and PTN-SEPs, have been reported by others.[33, 52]

SUMMARY

SEPs are a useful, reliable means of assessing somatosensory systems and gaining indirect information about motor systems in children. The factors of complex maturational changes in the CNS and body growth complicate the interpretation of SEPs. Thus, full understanding of factors that affect normative data in infants and children enhance clinical interpretation. SEPs in infancy and childhood in many clinical conditions have been useful in diagnosis and prognosis. The full extent of the clinical applications of SEPs is yet to be explored.

REFERENCES

1. Allison T: Scalp and cortical recordings of initial somatosensory cortex activity to median nerve stimulation in man. Ann NY Acad Sci 388:671–678, 1982
2. Allison T, Hume AL, Wood CC, et al: Developmental and aging changes in somatosensory, auditory, and visual evoked potentials. Electroencephalogr Clin Neurophysiol 58:14–24, 1984
3. American Electroencephalogram Society: Guideline for clinical evoked potential in studies. J Clin Neurophysiol 1:3–35, 1984
4. Barson AJ: The vertebral level of termination of the spinal cord during normal and abnormal development. J Anat (London) 106:489–497, 1970

5. Buchthal F, Rosenfalck A, Behse F: Sensory potentials of normal and diseased nerves. *In* Dyck PJ, Thomas PK, Lambert EH (eds): Peripheral Neuropathy. Philadelphia, WB Saunders, 1975, pp 442–464

6. Chiappa KH, Choi SK, Young RP: Short-latency somatosensory evoked potentials following median nerve stimulation in patients with neurological lesions. *In* JE Desmedt (ed): Clinical Uses of Cerebral, Brainstem, and Spinal Somatosensory Evoked Potentials, vol 7. Basel, Karger, 1980

7. Cracco JB, Bosch VV, Cracco RQ: Cerebral and spinal somatosensory evoked potentials in children with CNS degenerative disease. Electroencephalogr Clin Neurophysiol 49:437–445, 1980

8. Cracco JB, Cracco RQ: Spinal, brainstem, and cerebral SEP in the pediatric age group. *In* Cracco RQ, Bodis-Wollner I (eds): Evoked Potentials. New York, Alan R. Liss, 1986, pp 471–482

9. Cracco JB, Cracco RQ: Spinal somatosensory evoked potentials: Maturational and clinical studies. Ann NY Acad Sci 388:526–537, 1982

10. Cracco JB, Cracco RQ, Stolove R: Spinal evoked potentials in man: A maturational study. Electroencephalogr Clin Neurophysiol 46:58–64, 1979

11. Cracco J, Udani V, Cracco R: MN-SSEPs in Infants. American EEG Society Scientific Session. St. Louis, September 17, 1987

12. Cullity P, Franks CI, Duckworth T, et al: Somatosensory evoked cortical responses in normal infants. Dev Med Child Neurol 18:11–18, 1976

13. De Meirleir LJ, Taylor MJ: The prognostic utility of SEPs in comatose children. Pediatr Neurol 3:78–82, 1987

14. Desmedt JE, Brunko E, Debecker J: Maturation of the somatosensory evoked potentials in normal infants and children with special reference to the early N1 component. Electroencephalogr Clin Neurophysiol 40:43–58, 1976

15. Desmedt JE, Cheron G: Somatosensory evoked potentials in man: Subcortical and cortical components and their neural basis. Ann NY Acad Sci 388:388–411, 1982

16. Desmedt JE, Manil J: Somatosensory evoked potentials of the normal human neonate in REM sleep, in slow wave sleep and in waking. Electroencephalogr Clin Neurophysiol 29:113–126, 1970

17. Dobbing J, Smart JL: Vulnerability of developing brain and behavior. Br Med Bull 30:164–168, 1974

18. Dubowitz V, Whittaker GF, Brown BH, et al: Nerve conduction velocity. An index of neurological maturity of the newborn infant. Dev Med Child Neurol 10:741–749, 1968

19. Emerson RG, Seval M, Pedley TA: Somatosensory evoked potentials following median nerve stimulation. I. The cervical components. Brain 107:169–182, 1984

20. Fagan ER, Taylor MJ, Logan WJ: Somatosensory evoked potentials: Part II. A review of the clinical applications in pediatric neurology. Pediatr Neurol 3:249–255, 1987

21. Ferrington DG, Rowe MJ: Functional capacities of tactile afferent fibers in neonatal kittens. J Physiol (London) 307:335–353, 1980

22. Frank LM, Furgiuele TL, Etheridge JE: Prediction of chronic vegetative state in children using evoked potentials. Neurology 35:931–934, 1985

23. Gallai V: Maturation of SEPs in pre-term and full-term neonates. *In* Gallai V (ed): Maturation of the CNS and Evoked Potentials. Amsterdam, Elsevier, 1987, pp 95–106

24. Garg BP, Markand ON, DeMyer WE, et al: Evoked response studies in patients with adrenoleukodystrophy and heterozygous relatives. Arch Neurol 40:356–359, 1983

25. Georgesco M, Radiere M, Seror P, et al: Les potentiels cerebraux somesthesiques evoques a partir du membre inferieur chez le nouveau-ne le nourrisson. Rev EEG Neurophysiol 12:123–128, 1982

26. Gilles FH, Shankle EC, Dooling EC: Myelinated tracts: Growth patterns. *In* Gilles FH, Leviton A, Dooling EC (eds): The Developing Human Brain. Boston, John Wright, 1983, pp 117–183

27. Gilmore RL: Effects of sleep on central conduction time in infants and children. International EEG Congress Scientific Session. London, August 1985

28. Gilmore RL, Bass NH, Wright EA, et al: Development assessment of spinal cord and cortical evoked potentials after tibial nerve stimulation: Effects of age and stature on normative data during childhood. Electroencephalogr Clin Neurophysiol 62:241–251, 1985

29. Gilmore RL, Brock J, Hermansen MC, et al: Development of lumbar spinal cord and cortical evoked potentials after tibial nerve stimulation in the pre-term newborns: Effects of gestational age and other factors. Electroencephalogr Clin Neurophysiol 68:28–39, 1987

30. Gilmore RL, Hermansen M, Brock J, et al: Effect of sleep on cortical SSEP: Age dependency during growth and development. Electroencephalogr Clin Neurophysiol 64:42P, 1986

31. Gilmore RL, Lastimosa ACL: Determination of site and extent of brainstem gliomas using BAEPs and SSEPs. Electroencephalogr Clin Neurophysiol 56:5P, 1983

32. Gilmore RL, Nelson KR: Electrodiagnosis in Guillain-Barré syndrome in children: Comparison of somatosensory evoked potentials and F-wave studies. Electroencephalogr Clin Neurophysiol, abstract in press

33. Gilmore RL, Nelson KR: Electrodiagnosis in Guillian-Barré syndrome: Comparison of somatosensory evoked potentials and F-wave studies. Neurology 36(suppl 1):154, 1986

34. Goff WR, Shaywitz BA, Goff GD, et al: Somatic evoked potential evaluation of cerebral status in Reye syndrome. Electroencephalogr Clin Neurophysiol 55:388–398, 1983

35. Goldie W, McMahon A: The combined use of BAEPs and SSEPs in the assessment of brainstem dysfunction in children. Electroencephalogr Clin Neurophysiol 56:35, 1983

36. Goldie WD, McMahon A: The combined use of brainstem auditory and short-latency somatosensory evoked potentials in the assessment of brainstem dysfunction in children. Electroencephalogr Clin Neurophysiol 56:35P, 1983

37. Goldie WD, Spydell JD: Somatosensory evoked potentials following median nerve stimulation in infants: Normative and clinical studies. American EEG Society Workshop: EPs in Children. St. Louis, September 18, 1987

38. Gorke W: Somatosensory evoked cortical potentials indicating impaired motor development in infancy. Dev Med Child Neurol 28:633–641, 1986

39. Hashimoto T, Tayanama M, Hiura K, et al: Short latency somatosensory evoked potentials in children. Brain Dev 4:390–396, 1983

40. Hildebrand C, Skoglund S: Caliber spectra of some fiber tracts in the feline central nervous system during postnatal development. Acta Physiol Scand 364:5–41, 1971

41. Hrbek A, Karlberg P, Kjellmer I, et al: Clinical application of evoked electroencephalographic responses in newborn infants. I: Perinatal asphyxia. Dev Med Child Neurol 19:34–44, 1977

42. Hrbek A, Karlberg P, Olsson T: Development of visual and somatosensory evoked responses in pre-term newborn infants. Electroencephalogr Clin Neurophysiol 34:225–232, 1973

43. Hughes AF: The development of the dorsal funiculus in the human spinal cord. J Anat (London) 122:169–175, 1976

44. Laget P, Salbreux R, Raimbault J, et al: Relationship between changes in somesthetic evoked responses and electroencephalographic findings in the child with hemiplegia. Dev Med Child Neurol 18:620–631, 1976

45. Lastimosa ACB, Bass NH, Stanback K, et al: Lumbar spinal cord and early cortical evoked potentials after tibial nerve stimulation: Effects of stature on normative data. Electroencephalogr Clin Neurophysiol 54:499–507, 1982

46. Leuders H, Lesser R, Hahn J, et al: Subcortical somatosensory evoked potentials to median nerve stimulation. Brain 106:341–372, 1983

47. Lutschg J, Hanggeli C, Huber P: The evolution of cerebral hemispheric lesions due to pre- or perinatal asphyxia (clinical and neuroradiological correlation). Helv Paediatr Acta 38:245–254, 1983

48. Lutschg J, Pfenninger J, Ludin HP, et al: Brainstem auditory evoked potentials and early somatosensory evoked potentials in neurointensively treated comatose children. Am J Dis Child 137:421–426, 1983

49. Majnemer A, Rosenblatt B, Riley P, et al: Somatosensory evoked response abnormalities in high-risk newborns. Pediatr Neurol 3:350–355, 1987

50. Markand O, DeMyer W, Worth R, et al: Multi-modality evoked responses in leukodystrophies. In Courjon J, Mauguiere F, Revol M (eds): Clinical Applications of Evoked Potentials in Neurology (Advances in Neurology), vol 32. New York, Raven Press, 1982, pp 409–416

51. Merlob P, Sivan Y, Reisner SH: Lower limb standards in newborns. Am J Dis Child 138:140–142, 1984

52. Nelson KR, Gilmore RL, Massey A: Acoustic nerve conduction abnormalities in Guillain-Barré syndrome. Neurology 38:1263–1266, 1988
53. Ouvrier RA, McLeod JG, Conchin T: Morphometric studies of sural nerve in childhood. Muscle Nerve 10:47–53, 1987
54. Perot PL, Vera CL: Scalp recorded somatosensory evoked potentials to stimulation of nerves in the lower extremity in the evaluation of patients with spinal cord trauma. Ann NY Acad Sci 388:359–363, 1982
55. Rorke LB, Riggs HE: Myelination of the Brain in the Newborn. Philadelphia, Lippincott, 1969, pp 15, 18, 21, 23
56. Rossini PM, Zarola F, Di Capu M, et al: Somatosensory evoked potentials in neurodegenerative system disorders. In Gallai V (ed): Maturation of the CNS and Evoked Potentials. Amsterdam, Elsevier, 1986
57. Rowe MJ: Development of mammalian somatosensory pathways trends. Neuroscience 5:408–411, 1982
58. Roy MW, Gilmore R, Walsh JW: Somatosensory evoked potentials in tethered cord syndrome. Electroencephalogr Clin Neurophysiol 64:42P, 1986
59. Salamy A, Davis S, Eldredge L, et al: Neonatal status: An objective scoring method for identifying infants at risk for poor outcome. Early Human Development, in press
60. Schiff J, Cracco RQ, Rossini PM, et al: Spine and scalp somatosensory evoked potentials in normal subjects and patients with spinal cord disease. Evaluation of afferent transmission. Electroencephalogr Clin Neurophysiol 59:374–387, 1984
61. Schulte FJ, Michaelis R, Linke I, et al: Motor nerve conduction velocity for term, preterm and small-for-dates newborn infants. Pediatrics 42:17–26, 1968
62. Simpson JA: Fact and fallacy in measurement of conduction velocity in motor nerves. J Neurol Neurosurg Psychiatr 27:381–385, 1964
63. Taylor MJ, Chan-Lui WY, Logan WJ: Longitudinal evoked potential studies in hereditary ataxias. Can J Neurol Sci 12:100–105, 1985
64. Tobimatsu S, Fukui R, Kato M, et al: Multimodality evoked potentials in patients and carriers with adrenoleukodystrophy and adrenomyeloneuropathy. Electroencephalogr Clin Neurophysiol 62:18–24, 1985
65. Udani V, Cracco JB, Hittelman J, et al: Clinical and developmental evaluation, evoked potentials and MRI in pediatric AIDS. American EEG Society Scientific Session. St. Louis, September 18, 1987
66. Wagner AL, Buchthal F: Motor and sensory conduction in infancy and childhood: Reappraisal. Dev Med Child Neurol 14:189–216, 1972
67. White LE, Frank LM, Furguide TL, et al: Prognostic value of BAEP with near- and far-field SSEP in childhood coma. Neurology 35(suppl 1):199, 1985
68. Willis J, Seales D, Frazier E: Short latency somatosensory evoked potentials in infants. Electroencephalogr Clin Neurophysiol 59:366–373, 1984
69. Yakovlev P, Lecours A: The myelogenetic cycles of regional maturation of the brain. In Minkowski A (ed): Regional Development of the Brain in Early Life. Philadelphia, FA Davis, 1967, pp 3–69
70. Yamada S, Zinke DE, Sanders D: Pathophysiology of "tethered cord syndrome." J Neurosurg 54:494–503, 1981
71. Young RR, Shahani BT: Clinical value and limitations of F wave determination. Muscle Nerve 1:248–250, 1978

Department of Neurology MS 129
800 Rose Street
University of Kentucky Medical Center
Lexington, Kentucky 40536-0084

Use of Evoked Potentials for Diagnosis of Multiple Sclerosis

Keith H. Chiappa, MD*

Multiple sclerosis (MS) is a demyelinating disease of the central nervous system (CNS) characterized by foci of myelin destruction with relative preservation of axons and nerve cell bodies. Central myelin is formed by extensions of the cytoplasmic membrane of oligodendrocytes that wrap around the axon, resulting in concentric layers of lipid and protein. The acute MS plaque shows myelin breakdown and inflammation with perivenous infiltrates of mononuclear cells and lymphocytes; older lesions contain microglial phagocytes and reactive astrocytes. Inactive lesions (sclerotic plaques) contain relatively acellular fibroglial tissue (gliosis) and show loss of axis cylinders (see reference 59 for a review of the pathology of demyelination and remyelination). The pathogenesis of MS is unknown but this is a very active research area (see reference 63 for a review of related infectious and immunologic data).

The biochemistry and electrophysiology of nerve conduction with normal and abnormal myelination has been well studied, and Waxman,[115] Waxman and Ritchie,[116] Rasminsky,[91] Sears and Bostock,[100] and Sedgwick[101] provide excellent reviews of pertinent topics. Although these principles provide a starting point for understanding EP abnormalities seen in patients with demyelinating diseases, the generation of EPs often involves complex physiologic mechanisms whose response to partial anatomic and physiologic lesions is difficult, if not impossible, to predict or understand. These considerations will be discussed as they pertain to each EP modality.

The clinical utility of EPs in MS is based on their ability (1) to demonstrate abnormal sensory system function when the history and/or neurologic examination are equivocal, (2) to reveal the presence of clinically unsuspected malfunction in a sensory system when demyelinating disease

*Associate Professor of Neurology, Harvard Medical School; Director, EEG and Evoked Potentials Laboratory, Massachusetts General Hospital, Boston, Massachusetts

Portions of this article appear in *Advanced Evoked Potentials*, edited by H. Leuders, published by Martinus Nijhoff Publishing, and are reproduced with permission.

is suspected because of symptoms and/or signs in another area of the CNS, (3) to help define the anatomic distribution of a disease process, and (4) to monitor objective changes in a patient's status. Although some of the information they provide is similar to that elicitable at the bedside by an experienced clinician, these tests are very helpful in the evaluation of patients with suspected demyelinating disease because (1) they provide electrophysiologic data obtainable only with the use of amplifiers and oscilloscopes, (2) they quantify and objectify data that the clinician may only sense, and (3) they can localize lesions within a pathway whereas clinicians often cannot.

Pattern-shift visual (PSVEP), brain-stem auditory (BAEP), and short-latency somatosensory evoked potentials (SEPs) are the EP tests most commonly studied in patients suspected of having demyelinating disease. Latencies and amplitudes of the various waves provide numerical data; sometimes the absence of a wave or an abnormal configuration of its potential field also provides useful information.

PATTERN-SHIFT VISUAL EVOKED POTENTIALS

The pattern-shift visual EP (PSVEP) is obtained with a reversing checkerboard pattern and recorded from the scalp overlying visual cortex where a prominent positive peak appearing at about 100 msec in normal subjects (P100) is used for clinical interpretation. The major change associated with optic nerve demyelination is prolongation of P100 latency. The mean latency in MS patients in a representative study exceeded the normal mean by approximately 10 msec in patients with possible MS to 30 msec in patients with definite MS, and delays exceeding 100 msec have also been reported.[102]

Interocular latency difference is probably the most sensitive indicator of optic nerve dysfunction in the PSVEP and has been used to provide evidence of optic nerve pathology.[43, 102] Failure to utilize this parameter in a comparative study of flight of colors (FOC) testing versus PSVEPs[109] resulted in erroneously low sensitivity of the PSVEP. Rolak[97] used the interocular latency difference parameter and found that although FOC testing compared favorably with PSVEPs, it was less sensitive. Shahrokhi and colleagues[102] found that 8 of 100 ON and MS patients had abnormal PSVEPs according to this parameter alone.

Amplitude of P100 has not proven to be a reliable measure, presumably because of the relatively large normal variability of amplitude. Matthews and co-workers[67] reported that 3 of 110 definite MS patients had abnormal PSVEPs on the basis of amplitudes less than 4 mV. Shahrokhi and colleagues[102] found only 1 per cent of 149 patients who were abnormal in this measure. Halliday and associates[36] and Halliday and McDonald[35] noted that amplitude was correlated with visual acuity whereas latency was not.

The duration and shape of P100 has also been investigated.[17, 43, 102] Isolated abnormalities in these parameters are relatively uncommon and when present are usually associated with P100 latency abnormalities. An explanation for these findings has been provided by Riemslag and colleagues,[93] who stimulated different segments of the visual field with varying time separations between stimuli. When the stimulus onset asynchrony was 40 msec or fewer, no contribution from the second stimulus could be identified in the recorded response. This suggests that the relative preservation of P100 shape and duration in partial optic nerve demyelination is due to inhibition of the late arriving impulses that had traversed the abnormally conducting segments. In the experimental situation, even when the initial stimulus comprised only 25 per cent of the visual field and the later stimulus comprised 75 per cent, the first suppressed the second. Thus, in the partially demyelinated optic nerve, the healthiest fibers determine the latency and shape of the response and, if the response is delayed, a majority of the fibers must be involved.

PSVEPs provide a sensitive extension of the clinical examination and commonly used clinical tests (visual acuity, clinical and formal visual fields, pupillary responses, funduscopic examination, and red color desaturation). To demonstrate the relative sensitivity of the PSVEP, 198 patients with multiple sclerosis who had had PSVEP testing were studied retrospectively by extracting pertinent aspects of the neuro-ophthalmologic examination from their medical records.[7] When the PSVEP was normal, there was *never* an abnormality found on the clinical examination. Even when the PSVEP was abnormal, various clinical examinations were often normal. For example, in those patients with abnormal PSVEPs, the visual fields by usual clinical examination (confrontation) were normal in 96 per cent, formal fields were normal in 55 per cent, pupillary responses were normal in 74 per cent, fundus appearance was normal in 39 per cent, and there was no red color desaturation in 27 per cent (only 22 patients had this test reported). These figures convey the degree of sensitivity that the test can add to the routine clinical ophthalmologic examination. However, if the formal visual field examination is done carefully, a greater incidence of clinical abnormalities can be found even in asymptomatic patients,[54, 72, 77, 86, 113] although it never matches that of the PSVEP.

Despite the sensitivity of the PSVEP, the abnormalities produced by the demyelinating plaques of optic neuritis and MS are indistinguishable from abnormalities produced by many other retinal, compressive, and degenerative diseases. Thus, abnormal findings demonstrated by the PSVEP must be carefully integrated into the clinical situation by a physician familiar with the clinical use of this test. He or she must decide if other procedures (for example, electroretinography, formal visual fields, radiologic studies, subspecialty consultation) are indicated to differentiate the possible causes of the conduction delay. Blumhardt[4] has evaluated the role of PSVEPs in the early diagnosis of MS and has reiterated the point that the test provides a sensitive, objective extension of the clinical neurologic examination but is etiologically nonspecific.

A large number of clinical studies attest to the sensitivity of the PSVEP in revealing demyelinating lesions in the optic nerve, and in our experience, more than 95 per cent of patients who have a clear history of optic neuritis (ON) have abnormal PSVEPs. Of the more than 400 patients with optic neuritis presented in the literature, 89 per cent had PSVEP abnormalities; in some studies, the percentage is closer to 100 per cent. When there was no clinical evidence for optic nerve involvement, the incidence of PSVEP abnormalities was 51 per cent of 715 patients (see reference 12 for a complete review and references).

When the diagnosis of MS is suspected because of typical symptoms and/or signs referrable to other CNS locations, then the demonstration by an abnormal PSVEP of a clinically silent conduction defect in the optic nerve can further delineate the anatomic distribution of the disease process and thus narrow the range of diagnostic possibilities. Optic nerve demyelination is a common finding in autopsy material of MS patients,[60, 70] and this is paralleled by the incidence of PSVEP abnormalities, which ranges from a high of 96 per cent[34] to a low of 47 per cent.[43] In a large number of clinical studies encompassing almost 2,000 patients with all MS classifications, the average abnormality rate found was 63 per cent (see reference 12 for studies involved in that review). Of 464, 322, and 799 patients classified, respectively, as possible, probable, and definite MS, the average abnormality rates were 37 per cent, 58 per cent, and 85 per cent, respectively. These figures reflect the greater likelihood of optic nerve lesions with more definite clinical diagnoses. Of 744 patients reported as having no history or clinical findings of optic neuritis, 51 per cent had PSVEP abnormalities (ranging from a high of 93 per cent[36] to a low of 34 per cent[90]). The differences among studies are best explained by the different definitions of MS used, some studies being composed of a preponderance of one class of patients. Note also that screen and check sizes differed greatly among the studies previously mentioned. Contrasts, when reported, were all above 74 per cent. Luminance levels varied so much that the reliability of the measurements has to be doubted. Nuwer and co-workers[82] studied first-degree relatives of MS patients and found interocular latency difference abnormalities in 6 of 110, although absolute P100 latencies were normal. Shibasaki and associates[104] have found that Japanese patients with MS have a higher incidence of absent PSVEP responses than was seen in series reported from Western countries. Noseworthy and associates[80] found a greater number of PSVEP abnormalities in patients older than 50 years as compared with younger patients. (For a more detailed index to the literature on ON and MS, see references 12 and 34.)

P100 latency abnormalities are usually present whatever the time interval since the clinical episode of optic neuritis. Shahrokhi and associates[102] reported PSVEP abnormalities 5 years after the clinical episode, and Halliday and co-workers[66] reported patients who had abnormal PSVEPs 15 years later. Only about 5 per cent of patients with abnormal PSVEPs have the P100 latency return to normal even when followed for 10 to 15 years after visual acuity has returned to normal following an episode of optic neuritis. However, Matthews and Small[66] found a patient whose PSVEP, although still abnormal 3 years after an attack of optic neuritis, had returned to normal after another 3.5 years. They suggested that in some patients a very slow healing process might be at work. When the latency difference between the 2 eyes can be used for interpretation (sometimes patients have binocular PSVEP abnormalities when first studied), then the percentage of patients in whom the PSVEP returns to normal drops further. Thus, if optic neuritis is suspected and the patient complains of moderate to severe visual difficulty but the PSVEP is normal, that diagnosis is highly unlikely, especially in the acute situation.

Serial PSVEPs have been recorded in MS patients relative to both disease progression and therapeutic trials. These studies must be interpreted in light of the normal variability seen over time; Oken and colleagues[84] found absolute P100 latency shifts up to 11 msec and interocular latency difference changes up to 9 msec in 20 normal subjects tested 2 to 13 months apart. Halliday and co-workers[35] have followed patients with serial recordings over several years, noting steplike increases in latency associated with relapses characterized by visual impairment; if there was no visual system involvement, PSVEPs tended to remain unchanged. Matthews and Small[66] reported that 61 per cent of 39 eyes exhibited parallel latency and acuity improvements over an 18-month period, but they also found 9 eyes that had latency increases into an abnormal range, 6 of which had concurrent improvements in acuity. Aminoff and associates[1] found no relationship between changes in nonvisual clinical status and PSVEPs. Smith and colleagues[105] found no PSVEPs changes in eight patients treated with three days of high-dose methylprednisolone infusions (1 g daily). Gilmore and co-workers[31] saw transient PSVEP improvement in some patients given infusions of the calcium antagonist verapamil.

There have been various attempts to increase the sensitivity of the test in this clinical area. Phillips and associates[88] found that hyperthermia increased the incidence of PSVEP abnormalities. Oishi and colleagues[83] tested three different check sizes and found abnormalities more common with smaller checks (25 min), occasionally only with larger checks (100 min), and less often with 50-min checks. Using sinusoidal gratings and psychophysical techniques, spatial vision has been further studied in MS by several investigators.[18, 54, 76, 89, 92] Cant and colleagues[10] and Camisa and co-workers[9] found that lower luminance levels revealed more abnormalities and suggested routine use of more than one intensity level. However, this effect was not observed by others[24, 41] except for restricted foveal stimulation.[41] Hammond and Yiannikas[38] compared full, half, and central (4-degree field, 27-min checks) pattern stimulation and found the techniques complementary. Central stimulation was abnormal in 34 per cent of patients, confirming the preferential involvement of macular fibers in MS, and providing an alternative to half-field stimulation in evaluating full-field responses with abnormal waveforms. Mitchell and colleagues[75] studied the recovery cycle of PSVEPs in MS patients and found that there was no good correlation between conditioning (first) responses with abnormal latencies and abnormally delayed test (second) responses. They interpreted this as indicating that the conduction defects are in different locations. Kaufman and Celesia[47] used combined pattern electroretinograms and PSVEPs to localize the conduction defect in acute optic neuritis and patients with MS, usually finding normal P-ERGs and delayed PSVEPs. Long-standing disease with optic atrophy, presumably with axonal involvement and retrograde degeneration of retinal ganglion cells, may result in absence of P-ERGs, and this has been investigated as a prognostic tool.[11]

Patients with acute transverse myelitis show PSVEP abnormalities in only a small proportion of cases.[98, 118] Blumhardt and associates[4] studied 31 patients in whom the spinal cord symptoms developed over hours to days (nine of these were classified as transverse myelitis) and found PSVEP abnormalities in 10 per cent. Ropper and colleagues[98] found no PSVEP or BAEP abnormalities in 12 patients with acute transverse myelitis. The chronic, progressive myelopathies have a greater incidence of abnormal PSVEPs. The abnormality rates ranged from 76 per cent in the series of Bynke and co-workers[8] to 35 per cent in the 100 patients with disease of more than 6 months duration studied by Blumhardt and colleagues.[5]

It has been suggested that PSVEP data can be used clinically in the setting of undiagnosed spinal cord disease to help decide whether or not myelography is necessary.[62] Bynke and co-workers[8] suggested that if the clinical neuro-ophthalmologic examination and the PSVEP are abnormal, and the CSF shows oligoclonal IgG banding, then radiologic investigations can be limited or avoided.[8] However, the possibility of concurrent diseases dictates very careful assessment of the clinical situation before an abnormal PSVEP (with or without other tests) should be used as presumptive evidence of MS to delay myelography. In fact, Blumhardt and associates[5] found five patients with abnormal PSVEPs and abnormal myelograms. Three had only borderline narrowing of the cervical canals and spondylotic changes (two of these have subsequently developed further signs of MS), but two had cord compression caused by prolapsed intervertebral disks. After laminectomy one of these patients had little clinical change but the other had a marked improvement.

Conduction defects in the optic nerve secondary to demyelinating disease most commonly produce latency delays without much change in waveform configuration. With respect to considerations of the pathophysiology involved in PSVEP abnormalities, the effects of segmental demyelination have not been well studied in small myelinated axons like those in the optic nerves. McDonald[71] measured the length of 20 optic nerve plaques in 14 patients who died from multiple sclerosis; the length of the individual plaques varied from 3 to 30 mm, with a mean of 10.5 mm. Extrapolating from animal studies, he estimated that a demyelinated plaque of 10 mm in humans would correspond to 50 internodes. Using the conduction velocity of the fastest fibers in the monkey optic nerve (10 m/sec) and factoring in a twenty-fivefold slowing of conduction over the demyelinated segment, he arrived at an estimate of 25 msec for an average delay to be expected in MS patients. This is similar to the delays actually seen in the PSVEPs of these patients. McDonald was careful to point out the possible errors in this formulation, but it is an interesting series of speculations. Noel and Desmedt[78] have suggested that longer delays in the somatosensory system could be attributed to (1) more than one plaque, (2) larger plaques, and (3) the necessity for the low amplitude and desynchronized afferent volley to rely on temporal summation of synaptic potentials for eliciting the response from the next element in the pathway.

Also, the PSVEP P100 waveform is not the primary cortical response and delays in conduction through the optic nerve could have more complex effects on the sequence of signal processing along the visual pathways, that is, geniculate bodies, cortex, and thalamus. In this regard, Jacobson and colleagues[46] studied diphtheria toxin-induced optic nerve lesions in cats using square wave grating discrimination to follow the time course of recovery of spatial frequency perception. They found a hierarchical progression with medium spatial frequencies returning first (1 to 4 days); then low frequencies (1 to 2 months) and finally high frequencies (5 to 8 months) returning. These findings suggest that small checks might produce abnormal PSVEPs for a longer time than larger checks. They also found that the recovery time of pupillary reactivity to bright light and the length of recovery to spatial vision testing were both directly related to the magnitude of fiber loss. Furthermore, the anatomic findings suggested that the cat can have a 77 per cent loss of optic nerve fibers and still recover visual acuity and contrast sensitivity.

BRAIN-STEM AUDITORY EVOKED POTENTIALS

The brain-stem auditory evoked potential (BAEP) is recorded in response to a 10-sec click stimulus, most often using a vertex-to-earlobe derivation, and shows five peaks in the first 10 msec after the stimulus, arising in brain-stem auditory structures from eighth nerve to inferior colliculus. Its clinical utility stems from the close relationship between the EP waveforms and specific anatomic structures. This specificity allows localization of conduction defects in the brain stem to within a centimeter or so. In addition, BAEPs (and SEPs) are very resistant to alteration by anything other than structural pathology in the brain-stem auditory tracts. For example, barbiturate doses sufficient to render the EEG "flat" (isoelectric) and general anesthesia do not significantly affect BAEPs or SEPs. These factors of anatomic specificity and physiologic and metabolic immutability are the basis of the clinical utility of both BAEPs and SEPs.

Brain-stem auditory evoked potentials offer a look at "physiologic anatomy." They provide a sensitive tool for assessment of brain-stem auditory tracts and nearby structures. As with PSVEPs and SEPs, abnormalities demonstrated by BAEPs are etiologically nonspecific and must be carefully integrated into the clinical situation by a physician familiar with the clinical use of this test. He or she must decide if other procedures (for example, conventional audiometric studies, electrocochleography, electronystagmography, radiologic studies, subspecialty consultation) are indicated to differentiate the possible causes of the conduction delay.

There has been a large number of studies of BAEPs in patients with MS.[12] Of 1,000 patients in the literature with varying classifications of MS, 46 per cent had abnormal BAEPs. For patients classified as definite, probable, and possible MS, the average abnormality rates were 67 per cent, 41 per cent, and 30 per cent, respectively. Of patients reported as having no history or brain-stem findings, 38 per cent had BAEP abnormalities; abnormality rates varied from 21 per cent to 55 per cent. Thus, in one fifth to one half of MS patients without brain-stem symptoms or signs, BAEP testing will reveal evidence of clinically unsuspected lesions. Differences in definitions of MS, patient populations, and techniques account for the variations among studies. For example, Noseworthy and co-workers[80] have found a higher incidence of BAEP abnormalities in MS patients over 50 years of age as compared with younger patients. Hammond and Yiannikas[37] found a correlation between BAEP abnormality rates and disability.

In a large group of MS patients, the reliability of BAEP techniques was demonstrated by the fact that all parameters in the MS patients with BAEPs interpreted as normal (the BAEP-normal MS group) showed no statistical differences from the normal values.[14] Those MS patients who had BAEPs with abnormal interwave separations had latency values that were a mean of 4.9 SDs above the normal mean, and those MS patients who were determined to have abnormal BAEPs on the basis of an abnormal I/V amplitude ratio (17 per cent of the BAEP-abnormal MS group) had ratios that were a mean of 5.5 SDs above the normal mean. These facts, and the higher incidence of abnormalities in the definite MS group, suggest that the BAEP is a reliable test for clinical usage.

Although the normal mean plus 3 SDs was used in this study as the upper limit of normal, the BAEP-normal MS patients (including those in the definite MS group) had values for both interwave latency and amplitude parameters that were essentially identical to the normal values.[14] The fact that the values for the MS patients had a bimodal distribution (also noted for absolute wave V latency by Robinson and Rudge[96]), being either completely normal or markedly abnormal, suggests that the smallest MS plaques in this part of the auditory system are sufficient to produce a marked conduction abnormality.

A majority of the BAEP abnormalities in MS patients are wave V amplitude abnormalities (absence or abnormally low amplitude of wave V was seen in 87 per cent of the BAEP-abnormal MS patients).[14] The next most frequent abnormality, increased III–V Interpeak Latency (IPL), was seen in 28 per cent of the BAEP-abnormal MS patients. The presumed generators of waves III and V are the superior olivary complex and inferior colliculus, respectively; and thus the majority of the conduction abnormalities were found to occur between them, as would be expected because this is the longest segment of white matter in the tracts being tested. However, in those patients who had recognizable waves V, there was no significant correlation between the III–V separation and the wave I/V amplitude ratio, contrary to our expectations. In fact, in 17 per cent of the BAEP-abnormal MS patients the III–V separation was normal and the I/V amplitude ratio was abnormal. In addition, three patients had the unusual combination of no wave III, a recognizable wave V of normal amplitude, and an abnormal I–V separation. The disparity between these different kinds of abnormalities is not easily resolved merely by consideration of the known conduction deficits in demyelinated axons such as slow conduction across the demyelinated segment and increased refractory period. Multiplicity of lesions, possible contributions to the BAEP waveforms from conduction in separate but parallel tracts, and possible synchronous activation of different auditory tract structures need to be considered.

The importance of monaural stimulation is evident because 45 per cent of the BAEP abnormalities were seen with stimulation of one ear only.[14] The prevalence of monaural abnormalities suggests that, with respect to the BAEP waveform generators, there is relatively little bilateral conduction, although known anatomic features had suggested otherwise. Contralateral recordings have not been especially helpful in MS.[37]

Faster rates of stimulation alter all BAEP parameters, including interwave separations. It has been noted previously[95, 108] that increased click repetition rate revealed a higher incidence of abnormalities in the BAEPs of MS patients. However, in our group of MS patients, more BAEP abnormalities were not seen with 70 clicks/sec, although abnormalities seen at 10/sec were sometimes worse at 70/sec.[14] Elidan and colleagues[27] have reported similar findings. The relative difficulty of waveform recognition at 70/sec, with increased waveform duration and indistinct peaks, restricted the clinical utility of that stimulus rate. In a few patients with diseases other than MS we have noted the reverse situation, that is, the I–V separation was abnormal at 10/sec and normal at 70/sec. This "normalization" may be due to complete failure of conduction in the abnormal fibers at the faster rate, possibly owing to an increased refractory period. With their abnormal contribution removed from the resultant waveforms, the activity manifest is only that from the normally conducting fibers, hence the normal appearance. Although this effect was sought in the MS patients, it was not found. Phillips and associates[88] used hyperthermia but increased the yield of BAEP abnormalities by only one patient.

Emerson and colleagues,[28] Maurer,[69] and Hammond and co-workers[39] have noted that some patients with MS show BAEP abnormalities with only one click polarity, usually rarefaction clicks. The abnormality usually consists of a complete absence of wave V with one click polarity, and a normal wave V with the other. Decreasing click intensity results in a reappearance of wave V, and this might suggest a peripheral origin of the phenomenon. However, some of these patients have completely normal hearing on conventional audiometric tests, and this effect is not seen in normal subjects or patients with peripheral hearing disorders, so that it is presumably due to central conduction abnormalities, although firm human clinicopathologic evidence for this is lacking.

In spite of obvious abnormalities in the BAEP, none of the MS patients studied here had clinical complaints of hearing difficulties, and click thresholds were essentially normal (formal audiograms were rarely obtained but those obtained were normal). This is consistent with the findings of routine audiologic testing in MS patients[57] but detailed auditory and vestibular testing[79] and interaural time discrimination and auditory localization testing[40] may reveal functional abnormalities in MS patients. In the latter study almost all MS patients with abnormal BAEPs also had abnormal interaural time discrimination. Occasionally MS patients do have symptomatic hearing difficulties and abnormal BAEPs apparently related to the disease,[21, 44, 45, 56] but none were seen in our group. Presumably there are plaques of demyelination in the eighth nerve (its proximal portion contains central myelin) or close to the cochlear nuclei in the lower pons. The occurrence of grossly abnormal BAEPs in conjunction with subjectively normal hearing may reflect the production of BAEP abnormalities by temporal dispersion of the click-induced volley as it ascends the affected tracts. It may be that, although these asynchronous potentials do not sum to generate a discrete peak of activity discernible at the scalp, the integrity of conduction, albeit deranged, is sufficient to sustain functionally normal hearing. However, this does not explain those cases where the amplitude and waveform shape are essentially normal and there is an abnormally large interwave separation. Perhaps in these cases the demyelination involves a majority of the fibers equally. Also, of course, BAEP waveform generation might have little to do with functional hearing.

The consistency of the BAEP when followed over time in normals suggests that it could be used to follow the activity of lesions affecting these tracts, and might possibly provide assistance in evaluating the effectiveness of therapeutic measures, although one study has suggested that the main value of BAEPs in patients with MS was to indicate clinically silent lesions and that its value in monitoring the clinical condition of the individual patient was less.[52] Matthews and colleagues[68] followed for 38 months after BAEP testing 84 patients in whom the diagnosis of MS was under consideration. In nine of these patients an abnormal BAEP at initial presentation subsequently proved to be of diagnostic value in that it revealed a separate, clinically silent lesion, indicating a multifocal disease (and the patient on follow-up proved to have MS). Aminoff and associates[1] noted a significant increase in variability in the BAEP between tests in patients with clinical exacerbations of brain-stem or cerebellar disease, but they also occasionally found a marked discrepancy between clinical and BAEP changes. Smith and co-workers[105] found no BAEP changes in MS patients following high-dose methylprednisolone therapy, whereas Gilmore and colleagues[31] noted some shortening of interpeak latencies following infusion of the calcium antagonist verapamil.

It should be reiterated here that a large part of the clinical utility of the BAEP lies in its ability not only to reveal unsuspected, and thereby multiple, lesions, but also to document clinically equivocal findings. For example, some of our patients with MS initially presented with symptoms and/or signs that could have been produced by disease in the labyrinths. Other than absence of wave I in 3 of the patients with Meniere's disease, no abnormalities of interwave separations or amplitude ratios in the BAEP were seen in those 21 patients with labyrinthine diseases.[14] Thirty-seven per cent of the MS patients who presented with nystagmus at the time of testing had BAEP abnormalities. Similarly, van Buggenhout and co-workers[113] found BAEP abnormalities in half their patients who had vestibular lesions. Thus the BAEP can be helpful in this setting: if abnormal, then the lesion is clearly centrally rather than peripherally located. Conversely, 56 per cent of the patients with an internuclear ophthalmoplegia (INO) at the time of testing had abnormal BAEPs,[14] so that the BAEP does not help to distinguish MS from the other causes of an INO (for example, infarction and tumor,[16] which might also affect both medial longitudinal fasciculus and auditory tracts).

The BAEP is abnormal in some patients with system disorders affecting cerebellar function, particularly those who have spasticity, and thus is not helpful in differentiating possible MS in that setting.

Amyotrophic lateral sclerosis (ALS) sometimes presents initially with symptoms and/or signs that might be suggestive of MS; in our 26 patients with ALS none had abnormal BAEPs.[14] ON and cervical transverse myelitis may have etiologies closely related or identical to that of MS; all the patients in those groups had normal BAEPs, and the ON patients tested also had normal SEPs (the cervical transverse myelitis patients all had abnormal SEPs). Also, in a different study 12 consecutive patients with inflammatory acute transverse myelitis (virtually or completely transverse lesions) had normal BAEPs.[98] Trigeminal neuralgia has also been associated with MS; in our 15 patients with trigeminal neuralgia none had abnormal BAEPs. Thus, as is also the case clinically, at the time of onset of ON, cervical transverse myelitis, and trigeminal neuralgia, there may be no EP evidence of lesions elsewhere in the CNS.

SHORT-LATENCY SOMATOSENSORY EVOKED POTENTIALS

Short-latency somatosensory EPs (SEPs) are usually evoked with a 2/sec to 5/sec brief electrical pulse delivered transcutaneously to median, tibial, or other nerves, and recorded at several points along the sensory pathway (for example, for upper-limb testing, over the brachial plexus, dorsal column tracts and nuclei, and somatosensory cortex). The peak labeled EP is generated in the brachial plexus, P/N13 in the upper cervical cord and lower medulla, and N19–P22 in the thalamus-cortex. The clinical utility of SEPs is related to the same factors of anatomic specificity and physiologic and metabolic immutability as were discussed above for BAEPs. SEPs offer a look at "physiologic anatomy" and thus provide a sensitive tool for assessment of spinal cord, brain stem (posterior columns and medial lemniscal tracts), and nearby structures. Again, abnormalities demonstrated by SEPs are etiologically nonspecific. They must be carefully integrated into the clinical situation by a physician familiar with the clinical use of this test who can decide whether or not other procedures (for example, electromyography, radiologic studies, subspecialty consultation) are indicated to differentiate the possible causes of the conduction delay or absence of an obligatory potential.

There has been a large number of studies of SEPs in patients with MS.[12] Of 1,000 patients with varying classifications of MS reported in the literature, 58 per cent had abnormal median/digital SEPs and 76 per cent had abnormal peroneal/tibial SEPs. In patients classified as definite, probable, or possible MS, the average abnormality rates were 77 per cent, 67 per cent, and 49 per cent, respectively.

Although the effect of stimulus rate has been studied in normals, there has been no study of rate effects in patients with MS. Smith and colleagues[105] saw no change in median and tibial SEPs with infusion of high-dose methylprednisolone. Nuwer and co-workers[82] studied first-degree relatives of MS patients and found some abnormal interarm Erb's point to N18 latency differences, although all other SEP parameters were normal. In published studies on the relationship between clinical sensory findings and SEPs in patients with MS, 42 per cent (249/598) of patients reported to have no symptoms or signs referable to the sensory system had abnormal SEPs, whereas 75 per cent (250/335) of patients with sensory system symptoms and/or signs had abnormal SEPs (both upper and lower limbs included). There is about a 10 per cent higher incidence of clinically silent SEP abnormalities found on testing the lower limbs (as compared with the upper limbs).

Data from a group of 114 MS patients seen in our laboratory exemplify the findings that can be expected when using SEPs to test patients with MS or suspected of having MS. Twenty-nine per cent of the patients had completely normal tests (both upper and lower limb). Upper-limb SEPs were abnormal in 54 per cent of patients, lower-limb SEPs in 64 per cent. In 18 per cent of the patients, upper-limb SEPs were normal when lower-limb SEPs were abnormal, whereas the converse was true in 7 per cent. Only 2 per cent of patients had bilaterally abnormal upper-limb and bilaterally normal lower-limb SEPs, but the reverse was found in 11 per cent of the patients. Thirty-seven per cent of normal upper-limb SEPs were associated with abnormal lower-limb SEPs on the same side, whereas only 12 per cent of normal lower-limb SEPs were associated with abnormal upper-limb SEPs ipsilaterally. Some of the conclusions that may be drawn from these results are (1) when lower-limb testing is normal, upper-limb testing will reveal abnormalities in an additional, although small, group of patients, (2) SEP abnormalities in one limb (upper or lower) are not necessarily associated with SEP abnormalities in the other limb on the same side, although lower-limb abnormalities will be more commonly associated with upper-limb abnormalities than vice versa. Others have had similar results, the yield of abnormalities being greater with lower-limb stimulation.[26, 50, 103, 112]

Patients with suspected MS have been tested and the finding of all EPs normal except for SEPs pointing to an upper cervical cord conduction defect has prompted a myelogram that revealed significant cervical cord compression from spondylotic bars; some of these patients have improved with surgical decompression. Conversely, of course, multiple EP abnormalities do not necessarily indicate MS.

Although every conceivable abnormality is seen in the SEPs of the MS patients, the most interesting is the absence of P/N13 (lower medullary component) with preservation of N19–P23 (thalamus-cortex) and a normal brachial plexus to N19 separation. The pathophysiology of such a finding and how it relates to the generation of the SEP waveforms are matters of pure speculation. In our group of patients, 30 per cent of the abnormalities were unilateral and 70 per cent were bilateral, an incidence quite similar to the average in the literature. Of the bilateral abnormalities, 79 per cent were identical and 21 per cent were different on the two sides.[12] Roberts and associates[94] have used the dispersion of the thalamocortical waveforms, as determined by Fourier analysis, as an additional analysis parameter. Rossini and colleagues[99] registered SEP short-latency wavelets using restricted band-pass digital filtering and thereby increased the yield of abnormalities. Yamada and co-workers[119] studied long-latency in addition to short-latency SEP components and found additional abnormalities; they also felt that the long-latency components helped to resolve interpretive difficulties encountered with short-latency testing, especially when bilateral stimulation was used. Delwaide and colleagues[23] studied lumbosacral spinal

SEPs in MS patients and noted a correlation between intensity of spasticity and some elements of the EP waveform.

Matthews and associates[68] followed for 38 months after SEP testing 84 patients in whom the diagnosis of MS was under consideration. In only three of these patients an abnormal SEP at initial presentation subsequently proved to be of diagnostic value in that it revealed a separate, clinically silent lesion, indicating multifocal disease (and the patient on follow-up proved to have MS). Davis and co-workers[22] found that clinical motor and sensory findings in MS patients in the corresponding limb frequently correlated with abnormalities of the median nerve SEP cervical response. When new clinical features appeared, the SEP deteriorated in some patients but improved in others, and overall disability sometimes increased despite improved SEPs. Most SEP changes were not accompanied by clinical changes.

Ropper and colleagues[98] studied EP abnormalities in 12 consecutive patients with inflammatory acute transverse myelopathy (ATM) as their first neurologic illness. All nine patients tested with median SEPs had normal findings, the lesions being below cervical levels mediating that response. Five of six patients tested with peroneal SEPs had abnormal findings (the sixth was tested 8 months after onset when there was no residual neurologic deficit). All these patients had normal PSVEPs and BAEPs and none developed new neurologic signs during 18 months mean follow-up. The authors felt that the lack of other lesions by EP testing and the failure to develop new clinical lesions indicates that ATM, when defined as a virtually or totally complete transverse inflammatory lesion of the cord, is a different process from MS.

Attempts have been made to use SEPs—and other EPs—to gauge the effectiveness of plasmapheresis therapy in MS but only a few patients have been studied so far.[22, 117] It is not yet possible to draw conclusions.

Effects on SEPs of raising body temperature in patients with MS have been studied by Matthews and associates[64] and Kazis and co-workers.[49] The latter authors used intercurrent extra-CNS infection (viral or bacterial) as the hyperthermic agents, and the effect of toxins cannot be discounted as the cause of the observed SEP changes. Matthews and associates[64] used external heat to raise the body temperature of their subjects and found that P/N13 amplitude was markedly diminished by the temperature increase. Phillips and colleagues[88] found that hyperthermia increased the yield of peroneal SEP abnormalities in MS patients.

COMBINED EVOKED POTENTIAL STUDIES

The comparative utility of PSVEPs, BAEPs, and SEPs have been studied in several groups of patients.[14, 33, 50, 53, 62, 68, 88, 90, 110, 112] As might be postulated on the basis of length of white matter tracts involved, the order of relative utility of the tests in revealing evidence of clinically unsuspected lesions was SEP, PSVEP, and BAEP. These data suggest that there is not a specific differential susceptibility to demyelination in the systems involved in the tests. Rather, it is the length and amount of white matter tracts being tested that determine the likelihood of detection of a lesion in a given system.[88]

Bottcher and colleagues[6] followed patients for 2 to 4 years after PSVEP, SEP, and CSF immunoglobulin G testing and found that 81 per cent of those in whom both the EPs and the IgG index were abnormal initially had entered a higher MS diagnostic class at the later evaluation. Those patients in whom either the EPs or IgG index were normal initially remained in the same diagnostic class. Walsh and co-workers[114] followed 56 patients for 2.5 years and found an increased number of abnormalities in multimodality EPs that was paralleled by an increase in overall clinical disability. However, Aminoff and associates[1] noted that the correlation between changes in specific clinical features and EPs may be poor.

Noseworthy and colleagues[80] have studied PSVEP, BAEP, and blink reflexes in patients presenting after age 50 with suspected MS. They found both the EPs and CSF electrophoresis to have high diagnostic yield in this difficult diagnostic group.

Nuwer and co-workers[81] performed EPs annually during a 3-year, double-blind, placebo-controlled study of azathioprine with or without steroids in chronic progressive MS. Treatment-related visual and somato-sensory EP changes became statistically different 1 year before corresponding differences were seen in the Standard Neurological Examination scores, and the statistical significance of the EP changes was substantially greater than seen for changes in other clinical scales. The degree of significance was increased by using EP latency values, rather than simple criteria for change. Anderson and co-workers[2] were less impressed with EP utility in clinical MS trials.

MOTOR EVOKED POTENTIALS

Transcranial stimulation (electrical and magnetic) of the motor cortex is a subject of much current interest.[120] Mills and Murray[74] stimulated electrically over the arm area of the motor cortex, over the C7 vertebral level, and in the axilla, and recorded the evoked muscle action potentials of forearm flexor muscles in healthy controls and patients with MS. In the patients the cord-to-axilla conduction times were normal, whereas central conduction times (cortex to cord) were either markedly prolonged or absent. Snooks and Swash[106] used a similar stimulation technique to study spinal cord conduction velocities and found slowed motor conduction velocities between C6 and L1 in four of five patients with MS, all of whom had corticospinal signs in the legs. Cauda equina conduction was normal. Hess and associates[42] used magnetic stimulation to study central motor conduction in 83 MS patients and found abnormalities in 72 per cent, usually in those with brisk finger jerks, sometimes in the presence of a normal neurologic examination and sensory EPs. Thus, these motor evoked potentials provide a tool for the objective study of motor system abnormalities in MS (and many other diseases) and may afford closer clinical-electrophysiologic correlations.

MAGNETIC RESONANCE IMAGING AND EVOKED POTENTIALS

Magnetic resonance imaging (MRI) is proving to be an invaluable tool in the investigation of patients with suspected demyelinating disease, especially the T2-weighted images.[25] Immediate postmortem studies have shown that demyelinated lesions 3 mm in diameter are seen, and that the apparent lesion size on MRI is accurate.[107] Where signal intensity varied, so did the degree of inflammation, demyelination, and gliosis, and it was thought that MRI could distinguish gliotic and nongliotic demyelinated lesions. Serial MRI scans show the appearance and evolution of asymptomatic lesions[87] and enhancement may afford a measure of activity.[32] MRI has been shown to be better than EPs and CT in revealing multiple lesions in the CNS,[19, 29, 51, 85] including the spinal cord, but, of course, MRI is little more specific than EPs with respect to etiology. However, in the brain stem, EPs reveal a significant number of conduction defects not seen by MRI.[3, 19, 30, 51] Similarly, it can be expected that optic nerve lesions will be detected more reliably by EPs than MRI, although Miller and co-workers[73] recently suggested an improved MRI technique for searching for demyelinating lesions in the optic nerve. Thus, although as a general statement it can be said that the general neurologic evaluation of the patient suspected of having demyelinating disease is better served by MRI (and most patients with MS will eventually have an MRI scan), in selected cases specific questions are better answered by EPs, and some anatomic areas are better tested by EPs.

REFERENCES

1. Aminoff MJ, Davis SL, Panitch HS: Serial evoked potential studies in patients with definite multiple sclerosis. Arch Neurol 41:1197–1202, 1984
2. Anderson DC, Slater CE, Sherman R, et al: Evoked potentials to test a treatment of chronic multiple sclerosis. Arch Neurol 44:1232–1236, 1987
3. Baumhefner RW, Tourtellotte WW, Ellison G, et al: Multiple sclerosis: Correlation of magnetic resonance imaging with clinical disability, quantitative evaluation of neurologic function, evoked potentials and intra-blood-brain-barrier IgG synthesis. Neurology 36(1):283, 1986
4. Blumhardt LD: Do evoked potentials contribute to the early diagnosis of multiple sclerosis? In Warlow C, Garfield J (eds): Dilemmas in the Management of the Neurological Patient. Edinburgh, Churchill Livingstone, 1984, pp 18–42
5. Blumhardt LD, Barrett G, Halliday AM: The pattern visual evoked potential in the clinical assessment of undiagnosed spinal cord disease. In Courjon J, Mauguiere F, Revol M (eds): Clinical Applications of Evoked Potentials in Neurology. New York, Raven Press, 1982, pp 463–471
6. Bottcher J, Trojaborg W: Follow-up of patients with suspected multiple sclerosis: A clinical and electrophysiological study. Neurol Neurosurg Psychiatry 45:809–814, 1982
7. Brooks EB, Chiappa KH: A comparison of clinical neuro-ophthalmological findings and pattern shift visual evoked potentials in multiple sclerosis. In Courjon JJ, Mauguiere F, Revol M (eds): Clinical Applications of Evoked Potentials in Neurology. New York, Raven Press, 1982, pp. 435–437
8. Bynke H, Olsson JE, Rosen I: Diagnostic value of visual evoked response, clinical eye examination and CSF analysis in chronic myelopathy. Acta Neurol Scand 56:55–69, 1977
9. Camisa J, Bodis-Wollner I, Mylin L: Luminance-dependent pattern VEP delay in human demyelinating disease. Soc Neurosci Abstracts 6:596, 1980

10. Cant BR, Hume AL, Shaw NA: Effects of luminance on the pattern visual evoked potential in multiple sclerosis. Electroencephalogr Clin Neurophysiol 45:496–504, 1978

11. Celesia GG, Kaufman D, Cone SB: Simultaneous recording of pattern electroretinography and visual evoked potentials in multiple sclerosis. Ann Neurol 43:1247–1252, 1986

12. Chiappa KH: Evoked Potentials in Clinical Medicine. New York, Raven Press, 1983

13. Chiappa KH: Pattern shift visual, brainstem auditory, and short-latency somatosensory evoked potentials in multiple sclerosis. Neurology 30:110–123, 1980

14. Chiappa KH, Harrison JL, Brooks EB, et al: Brainstem auditory evoked responses in 200 patients with multiple sclerosis. Neurol 7:135–143, 1980

15. Chiappa KH, Ropper AH: Evoked potentials in clinical medicine. Engl J Med 306:1140–1150, 1205–1211, 1982

16. Cogan DG, Wray SH: Internuclear ophthalmoplegia as an early sign of brainstem tumors. Neurology 20:629–633, 1970

17. Collins DWK, Black JL, Mastaglia FL: Pattern reversal visual evoked potential. J Neurol Sci 36:83–95, 1978

18. Coupland SG, Kirkham TH: Orientation-specific visual evoked potential deficits in multiple sclerosis. Can J Neurol Sci 9:331–337, 1982

19. Cutler JR, Aminoff MJ, Brant-Zawadzki M: Comparative value of MRI and evoked potential studies in multiple sclerosis. Neurology 36(1):156, 1986

20. Dau PC, Petajan JH, Johnson KP, et al: Plasmapheresis in multiple sclerosis: Preliminary findings. Neurology 30:1023–1028, 1980

21. Daugherty WT, Lederman RJ, Nodar RH, et al: Hearing loss in multiple sclerosis. Arch Neurol 40:33–35, 1983

22. Davis SL, Aminoff MJ, Panitch HS: Clinical correlations of serial somatosensory evoked potentials in multiple sclerosis. Neurology 35:359–365, 1985

23. Delwaide PJ, Schoenen J, DePasqua V: Lumbosacral spinal evoked potentials in patients with multiple sclerosis. Neurology 35:174–179, 1985

24. Diener H, Koch CW, Dichgons J: The significance of luminance on visual evoked potentials in diagnosis of MS. Archiv Psychiatrie Nervenkrankheiten 231:149–154, 1982

25. Drayer BP, Barrett L: Magnetic resonance imaging and CT scanning in multiple sclerosis. Ann NY Acad Sci 436:294–314, 1984

26. Eisen A, Odusote K: Central and peripheral conduction times in multiple sclerosis. Electroencephalogr Clin Neurophysiol 48:253–265, 1980

27. Elidan J, Sohmer H, Gafni M, et al: Contribution of changes in click rate and intensity on diagnosis of multiple sclerosis by brainstem auditory evoked potentials. Acta Neurol Scand 65:570–585, 1982

28. Emerson RG, Brooks EB, Parker SW, et al: Effects of click polarity on brainstem auditory evoked potentials in normal subjects and patients: Unexpected sensitivity of wave V. Ann NY Acad Sci 388:710–721, 1982

29. Gebarski SS, Gabrielsen TO, Gilman S, et al: The initial diagnosis of multiple sclerosis: Clinical impact of magnetic resonance imaging. Ann Neurol 17:469–474, 1985

30. Geisser BS, Kurtzberg D, Arezzo JC, et al: Trimodal evoked potentials compared with magnetic resonance imaging in the diagnosis of multiple sclerosis. Neurology 36(1):158, 1986

31. Gilmore RL, Kasarskis EJ, McAllister RG: Verapamil-induced changes in central conduction in patients with multiple sclerosis. J Neurol Neurosurg Psychiatry 48:1140–1146, 1985

32. Gonzalez-Scarano F, Grossman RI, Galetta SL, et al: Enhanced magnetic images in multiple sclerosis. Neurology 36(1):285, 1986

33. Green JB, Price R, Woodbury SG: Short-latency somatosensory evoked potentials in multiple sclerosis. Comparison with auditory and visual evoked potentials. Arch Neurol 37:630–633, 1980

34. Halliday AM: The visual evoked potential in the investigation of diseases of the optic nerve. In Halliday AM (ed): Evoked Potentials in Clinical Testing. New York, Churchill Livingstone, 1982, pp 187–234

35. Halliday AM, McDonald WI: Visual evoked potentials. In Stalberg E, Young RR (eds): Neurology I: Clinical Neurophysiology. London, Butterworths, 1981, pp 228–258

36. Halliday AM, McDonald WI, Mushin J: Visual evoked responses in the diagnosis of multiple sclerosis. Br Med J 4:661–664, 1973
37. Hammond SR, Yiannikas C: The relevance of contralateral recordings and patient disability to assessment of brain-stem auditory evoked potential abnormalities in multiple sclerosis. Arch Neurol 44:382–387, 1987
38. Hammond SR, Yiannikas C: Contribution of pattern reversal foveal and half-field stimulation to analysis of VEP abnormalities in multiple sclerosis. Electroencephalogr Clin Neurophysiol 64:101–118, 1986
39. Hammond SR, Yiannikas C, Chan YW: A comparison of brainstem auditory evoked responses by rarefaction and condensation stimulation in control subjects and in patients with Wernicke-Korsakoff Syndrome and multiple sclerosis. J Neurol Sci 74:177–190, 1986
40. Hausler R, Levine RA: Brain stem auditory evoked potentials are related to interaural time discrimination in patients with multiple sclerosis. Brain Res 191:589–594, 1980
41. Hennerici M, Wist ER: A modification of the visual evoked response method involving small luminance decrements for the diagnosis of demyelinating disease. In Courjon J, Mauguiere F, Revol M (eds): Clinical Applications of Evoked Potentials in Neurology. New York, Raven Press, 1982, 433–441
42. Hess CW, Mills KR, Murray NMF, et al: Magnetic brain stimulation: Central motor conduction studies in multiple sclerosis. Ann Neurol 22:744–752, 1987
43. Hoeppner T, Lolas F: Visual evoked responses and visual symptoms in multiple sclerosis. J Neurol Neurosurg Psychiatry 41:493–498, 1978
44. Hopf HC, Maurer K: Wave I of early auditory evoked potentials in multiple sclerosis. Electroencephalogr Clin Neurophysiol 56:31–37, 1983
45. Jabbari B, Marsh EE, Gunderson CH: The site of the lesion in acute deafness of multiple sclerosis—Contribution of the brain stem auditory evoked potential test. Clin Electroencephalogr 13:241–244, 1982
46. Jacobson SG, Eames RA, McDonald WI: Optic nerve fiber lesions in adult cats: Pattern of recovery of spatial vision. Exp Brain Res 36:491–508, 1979
47. Kaufman D, Celesia GG: Simultaneous recording of pattern electroretinogram and visual evoked responses in neuro-ophthalmologic disorders. Neurology 35:644–651, 1985
48. Kayamori R, Dickins S, Yamada T, et al: Brainstem auditory evoked potential and blink reflex in multiple sclerosis. Neurology 34:1318–1323, 1984
49. Kazis A, Vlaikidis N, Xafenios D, et al: Fever and evoked potentials in multiple sclerosis. J Neurol 227:1–10, 1982
50. Khoshbin S, Hallett M: Multimodality evoked potentials and blink reflex in multiple sclerosis. Neurology 31:138–144, 1981
51. Kirshner HS, Tsai SI, Runge VM, et al: Magnetic resonance imaging and other techniques in the diagnosis of multiple sclerosis. Arch Neurol 42:859–863, 1985
52. Kjaer M: Variations of brain stem auditory evoked potentials correlated to duration and severity of multiple sclerosis. Acta Neurol Scand 61:157–166, 1980
53. Kjaer M: The value of brainstem auditory, visual and somatosensory evoked potentials and blink reflexes in the diagnosis of multiple sclerosis. Acta Neurol Scand 62:220–236, 1980
54. Kupersmith MJ, Nelson JI, Seiple WH, et al: The 20/20 eye in multiple sclerosis. Neurology 33:1015–1020, 1983
55. Lacquaniti F, Benna P, Gilli M, et al: Brainstem auditory evoked potentials and blink reflex in quiescent multiple sclerosis. Electroencephalogr Clin Neurophysiol 47:607–610, 1979
56. Lederman RJ, Nodar RH, Conomy JP, et al: Hearing loss in multiple sclerosis. Neurology 28:406, 1978
57. LeZak RJ, Selhub B: On hearing in multiple sclerosis. Ann Otol Rhinol Laryngol 75:1102–1110, 1966
58. Lowitzsch K, Kuhnt U, Sakmann C, et al: Visual pattern evoked responses and blink reflexes in assessment of MS diagnosis. J Neurol 213:17–32, 1976
59. Ludwin SK: Pathology of demyelination and remyelination. In Waxman SG, Ritchie JM (eds): Demyelinating Disease: Basic and Clinical Electrophysiology. New York, Raven Press, 1981, pp 123–168
60. Lumsden CE: The neuropathology of multiple sclerosis. In Handbook of Clinical Neurophysiology, vol. 9. Amsterdam, North-Holland, 1970, pp 175–234

61. Maravilla KR, Weinreb JC, Suss R, et al: Magnetic resonance demonstration of multiple sclerosis plaques in the cervical cord. Am J Rad 144:381–385, 1985
62. Mastaglia FL, Black JL, Collins DWK: Visual and spinal evoked potentials in the diagnosis of multiple sclerosis. British Medical Journal 2:732, 1976
63. Matthews WB, Acheson ED, Batchelor JR, et al (eds): McAlpine's Multiple Sclerosis. London, Churchill Livingstone, 1985
64. Matthews WB, Read DJ, Pountney E: Effect of raising body temperature on visual and somatosensory evoked potentials in patients with multiple sclerosis. J Neurol Neurosurg Psychiatry 42:250–255, 1979
65. Matthews WB, Small M: Prolonged follow-up of abnormal visual evoked potentials in multiple sclerosis: Evidence for delayed recovery. J Neurol Neurosurg Psychiatry 46:639–642, 1983
66. Matthews WB, Small DG: Serial recording of visual and somatosensory evoked potentials in multiple sclerosis. J Neurol Sci 40:11–21, 1979
67. Matthews WB, Small DG, Small M, et al: Pattern reversal evoked visual potentials in the diagnosis of multiple sclerosis. J Neurol Neurosurg Psychiatry 40:1009–1014, 1977
68. Matthews WB, Wattam-Bell JRB, Pountney E: Evoked potentials in the diagnosis of multiple sclerosis: A follow-up study. J Neurol Neurosurg Psychiatry 45:303–307, 1982
69. Maurer K: Uncertainties of topodiagnosis of auditory nerve and brain-stem auditory evoked potentials due to rarefaction and condensation stimuli. Electroencephalogr Clin Neurophysiol 62:135–140, 1985
70. McAlpine D, Lumsden CE, Acheson ED (eds): Multiple Sclerosis: A Reappraisal. Edinburgh, Churchill Livingstone, 1972
71. McDonald WI: Pathophysiology of conduction in central nerve fibers. In Desmedt JE (ed): Visual Evoked Potentials in Man: New Developments. Oxford, Clarendon Press, 1977, pp 427–437
72. Meienberg O, Flammer J, Ludin HP: Subclinical visual field defects in multiple sclerosis. J Neurol 227:125–133, 1982
73. Miller DH, Johnson G, McDonald WI, et al: Detection of optic nerve lesions in optic neuritis with magnetic resonance imaging. Lancet 1490–1491, June 28, 1986
74. Mills KR, Murray MMF: Corticospinal tract conduction time in multiple sclerosis. Ann Neurol 18:601–605, 1985
75. Mitchell JD, Hansen S, McInnes A, et al: The recovery cycle of the pattern visual evoked potential in normal subjects and patients with multiple sclerosis. Electroencephalogr Clin Neurophysiol 56:309–315, 1983
76. Neima D, Regan D: Pattern visual evoked potentials and spatial vision in retrobulbar neuritis and multiple sclerosis. Arch Neurol 41:198–201, 1984
77. Nikoskelainen E, Falck B: Do visual evoked potentials give relevant information to the neuro-ophthalmological examination in optic nerve lesions? Acta Neurol Scand 66:42–57, 1982
78. Noel P, Desmedt JE: Cerebral and far-field somatosensory evoked potentials in neurological disorders involving the cervical spinal cord, brainstem, thalamus and cortex. Prog Clin Neurophysiol 7:205–230, 1980
79. Noffsinger D, Olsen WO, Carhart R, et al: Auditory and vestibular aberrations in multiple sclerosis. Acta Otolarygol (suppl 303):4–63, 1972
80. Noseworthy J, Paty D, Wonnacott T, et al: Multiple sclerosis after age 50. Neurology 33:1537–1544, 1983
81. Nuwer MR, Packwood JW, Myers LW, et al: Evoked potentials predict the clinical changes in a multiple sclerosis drug study. Neurology 37:1754–1761, 1987
82. Nuwer MR, Visscher BR, Packwood JW, et al: Evoked potential testing in relatives of multiple sclerosis patients. Ann Neurol 18:30–34, 1985
83. Oishi M, Yamada T, Dickins S, et al: Visual evoked potentials by different check sizes in patients with multiple sclerosis. Neurology 35:1461–1465, 1985
84. Oken BS, Chiappa KH, Gill E: Normal temporal variability of P100 latency. Electroencephalogr Clin Neurophysiol 68:153–156, 1987
85. Ormerod IEC, McDonald WI, du Boulay GH, et al: Disseminated lesions at presentation in patients with optic neuritis. J Neurol Neurosurg Psychiatry 49:124–127, 1986
86. Patterson VH, Heron JR: Visual field abnormalities in multiple sclerosis. J Neurol Neurosurg Psychiatry 43:205–208, 1980
87. Paty DW, Isaac CD, Grochowski E, et al: Magnetic resonance imaging in multiple

sclerosis: A serial study in relapsing and remitting patients with quantitative measurements of lesion size. Neurology 36(1):177, 1986

88. Phillips KR, Potvin AR, Syndulko K, et al: Multimodality evoked potentials and neurophysiological tests in multiple sclerosis. Effect of hyperthermia on test results. Arch Neurol 40:159–164, 1983

89. Plant GT: Transient visually evoked potentials to sinusoidal gratings in optic neuritis. J Neurol Neurosurg Psychiatry 46:1125–1133, 1983

90. Purves SJ, Low MD, Galloway J, et al: A comparison of visual, brainstem auditory, and somatosensory evoked potentials in multiple sclerosis. Can J Neurol Sci 8:15–19, 1981

91. Rasminsky M: Hyperexcitability of pathologically myelinated axons and positive symptoms in multiple sclerosis. In Waxman SG, Ritchie JM (eds): Demyelinating Disease: Basic and Clinical Electrophysiology. New York, Raven Press, 1981, pp 289–298

92. Regan D, Bartol S, Murray TJ, et al: Spatial frequency discrimination in normal vision and in patients with multiple sclerosis. Brain 105:735–754, 1982

93. Riemslag FCC, Spekreijse H, Van Wessem TN: Responses to paired onset stimuli: Implications for the delayed evoked potentials in multiple sclerosis. Electroencephalogr Clin Neurophys 62:155–166, 1985

94. Roberts KB, Lawrence PD, Eisen A: Dispersion of the somatosensory evoked potential in multiple sclerosis. Institute of Electrical and Electronic Engineers Transactions in Biomedical Engineering 30:360–364, 1983

95. Robinson K, Rudge P: The use of the auditory evoked potential in the diagnosis of multiple sclerosis. J Neurol Sci 45:235–244, 1980

96. Robinson K, Rudge P: Abnormalities of the auditory evoked potentials in patients with multiple sclerosis. Brain 100:19–40, 1977

97. Rolak LA: The flight of colors test in multiple sclerosis. Arch Neurol 42:759–760, 1985

98. Ropper AM, Miett T, Chiappa KH: Absence of evoked potential abnormalities in acute transverse myelopathy. Neurology 32:80–82, 1982

99. Rossini PM, Basciani M, DiStefano E, et al: Short-latency scalp somatosensory evoked potentials and central spine to scalp propagation characteristics during peroneal and median nerve stimulation in multiple sclerosis. Electroencephalogr Clin Neurophysiol 60:197–206, 1985

100. Sears TA, Bostock H: Conduction failure in demyelination: Is it inevitable? In Waxman SG, Ritchie JM (eds): Demyelinating Disease: Basic and Clinical Electrophysiology. New York, Raven Press, 1981, pp 357–376

101. Sedgwick EM: Pathophysiology and evoked potentials in multiple sclerosis. In Hallpike JF et al (eds): Multiple Sclerosis: Pathology, Diagnosis and Management. Baltimore, Williams and Wilkins, 1983

102. Shahrokhi F, Chiappa KH, Young RR: Pattern shift visual evoked responses: Two hundred patients with optic neuritis and/or multiple sclerosis. Arch Neurol 35:65–71, 1978

103. Shibasaki H, Kakigi R, Tsuji S, et al: Spinal and cortical somatosensory evoked potentials in Japanese patients with multiple sclerosis. J Neurol Sci 57:441–453, 1982

104. Shibasaki H, Kuroiwa Y: Pattern reversal visual evoked potentials in Japanese patients with multiple sclerosis. J Neurol Neurosurg Psychiatry 45:1139–1143, 1982

105. Smith T, Zeeberg I, Sjo O: Evoked potentials in multiple sclerosis before and after high-dose methylprednisolone infusion. Eur Neurol 25:67–73, 1986

106. Snooks SJ, Swash M: Motor conduction velocity in the human spinal cord: Slowed conduction in multiple sclerosis and radiation myelopathy. J Neurol Neurosurg Psychiatry 48:1135–1139, 1985

107. Stewart WA, Hall LD, Berry K, et al: Magnetic resonance imaging (MRI) in multiple sclerosis (MS): Pathological correlation studies in eight cases. Neurology 36(1):320, 1986

108. Stockard JJ, Rossiter VS: Clinical and pathologic correlates of brain stem auditory response abnormalities. Neurology 27:316–325, 1977

109. Swart S, Millac P: A comparison of flight of colours with visually evoked responses in patients with multiple sclerosis. J Neurol Neurosurg Psychiatry 43:550–551, 1980

110. Tackmann W, Strenge H, Barth R, et al: Evaluation of various brain structures in multiple sclerosis with multimodality evoked potentials, blink reflex and nystagmography. J Neurol 224:33–46, 1980

111. Tackmann W, Ettlin T, Strenge H: Multimodality evoked potentials and electrically elicited blink reflex in optic neuritis. J Neurol 227:157–163, 1982
112. Trojaborg W, Petersen E: Visual and somatosensory evoked cortical potentials in multiple sclerosis. J Neurol Neurosurg Psychiatry 42:323–330, 1979
113. van Buggenhout E, Ketelaer P, Carton H: Success and failure of evoked potentials in detecting clinical and subclinical lesions in multiple sclerosis patients. Clin Neurol Neurosurg 84:3–14, 1982
114. Walsh JC, Garrick R, Cameron J, et al: Evoked potential changes in clinically definite multiple sclerosis: A two-year follow-up study. J Neurol Neurosurg Psychiatry 45:494–500, 1982
115. Waxman SG: Clinicopathological correlations in multiple sclerosis and related diseases. In Waxman SG, Ritchie JM (eds): Demyelinating Disease: Basic and Clinical Electrophysiology. New York, Raven Press, 1981, pp 169–182.
116. Waxman SG, Ritchie JM: Electrophysiology of demyelinating diseases: Future directions and questions. In Waxman SG, Ritchie JM (eds): Demyelinating Disease: Basic and Clinical Electrophysiology. New York, Raven Press, 1981, pp 511–514
117. Weiner HL, Dawson DM: Plasmapheresis in multiple sclerosis: A preliminary study. Neurology 30:1029–1033, 1980
118. Wulff CH: Evoked potentials in acute transverse myelopathy. Dan Med Bull 32:282–287, 1985
119. Yamada T, Shivapour E, Wilkinson T, et al: Short- and long-latency somatosensory evoked potentials in multiple sclerosis. Arch Neurol 39:88–94, 1982
120. Young RR, Cracco RQ: Clinical neurophysiology of conduction in central motor pathways. Ann Neurol 18:606–610, 1985

Laboratory of Clinical Neurophysiology
Massachusetts General Hospital
Boston, Massachusetts 02114

0733–8619/88 $0.00 + .20

Use of Somatosensory Evoked Potentials for Intraoperative Monitoring of Cerebral and Spinal Cord Function

Marc R. Nuwer, MD, PhD*

Prevention of damage to the central nervous system is very important. Once damage has been done, it is often irreversible. In operations around the central nervous system, complications do sometimes occur. Monitoring the nervous system can identify complications early enough so that treatment or correction can be implemented before the impairment becomes permanent.

Evoked potentials (EPs) provide a method for intraoperative monitoring of the central nervous system. Somatosensory evoked potentials (SEPs) are able to monitor the posterior column pathways and their rostral connections up to and into the central region of cerebral cortex. Monitoring these somatosensory pathways also provides an indirect way to monitor adjacent motor pathways because most acute impairment affects function of many adjacent pathways, not just the posterior columns alone. In this way, somatosensory monitoring really provides information about the status of the whole spinal cord, plus information about substantial portions of the brain stem and the central regions of the hemispheres. Several different techniques are available for such somatosensory monitoring, differing in their recording electrode placement, settings of filters, and the like.

Situations for such monitoring vary considerably. Intraoperative somatosensory monitoring is probably most frequently used during placement of Harrington instrumentation or other similar apparatus for spinal stabilization in patients with scoliosis. These EP techniques have also been employed in various neurosurgical procedures. Thoracic surgeons have used EP monitoring during crossclamping of the thoracic aorta, to measure whether the spinal cord becomes dangerously ischemic. Monitoring hemisphere function can be useful during carotid endarterectomy, or during

---

*Associate Professor, UCLA Department of Neurology, Reed Neurological Research Center, Los Angeles, California

repair of carotid circulation aneurysms. At a few centers, EPs have also been used during cardiopulmonary bypass to assess the adequacy of cerebral perfusion. Finally, recordings directly from exposed cortex can help localize the motor gyrus.

EPs can also provide services beyond the identification of specific central nervous system impairment. Intraoperative EPs are sensitive to new systemic impairment such as hypoxia or hypotension when those factors are severe enough to alter central nervous system function. Occasionally, EP changes have been the earliest sign of such a systemic impairment. Monitoring can provide reassurance to the surgeon during the course of an operation, indicating that complications are unlikely to have occurred up to that point. This information can allow the surgeon to proceed further, providing patients with a greater degree of surgical intervention than they would have had in the absence of monitoring. Some high-risk patients may be considered for a surgical procedure only with monitoring, including patients who otherwise would have been ineligible for that surgical procedure because of the relative risks of adverse outcome. One should also consider the psychological benefits in providing some reassurance to patients, families, and physicians.

Monitoring EPs intraoperatively is still an imperfect technique. The potentials are small and can be sensitive to a variety of factors. Anesthetic agents themselves can cause significant changes. The intraoperative setting is often foreign to EEG technologists and neurologists, and recordings in those areas can be more difficult than in the outpatient laboratory area. Nevertheless, with some understanding of the relevant physiology, EP technology and anesthetic effects, most neurologists and EEG technologists will be able to go into the operating room and provide significant, valuable services for the surgical team in selected cases.

SPINAL SURGERY

Recording Techniques

Monitoring from the Scalp. The most straightforward way for measuring intraoperative SEPs is quite similar to the EP technique used in outpatient settings. Stimulating electrodes are placed over the posterior tibial nerve at the ankle and recording electrodes are placed over the scalp or neck. Additional recording electrodes can be placed at the knee, upper leg, or low back. Alternate stimulating sites include the peroneal nerve at the knee and the tibial nerve in the popliteal fossa. However, the ankle is usually preferred because of its accessibility under the surgical drapes if questions arise whether the electrode has become dislodged. It is much more difficult to check the knee under the surgical drapes. Needle electrodes are often employed at sites under the drapes, because paste or gel tends to dry over several hours.

Bilateral leg stimulation is advantageous because it allows monitoring of both halves of the spinal cord. But if both legs were stimulated simultaneously, the EP signals from the two separate stimulation sites

Figure 1. Effects of increasing the rate of stimulus presentation in one patient, for posterior tibial stimulation and scalp recordings. As rate is increased, EP amplitude decreases. The product rate × amplitude helps compare the advantageous increase in speed of testing and the disadvantageous loss of amplitude. In the patient the rate 5.1/sec appeared to be the best compromise between speed and attenuation. (*From* Nuwer MR, Dawson E: Intraoperative evoked potential monitoring of the spinal cord: Enhanced stability of cortical recordings. Electroencephalogr Clin Neurophysiol 59:318–327, 1984; with permission.)

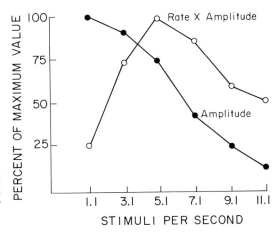

would become indistinguishable. The loss of the signal from one leg might be missed because the other is still intact. Such has actually happened.[33] Monitoring of both the left- and the right-sided pathways should be done by stimulation to the two legs delivered at separate times, such as alternating left and right. Automated monitoring programs on commercial equipment are available to perform interleaved stimulating procedure, providing simultaneous but separated monitoring of the two sides. This technique has been termed asynchronous parallel averaging.[38]

Stimulus intensity needs to be adjusted to a point well above the motor threshold for eliciting a twitch at the foot muscles. Neuromuscular junction blocking agents prevent this twitch during monitoring. Assessment of the motor threshold can be carried out prior to such use of such blocking agents, or else a relatively high typical stimulus intensity of 20 to 30 mA could be employed. Lower stimulus intensities produce smaller EP amplitudes.

Setting the stimulus rate involves a trade-off. The faster the rate, the lower the EP amplitude (Fig. 1). The slower the rate, the longer each EP takes to collect. A typical, optimal trade-off point is about five stimuli per sec.[39] For patients who have a very low EP amplitude, amplitude can be increased by slowing the stimulus rate. For patients with a particularly tall EP amplitude, a stimulus rate greater than five per second could be employed to speed up the EP collection process.

Filters are usually set to 30 Hz for the low filter and 3000 Hz for the high filter. The low-filter setting is important for reducing the background variability and irreproducibility of the EP signal. Low settings of the low filter, for example, 1 Hz, lead to unwanted EP variability. Moving the low filter to a higher setting, for example, 75 Hz, leads to an unacceptable decrease in EP amplitude in many cases. The optimal trade-off for most patients is around 30 Hz, which decreases background variability without sacrificing too much EP amplitude[39, 40] (Fig. 2).

The 60 Hz notch filter is left off. This is necessary during most SEP testing. The use of such filter would cause ringing, an exponentially

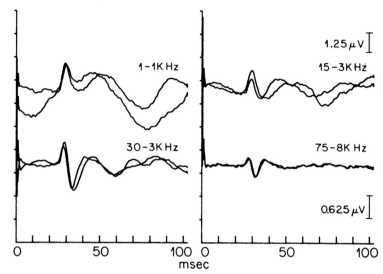

Figure 2. Effects of four different filter settings during intraoperative recordings in 1 patient, taken from a single scalp channel (Cz–Pz). Variability is greatest in the 1 Hz channel and is reduced by higher filter settings. The 30 Hz filters yields good reproducibility. The 75 Hz filter causes a substantial amplitude loss for the early peaks. Each pair of EPs is a typical set of two consecutive recordings. The amplitude scale is doubled for the lower two EPs. (*From* Nuwer MR, Dawson E: Clinical Orthopaedics and Related Research. Philadelphia, J. B. Lippincott, 1984; with permission.)

decreasing sinusoidal artifact that can be confused with a real EP.[38] The presence of 60 Hz noise in a signal should be dealt with by removing the source of that noise and by proper grounding techniques rather than by use of the 60 Hz filter.

Recording electrodes can be placed at the low back and at the scalp. Electrodes at the lumbar region, or even at the knee, are used to ascertain that the stimulus itself is delivering an unchanged signal to the lumbar spinal cord. A change in this peripheral signal would indicate a malfunction of the stimulator, dislodgement of the stimulating electrodes, or some local clinical change in the limb. More rostrally, electrodes are placed near the scalp vertex, optimally near the midline at a site between Cz and Pz of the International 10–20 system. The site halfway between those two electrodes has been called Ez.[37] Another site sometimes used is Cz′, located 2 cm behind Cz. Because the scalp region of maximum amplitude varies in location by several centimeters or more, additional electrode sites E1 and E2 off the midline can be useful. A reference electrode is used at the forehead, ears, or neck. The use of forehead sites Fz or Fpz helps reduce noise from muscle and movement artifacts. The neck as a reference is used sometimes, because it helps bring out the earliest potentials that may be generated at a subcortical level.

Scalp-recording technical parameters are summarized in Table 1.

Spinal-Recording Techniques. Spinal potentials can be recorded from electrodes situated in the epidural space or in the intervertebral ligaments. The epidural catheter electrodes can record particularly tall, well-defined

Table 1. *Simplified Setup for Scalp Recordings*

Stimulation	
Nerves	posterior tibial at ankle
Side	alternate left and right
Intensity	above motor threshold
Electrodes	subdermal needles
Pulse width	200 µsec
Repetition rate	5.1/sec at each leg
Recording	
Channels	E1–E2
	Ez–Fpz
	lumbar–sacral
Available alternative channels	cervical–Fpz
Filters	30–3000 Hz
60 Hz filter	off
Time base	60 msec
Sample size	300–500 accepted stimuli
Measure	latencies and amplitudes of most prominent peaks between 30 and 50 msec

potentials.[16] These electrodes can be placed once the surgical site is opened or preoperatively using a Tuohy needle, with a technique similar to that used for epidural anesthesia. Alternatively, simple needle electrodes in the intervertebral ligaments can be used,[25] but these can be placed only after opening the back. There have been no reports of complications due to these two types of spinal electrodes. Other, more complex recording techniques are available but are beyond the scope of this article.[27, 44]

The cortical and spinal recording techniques can be compared in several ways (Table 2). Scalp recordings seem satisfactory for many settings, including in scoliosis surgery that is probably the most common intraoperative setting. The cortical monitoring technique does poorly in the elderly, in patients with pre-existing central nervous system impairment, or in patients requiring inhalation anesthetic agents like isoflurane. In some instances, the scalp- and spinal-recording techniques can be used together: For example, the cortical monitoring can be used during the opening and closing portions of an operation, prior to placement of or after removal of spinal electrodes, thus providing continuous monitoring for the entire procedure.

Table 2. *Comparison of Recording Techniques*

	SCALP ELECTRODES	INVASIVE ELECTRODES
Minimum time to produce each EP	1–2 min	10–30 sec-epidural 1–2 min–ligamental
Forane 0.5%	usually gone	usually preserved
Can monitor caudal to surgery too	yes	yes
Begin monitoring	at or before induction	after opening
Discontinue monitoring	after awakening	during closing
Wires	hidden	in surgical field
Risk of damage	none	epidural–small, ligamental–none

Cervical Cord Monitoring. When monitoring procedures of this cervical spinal cord, the median or ulnar nerve pathways may be most advantageous. Stimulation and recording parameters are similar to those used for the posterior tibial nerve. However, the ulnar and median nerves yield taller, more easily defined scalp evoked potentials, and so these pathways should be used in preference to lower-extremity stimulation whenever possible. Median and ulnar nerve stimulation is usually delivered at the wrist. Recording is made from C3' or C4' over the contralateral scalp. Simultaneous monitoring of both arms is possible. Recording sites at Erb's point on the shoulder can help control for peripheral stimulation changes. When a C3' or C4' electrode is referred to the contralateral Erb's point electrode, the set of cervical evoked potentials is usually well seen along with the Erb's point and thalamocortical potentials. Monitoring in this way can help define the anatomic level at which any new impairment has occurred. This would be sensitive not only to changes at the cervical spinal cord level, but also can be used for monitoring changes at a thalamocortical level owing to hemispheric ischemia or other factors.

Patient-Related Factors

Somatosensory monitoring can be obtained from patients at almost any age; particularly young patients have evoked potentials that occur at somewhat longer latencies than those seen in adults. Elderly patients have small cortical EPs under anesthesia, sometimes so small as to make monitoring difficult. Otherwise, monitoring is similar across age groups.

Temperature can substantially change these potentials. With deliberate hypothermia to 30°C these potentials can become very low in amplitude or disappear. Median nerve EPs are somewhat easier to record at very low temperatures, leading to their use in some settings with cardiopulmonary bypass and hypothermia. Over the course of an operation it is common for the patient's core temperature to drop 1 degree or more. Limb temperature often drops even more. These changes do affect the latencies of the evoked potentials and need to be taken into account in interpretation of gradual intraoperative changes. The effects of limb temperature per se can usually be deduced from gradual changes in the lumbar or Erb's point peak latencies.

Deliberate hypotension can cause some changes in these potentials. EPs seem relatively stable at systolic blood pressures as low as 80 mm Hg, and can be stable and recorded at somewhat lower amplitudes at even lesser pressures. Fluctuating hypotension can cause fluctuating amplitudes.

Drugs and anesthesia can cause significant changes. As previously mentioned, isoflurane can abolish cortical potentials. Other halogenated anesthetic agents can do the same, such as halothane and enflurane. Nitrous oxide and narcotic-balanced anesthesia does cause some loss of amplitude of cortical potentials, often about 50 per cent, but this is nevertheless the usual anesthetic approach employed with cortical monitoring techniques. Acute boluses of barbiturates or other central active drugs can cause transient changes in EP amplitudes and latencies. Boluses of such medication are discouraged, and continuous drip techniques should be employed if possible. Neuromuscular junction blocking agents are often used, which are advantageous for the monitoring team because they remove substantial amounts of unwanted muscle artifact. If muscle artifacts appear to increase gradually over time, additional doses of these blocking agents can be very helpful.

Pre-existing neurologic deficits can substantially interfere with EPs. Even mildly to moderately abnormal preoperative cortical EPs can disappear completely under anesthesia. This is seen especially for patients with scoliosis associated with cerebral palsy and in some patients monitored for neurosurgic disorders. Some pre-existing neurologic disorders also abolish the spinal EPs, for example, in scoliosis associated with Friedreich's ataxia.

Clinical Settings

Scoliosis. Paraplegia is one of the most feared complications during orthopedic surgery for chronic spinal deformities. For adults undergoing operative correction of scoliosis, loss of motor function in the lower extremities occurs in approximately 1.7 per cent of cases done at expert institutions.[28] This is a common setting for employing SEP monitoring intraoperatively. In several clinical series, SEPs have accurately predicted future occurrence of major neurologic sequelae, which were usually accompanied by a complete loss of the EPs.[5, 17, 35, 46] Loss of EPs usually led to interventions by the surgeons and wake-up tests. In some cases, the EPs returned after an intervention and the patient awoke without a new neurologic deficit. In one case of lost EPs, the wake-up test was normal so no further intervention was made, but the patient awoke paraparetic.

During scoliosis surgery, the time of maximum risk is at distraction (mechanical straightening) or during the subsequent closing period. EP amplitudes usually remain stable, varying less than 20 per cent. If cortical EP amplitudes drop by more than 35 per cent, or if latencies increase by more than 1 msec, concern should be raised about occurrence of a potential neurologic complication.[34] This is especially true if the EP amplitude drops by more than 50 per cent. In many cases, neurologic complications have caused a complete loss of EPs.

Spinal Tumors and Malformations. Monitoring during various neurosurgical procedures is a common intraoperative use of SEPs. Several series of patients have been reported in which the SEPs did correctly predict which patients had postoperative changes. Some EP changes occur with cooling of the cord, as well as with compression, ischemia, traction, or other manipulations. Removal of an extra-axial tumor has resulted in improved amplitudes and conduction latencies.[29] Monitoring during ligation of feeding vessels to an arteriovenous malformation can help assess whether excessive ischemia to the cord is induced by the changing vascular flow patterns associated with the ligations[40] (Fig. 3). One set of surgeons reported that "the demonstration of axonal conduction through the operative field allowed us to sacrifice many feeding arteries which, on the basis of microsurgical inspection alone, we could not have done with confidence."[41] Sometimes the complications detected by EPs are not only unexpected but also are out of the surgeon's immediate operative field. In one circumstance, a loss of EPs over several minutes caused the monitoring team to rule out any obvious compression, anesthetic affect, or technical problem. Nothing

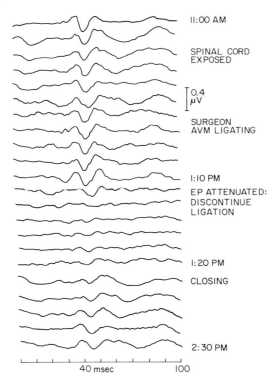

11:00 AM

SPINAL CORD
EXPOSED

0.4
μV

SURGEON
AVM LIGATING

1:10 PM

EP ATTENUATED:
DISCONTINUE
LIGATION

1:20 PM

CLOSING

2:30 PM

40 msec   100

Figure 3. Disappearance of EPs in this patient warned the surgeon against further ligation of a thoracic cord AVM. When the EP disappeared most, the proposed ligation had been accomplished; further intervention was stopped. EPs returned to normal amplitudes in about 1 hr, although latencies remained more delayed. The baseline EP in this patient had an abnormal delay in latencies, probably due to the AVM. These EPs showed more variability (30 per cent) than was seen in most patients. Stimulation was to one peroneal nerve. The patient awoke without any new neurologic impairment. (*From* Nuwer MR, Dawson E: Intraoperative evoked potential monitoring of the spinal cord: Enhanced stability of cortical recordings. Electroencephalogr Clin Neurophysiol 59:318–327, 1984; with permission.)

was found and so a further search was undertaken, which uncovered a 1 cm free fragment of nucleus pulposus extradurally in an area of tight stenosis two vertebral segments below the level of the operation. After removal of that fragment, the EPs returned within 2 minutes and eventually returned to near baseline latency and amplitude values; the patient awoke without a change in neurologic status.[32]

Crossclamping the Aorta. Crossclamping the aorta is used primarily during procedures to repair a coarctation or an aortic aneurysm. Upon crossclamping, the spinal cord may become acutely ischemic. If EPs disappear abruptly upon crossclamping, the risk of neurologic postoperative complications is high.[18, 21, 22] If the EPs disappear only very gradually, for example, over more than 30 minutes, the changes may be due to just the effects of a distal aortic ischemia on the peripheral portion of the monitored pathway. EPs can influence the surgeons about the need to place a vascular shunt to maintain distal perfusion, or about the need to identify any intercostal arteries critical for proper spinal cord perfusion. Loss of EPs during crossclamping is usually associated with distal aortic pressures below 40 mm Hg. If this causes cord ischemia, neurologic complications are common if perfusion is not restored within 15 to 30 minutes.

Animal Models

Lesion Studies of Spinal Cord Tract. Several animal studies have investigated which spinal cord tract carries the intraoperative EP signals.

Stimulation and recording methods employed in cats by Cohen and colleagues[6] were similar to those used in intraoperative cortical SEP monitoring, with recording electrodes placed on the scalp overlying somatosensory cortex. The integrity of the posterior columns was both necessary and sufficient to conduct a normal-appearing early positive cortical SEP. The lateral columns may carry some longer latency components. The ventral columns appeared to carry no significant component of the EP. Separate monitoring of each posterior column was useful for detecting injuries that asymmetrically affected the posterior portions of the spinal cord.

Powers and co-workers[42] found that the posterior columns also contributed to early and late waves recorded at a spinal level, but the ipsilateral dorsal spinocerebellar tract also contributed the early spinal EPs. This is consistent with observations made with human epidural spinal cord monitoring studies,[16, 45] in which the spinocerebellar tract was thought to generate the earliest of the spinal-recorded EP peaks.

Spinal Cord Ischemia. Somatosensory EPs are sensitive indicators of significant spinal cord ischemia. In a variety of animal studies, significant neurologic deficits did not occur from ischemia unless the SEPs were significantly changed.[2, 7, 22] A normal, stable EP always predicted a good neurologic outcome. When EPs were lost briefly (fewer than 5 minutes), the risk of significant neurologic deficits was quite small. When EPs were lost for a longer time (15 minutes or more), the risk of neurologic postoperative impairment was quite high unless the subject was protected by special techniques such as hypothermia.

In both human experience and animal models, paraplegia or paraparesis and associated cord pathology occur from acute compression, distraction, or other mechanical injury only when the EP has become substantially changed.[9, 11, 31, 36] This parallel between EPs and major motor impairment occurs despite the fact that the major EP transmission is up the posterior columns. Considerable reduction of spinal canal (more than 50 per cent) is usually needed to cause both an EP change and major motor impairment.[20] Motor impairment can still be avoided with such compression if the compression is reversed promptly, for example, within 15 minutes. Hypotension exacerbates the EP changes occurring during compression, and raising the blood pressure can correct an altered EP and probably helps to avoid major motor complications.[4, 14]

The EP can be recorded from a cortex or the spinal cord. In several animal models, the difference between the two methods appears rather small. The slow, late EPs at the cortex might be the least sensitive indicators of all, but the early cortical EPs produce results similar to spinal EP tests.[2, 43]

Unusual potentials can occur around the region of spinal compression. These injury potentials can mimic EPs and can even be larger than the original baseline normal EPs.[8, 43] However, their waveshape differs substantially from the shape of the original spinal EPs. As a result, it is necessary to pay close attention to the amplitude, latency, and overall waveshape of spinal EPs. Only in doing so can the monitoring team help to differentiate between large acute injury potentials and original baseline normal EPs.

Blood flow changes can interact additively or synergistically with the effects of compression. Perfusion effects may be important in many clinical settings. However, several animal models do suggest that it is the pathologic distraction (pulling in opposite directions) or flexion of the spinal cord that often causes the physical damage to axons. This mechanical mechanism of damage may actually be more important than ischemia for causing permanent damage in some surgical or trauma settings.

What to Think When the EP Changes

Changes in EPs intraoperatively can be from a variety of causes. Technically, the equipment may suddenly fail to work correctly. Modern monitoring equipment is based on computer technology that can occasionally fail for no apparent reason. Also, in the setting of surgery, many wires have to be strung across the room. Wires can be cut or become dislodged. The disappearance of an EP may be due to nothing more than the unplugging of a stimulus wire. The use of channels over the lower spinal column or the upper leg can be helpful in deciding whether the stimulus is still being delivered properly.

Anesthetic effects can cause acute or chronic changes in the EPs. Deepening anesthesia can result in loss of EP amplitude or slight delays in latency. Acute boluses of medication can substantially change the EPs, especially for drugs known to have central nervous system effects. Deliberate raising and lowering of the blood pressure might contribute some small amount of effect, especially if the systolic pressure is hovering at a rather low level.

Temperature can cause a slow change in EPs as the body's core temperature slowly drops during surgery. Limb temperature often drops even further than core temperature, and this can produce an extra degree of slowing in the peripheral portion of the pathways. This is accounted for by watching the patient's temperature, and using the lumbar electrode channels to discount the extra degree of peripheral slowing.

Acute systemic clinical changes can also affect EPs. Acute hypoxia from any cause can result in EP changes. Occasionally the EPs have been the earliest warning signal of such acute changes. Acute hypotension from bleeding or medications can also cause acute EP changes, especially if the hypotension reaches clinically significant degrees.

Surgical complications can also cause acute EP changes. This includes various types of compression of either the nervous system structures themselves or their vascular supply, as well as distraction, blunt injury, laceration, or other similar problems (Fig. 4). Sometimes the problem may be corrected as simply as changing the position of a retractor.

False-positive monitoring also occurs. A false positive would represent a setting in which EPs changed significantly without any apparent technical, anesthetic-related, systemic, or surgical problem. Such false-positive fluctuations usually reverse by themselves, often within a few minutes. It is possible that some of these false-positive events really represent true-positive monitoring identification of central nervous system physiologic impairment that was from an obscure cause. With good monitoring techniques, the rate of false-positive changes can be kept low.[34]

False-negative monitoring is also of great concern.[13, 24] This represents

Figure 4. Median nerve EP cortical peak amplitude loss and latency delay during Luque wire instrumentation of an unstable cervical spinal column. When at 11:00 AM the amplitude decreased to less than 50 per cent baseline and the latency increased further, the wiring was partly removed. EP deterioration abated. The surgeon then carefully replaced the wiring, while the EPs remained relatively stable. The patient awoke with transient weakness and sensory changes in one arm. (*From* Nuwer MR: Evoked Potential Monitoring in the Operating Room. New York, Raven Press, 1986; with permission.)

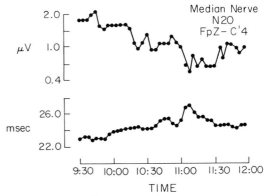

situations where the EPs remain stable despite serious postoperative neurologic impairment. To date there has not been any report of serious motor impairment postoperatively in any situation in which the intraoperative EPs continued to be normal and stable at the time of the motor impairment. This is reassuring because it suggests that somatosensory EPs can detect essentially all significant acute complications of the spinal cord including impairment mainly in the motor tracts. However, one must be cautious in understanding this general rule. There have been a number of reports of significant "misses" of monitoring. These have involved several types of situations. One report has been of a lesion occurring at a thoracic level while the median nerve pathways were being monitored. Another report was of the onset of complications several hours postoperatively. It is possible to do an anterior cordotomy for pain and still spare the posterior columns and spare the SEPs. In another report, the EPs were substantially altered in latency and wave shape from earlier recordings under anesthesia, but the surgical team did not interpret these as a warning of possible impairment. In that case, the surgical team's lack of response was because the EPs did not completely disappear, and they interpreted the preservation of some EPs as being reason to believe that the pathway was still intact. All these individual reports should caution the monitoring team about placing too much emphasis on the results of the EP monitoring. The EPs may miss lesions occurring far away from the monitored pathways. They cannot predict whether further impairment will occur during the immediate postoperative period. Substantial changes in the EPs can be a sign of significant impairment, even if some of the EP is still preserved.

MONITORING THE CEREBRAL HEMISPHERES

Techniques

Ordinary median nerve somatosensory monitoring can be used to assess the functional status of the hand region of the somatosensory cortex. The general techniques are similar to those described above for monitoring of the cervical spinal cord. The median nerve is usually chosen, because its cortical representation includes the thumb area, which is disproportionately large. The effects of various patient-related factors are also similar to that described above for spinal cord monitoring: The monitoring team needs to assess the relative effects of preoperative drugs, depth of anesthesia, temperature effects, effects of significant hypotension, and pre-existing neurologic impairment.

Cerebral and Systemic Ischemia

Ischemia causes a decreased cortical EP amplitude when the cortical blood flow falls below approximately 20 ml per 100 g per min and a loss of the EP at 15 ml per 100 g per min, rates that are near but not quite at the critical levels for cortical perfusion.[23] Subcortical and spinal EP recordings are more resistant to ischemia.[19] These latter tests may continue to show measurably electrical signals, even after blood flow to their generators has ceased for several minutes. Not only do cortical amplitudes change during cortical ischemia, but also the cortical latencies systematically lengthen. The worse the EP changes, the worse the deficit postoperatively. These findings seem to be relatively independent of the several types of animal models used to study them. Many separate investigators agree that cortical EPs are a relatively safe, sensitive, reproducible tool for detecting systemic or carotid distribution hypotension (and probably hypoxia). The EPs change at just about the right point in time, when moderately severe central nervous system ischemia is occurring, but before the damage has become sufficiently critical to produce permanent damage.

Clinical Settings

Carotid Endarterectomy and Aneurysms. During crossclamping of the internal carotid artery, significant ischemia can occur to the ipsilateral cerebral hemisphere. The degree of ischemia can be assessed in several ways. Ordinary EEG monitoring can show evidence of increased slowing or in a more severe ischemia, decrease in all frequencies in the ischemic region. SEPs can help to monitor the same type of ischemic impairment. The somatosensory pathways are specific to the central region of cortex. EEG is therefore superior in giving a much wider coverage of the hemisphere. EPs, however, tend to change at a level of ischemia that is closer to the critical level. Compared with EEG, EPs change and disappear at about 20 per cent lower perfusion. As such, EPs may have fewer false-positive changes than does EEG. It is possible that the two tests could best be used together: the EEG to give better, wider coverage, and the EPs to indicate the severity of the ischemia when it is nearing a critical level. Monitoring both the operated and the nonoperated hemispheres can help differentiate the effects of local hypoperfusion from more general systemic hypotension. In some cases, bilateral hemispheric electrophysiologic impairment is seen because of the coexistence of bilateral vascular disease. In any case, generalized electrophysiologic changes are an indication of a need for raising the cerebral perfusion pressure either by placing a vascular shunt or by raising the systemic blood pressure.

Some individual cases have provided lessons about these EPs. In one carotid endarterectomy case, the rostral carotid stump back pressure was 90 mm Hg, which is well within the normal range. Yet the cortical EPs disappeared ipsilaterally, indicating a critical ischemia at the cortex. A delayed, low-amplitude cortical peak reappeared 10 min after reopening the carotid artery. The patient awoke with a moderate degree hemiparesis.[12] In another case in which an internal carotid aneurysm ruptured during clipping, the concomitant loss of ipsilateral EPs indicated to the surgeons that collateral flow was acutely insufficient to provide adequate cortical perfusion. This helped guide the speed needed for emergent repairs, and in the subsequent period it also helped guide blood pressure control with dopamine.[15]

Studies of lesser degrees of EP change during carotid crossclamping have uncovered correlations with lesser degrees of clinical cerebral damage. When EPs change significantly but the patient awakes without any gross stroke, some lesser amount of cerebral damage may nevertheless have occurred. In one pair of studies, this was indeed the case.[3, 10] Patients whose cortical EP amplitudes decreased more than 50 per cent performed substantially worse on their postoperative neuropsychological testing compared with patients who had had only slight or no EP attenuation.

Cardiopulmonary Bypass. The integrity of the spinal cord, brain stem, and cerebral hemispheres can be assured during cardiopulmonary bypass and profound hypothermic circulatory arrest by using EPs. The EPs can usually be successfully monitored when the vital signs are maintained at levels used during these types of procedures. The principal exceptions are cortical EP loss during actual circulatory arrest in infants, as would be expected, and also a loss of cortical EPs when profound hypothermia is used in some other cases. This use of EPs is still relatively new and not widely used by thoracic surgeons. There is still some controversy regarding its relative effectiveness or usefulness. In anecdotal circumstances, the EPs have been able to correctly predict the occurrence of neurologic impairment. Technically, among various types of EPs including visual, auditory, and somatosensory, the median nerve N18 or N20 peak is probably the most resistant to the effects of hypothermia, always recordable at temperatures as low as 25°C and usually persisting even at temperatures as low as 20°C.[30]

MOTOR CORTEX LOCALIZATION

It is sometimes advantageous to locate the motor cortex during neurosurgical procedures. This can be done using anatomical landmarks in some cases, but there can be difficulty using these landmarks because of anatomical variability, limited exposure during the craniotomy, or when the local tissues have been disrupted by pathology. Another approach has been electrical stimulation of the cerebral cortex, with observations of the movements of the limbs. This has the disadvantage of precluding the use of standard doses of neuromuscular junction blocking agents because movements must be observed. It also has the disadvantage that someone needs to watch under the drapes to note the results. Sometimes, patients

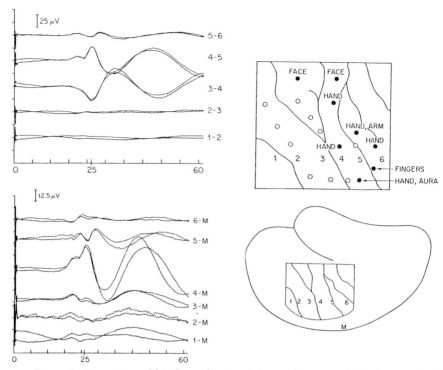

Figure 5. Comparison of bipolar and referential recordings recorded using a strip of electrodes lying 1 cm apart on the exposed cortex. The electrode locations are compared to locations where electrical stimulation caused sensations in this patient (operated on under local anesthesia). At one location, cortical stimulation also triggered the patient's typical epileptic aura. The reference electrode was in scalp muscle (M). (*From* Nuwer MR: Evoked Potential Monitoring in the Operating Room. New York, Raven Press, 1986; with permission.)

are tested in the awake state so that sensations can be directly reported for stimulation of sensory regions.

A promising improvement is provided by SEPs.[1, 26, 38] With median nerve stimulation, a prominent set of cortical potentials is recorded at around the central fissure at the hand level. These can be observed intraoperatively with the patient under general anesthesia and with neuromuscular junction blocking agents used as needed. These potentials can be recorded quite easily in most patients so that the technique might take as few as 5 to 10 min to carry out.

Technically, the procedure is very similar to ordinary median nerve stimulation at the wrist with recording from commercial electrodes designed for use in electrocorticography (Fig. 5). One version of these electrodes is a strip of platinum or stainless steel disks embedded in flexible silicone sheets or strips, with wires that can be plugged directly into EEG jackboxes. This strip is moved around on the exposed cortex until the region of the evoked potentials is found. This region is often rather small, sometimes extending no more than about 1 cm from the hand region of the central fissure.

A key in the interpretation of these is to look for the early negative and positive potentials, because various later potentials can be present across wider regions of the scalp. The earliest potential is usually a small negativity over the hand region of the postcentral cortex, accompanied by a positive potential on the motor side of the central fissure. Very shortly thereafter an even taller positive EP occurs over the postcentral hand region. The location of these potentials can be defined by comparing the electrical polarities at a series of recording sites, looking for the region at which the potentials have their maxima. Recordings can be made either in a bipolar or in a referential manner; bone or muscle makes a suitable site for a reference electrode in this technique. These techniques could also be adapted to identification of cortical regions corresponding to other body parts, for example, face or leg regions.

SUMMARY

EPs can be used in the operating room for monitoring the integrity of many levels of the central nervous system. SEPs can monitor the spinal cord, brain stem, and cerebral hemispheres. Such monitoring can alert the surgical team to the presence of complications, allowing prompt correction in some cases so as to prevent postoperative neurologic deficits.

Monitoring can be done from stimulation of either the lower or upper extremity. Recordings can be taken over the scalp or can be made from electrodes put into the surgical site itself. Monitoring of the spinal cord is most often done for surgery involving scoliosis, spinal tumors, or arteriovenous malformations, and during crossclamping of the thoracic aorta. Animal models and human surgical experience has shown that monitoring the posterior columns is an effective way to assess the status of the motor pathways of the spinal cord, because the two pathways are both affected in almost all acute circumstances.

Monitoring can also assess the functional status of the cerebral hemispheres. This is most often applied during carotid endarterectomy or repair of aneurysms of the carotid artery and its branches. Occasionally, this has also been applied to monitoring the cortex during cardiopulmonary bypass. Such EP monitoring does not cover the wide areas of cortex that can be monitored using EEG, but the EPs do tend to change and disappear at a level of ischemia nearer to the true critical level.

Intraoperative median nerve EPs can also be used to identify the hand level of the motor and somatosensory cortex. Such identification of motor cortex can help guide neurosurgeons in their choice of how or where to perform a biopsy, excision, and the like.

Overall, intraoperative evoked potential monitoring is becoming widespread because it is a practical way to help avoid neurologic complications, and it can be carried out using equipment already available in many hospitals. A substantial further review in this field can be found in *Evoked Potential Monitoring in the Operating Room.*[38]

REFERENCES

1. Allison T, Goff WR, Williamson PD, et al: On the neural origin of early components of

the human somatosensory evoked potentials. *In* Desmedt JE (ed): Clinical Uses of Cerebral, Brainstem and Spinal Somatosensory Evoked Potentials. Progress in Clinical Neurophysiology, vol. 7. Basel, Karger, 1980, pp 51–68

2. Bennett MH: Effects of compression and ischemia on spinal cord evoked potentials. Exp Neurol 80:508–519, 1983

3. Brinkman SD, Braun P, Ganji S, et al: Neuropsychological performance one week after carotid endarterectomy reflects intra-operative ischemia. Stroke 15:497–503, 1984

4. Brodkey JS, Richards DE, Blasingame JP, et al: Reversible spinal trauma in cats: Additive effects of direct pressure and ischemia. J Neurosurg 37:591–593, 1972

5. Brown RH, Nash CL Jr: Current status of spinal cord monitoring. Spine 4:466–470, 1979

6. Cohen AR, Young W, Ransohoff J: Intraspinal localization of the somatosensory evoked potential. Neurosurgery 9:157–162, 1981

7. Coles JG, Wilson GJ, Sima SF, et al: Intraoperative detection of spinal cord ischemia using somatosensory cortical evoked potentials during thoracic aortic occlusion. Ann Thorac Surg 34:299–306, 1982

8. Cracco RQ, Evans B: Spinal evoked potential in the cat: Effects of asphyxia, strychnine, cord section, and compression. Electroencephalogr Clin Neurophysiol 44:187–201, 1978

9. Croft TJ, Brodkey JS, Nulsen FE: Reversible spinal cord trauma. A model for electrical monitoring of spinal cord function. J Neurosurg 36:402–406, 1972

10. Cushman L, Brinkman SD, Ganji S, et al: Neuropsychological impairment after carotid endarterectomy correlates with intraoperative ischemia. Cortex 20:403–412, 1984

11. D'Angelo CM, VanGilder JC, Taub A: Evoked cortical potentials in experimental spinal cord trauma. J Neurosurg 38:332–336, 1973

12. Gigli GL, Caramia M, Marciani MG, et al: Monitoring of subcortical and cortical somatosensory evoked potentials during carotid endarterectomy: Comparison with stump pressure levels. Electroencephalogr Clin Neurophysiol 68:424–432, 1987

13. Ginsburg HH, Shetter AG, Raudzens PA: Postoperative paraplegia with preserved intraoperative somatosensory evoked potentials. J Neurosurg 63:296–300, 1985

14. Griffiths IR, Trench JG, Crawford RA: Spinal cord blood flow and conduction during experimental cord compression in normotensive and hypotensive dogs. J Neurosurg 50:353–360, 1979

15. Hyman SA, Skelley CC, Arendall R, et al: Median nerve somatosensory evoked potentials as an indicator of ischemia in a case involving an aneurysm of the internal carotid artery. Neurosurg 21:391–393, 1987

16. Jones SJ, Edgar MA, Ransford AO: Sensory nerve conduction in the human spinal cord: Epidural recordings made during scoliosis surgery. J Neurol Neurosurg Psychiatry 45:446–451, 1982

17. Jones SJ, Edgar MA, Ransford AO, et al: A system for the electrophysiological monitoring of the spinal cord during operations for scoliosis. J Bone Joint Surg Br 65B:134–139, 1983

18. Kaplan BJ, Friedman WA, Alexander JA, et al: Somatosensory evoked potential monitoring during repair of aortic coarctations. J Neurosurg 19:82–90, 1986

19. Kobrine AI, Evans DE, Rizzoli HV: Relative vulnerability of the brain and spinal cord to ischemia. J Neurol Sci 45:65–72, 1980

20. Kojima Y, Yamamoto T, Ogino H, et al: Evoked spinal potentials as a monitor of spinal cord viability. Spine 4:471–477, 1979

21. Krieger KH, Spencer FC: Is paraplegia after repair of coarctation of the aorta due principally to distal hypotension during aortic cross-clamping? Surgery 97:2–7, 1985

22. Laschinger JC, Cunningham JN, Catinella FP, et al: Detection and prevention of intraoperative spinal cord ischemia after cross-clamping of the thoracic aorta: Use of somatosensory evoked potentials. Surgery 92:1109–1117, 1982

23. Lesnick JE, Michele JJ, Simeone FA, et al: Alteration of somatosensory evoked potentials in response to global ischemia. J Neurosurg 60:490–494, 1984

24. Lesser RP, Raudzens P, Luders H, et al: Postoperative neurological deficits may occur despite unchanged intraoperative somatosensory evoked potentials. Ann Neurol 19:22–25, 1986

25. Lueders H, Gurd A, Hahn J, et al: A new technique for intraoperative monitoring of spinal cord function: Multichannel recording of spinal cord and subcortical evoked potentials. Spine 7:110–115, 1982

26. Lueders H, Lesser RP, Hahn J, et al: Cortical somatosensory evoked potentials in response to hand stimulation. J Neurosurg 58:885–894, 1983

27. Maccabee PJ, Levine DB, Pinkhasov EI, et al: Evoked potentials recorded from scalp and spinous processes during spinal column surgery. Electroencephalogr Clin Neurophysiol 56:569–582, 1983

28. MacEwen GD, Bunnell WP, Sriram K: Acute neurological complications in the treatment of scoliosis: A report of the scoliosis research society. J Bone Joint Surg (Am) 57A:404–408, 1975

29. Macon JB, Poletti CE, Sweet WH, et al: Spinal conduction velocity measurement during laminectomy. Sur Forum 31:453–455, 1980

30. Markand ON, Dilley R, Moorthy SS, et al: Somatosensory evoked responses (SERs) during carotid endarterectomy (CEA). Electroencephalogr Clin Neurophysiol 57:46P, 1984

31. Martin SH, Bloedel JR: Evaluation of experimental spinal cord injury using cortical evoked potentials. J Neurosurg 39:75–81, 1973

32. McPherson RW, North RB, Udvarhelyi GB, et al: Migrating disc complicating spinal decompression in an achondroplastic dwarf: Intraoperative demonstration of spinal cord compression by somatosensory evoked potentials. Anesthesiology 61:764–767, 1984

33. Molaie M: False negative intraoperative somatosensory evoked potentials with simultaneous bilateral stimulation. Clin Electroencephalogr 17:6–9, 1986

34. More RC, Nuwer MR, Dawson EG: True and false positive amplitude attenuations during cortical evoked potential spinal cord monitoring. *In* Ducker T, Brown R (eds): Neurophysiology and Standards of Spinal Cord Monitoring. New York, Springer-Verlag, in press

35. Mostegl A, Bauer R: The application of somatosensory-evoked potentials in orthopedic spine surgery. Arch Orthop Trauma Surg 103:179–184, 1984

36. Nordwall A, Axelgaard J, Harada Y, et al: Spinal cord monitoring using evoked potentials recorded from feline vertebral bone. Spine 4:486–494, 1979

37. Nuwer M: Recording electrode site nomenclature. J Clin Neurophysiol 4:121–133, 1987

38. Nuwer M: Evoked Potential Monitoring in the Operating Room. New York, Raven Press, 1986

39. Nuwer M, Dawson E: Intraoperative evoked potential monitoring of the spinal cord: Enhanced stability of cortical recordings. Electroencephalogr Clin Neurophysiol 59:318–327, 1984

40. Nuwer M, Dawson E: Intraoperative evoked potential monitoring of the spinal cord: A restricted filter, scalp method during Harrington instrumentation for scoliosis. Clin Orthop 183:42–50, 1984

41. Owen MP, Brown RH, Spetzler RF, et al: Excision of intramedullary arteriovenous malformation using intraoperative spinal cord monitoring. Surg Neurol 12:271–276, 1979

42. Powers SK, Bolger CA, Edwards MSB: Spinal cord pathways mediating somatosensory evoked potentials. J Neurosurg 57:472–482, 1982

43. Schramm J, Hashizume K, Fukushima T, et al: Experimental spinal cord injury produced by slow, graded compression: Alterations of cortical and spinal evoked potentials. J Neurosurg 50:48–57, 1979

44. Tamaki T, Noguchi T, Takano H, et al: Spinal cord monitoring as a clinical utilization of the spinal evoked potentials. Clin Orthop 184:58-64, 1984

45. Tsuyama N, Tsuzuki N, Kurokawa T, et al: Clinical application of spinal cord action potential measurement. Int Orthop 2:39–46, 1978

46. Wilbur RG, Thompson GH, Shaffer JW, et al: Postoperative neurological deficits in segmental spinal instrumentation. A study using spinal cord monitoring. J Bone Joint Surg (Am) 66A:1178–1187, 1984

UCLA Department of Neurology
Reed Neurological Research Center
710 Westwood Plaza
Los Angeles, California 90024

Intraoperative Monitoring of Auditory and Brain-Stem Function

Rodney A. Radtke, MD* and C. William Erwin, MD†

During the past several years, intraoperative monitoring of brain-stem auditory evoked potentials (BAEPs) has become routine practice in many medical centers.[1, 2, 8–13, 15–20, 27, 29–31] During posterior fossa surgical procedures, the continuous recording of BAEPs has allowed neurophysiologic assessment of auditory and brain-stem function in the anesthetized patient. The initial description of intraoperative use of BAEPs appeared in 1978, when Levine and co-authors[15] described their experience in a small number of patients. Subsequently, several larger series extended the experience with intraoperative BAEPs and were quickly followed by widespread use of the technique throughout the United States.[2, 10, 12, 18, 31]

BAEPs are ideally suited for use in the operating room because they are not significantly altered by the anesthetic agents or physiologic changes encountered during surgery.[26, 33, 38] Their use does not increase operative time or subject the patient to additional risk. The intraoperative BAEP is a robust response that can be reliably recorded in essentially all patients with adequate preoperative hearing function. The use of BAEPs allows rapid sampling of eighth nerve and brain-stem function. Intraoperative changes in the BAEP are frequently noted and adjustment of the surgical approach usually results in improvement in the response and a maintenance of function postoperatively. Recently, the use of intraoperative BAEPs was demonstrated to be associated with significantly reduced postoperative morbidity.[29, 30] As a result of all these factors, BAEPs are playing an increasingly important role in posterior fossa surgical procedures.

Table 1 lists the surgical procedures during which BAEP monitoring is commonly employed.[1, 2, 5, 8–13, 17–20] The main application has been in the surgical approach to the cerebellopontine angle (CPA). This approach primarily threatens auditory function due to injury of the eighth nerve or

---

*Assistant Professor of Medicine (Neurology)
†Assistant Professor of Medicine (Neurology) and Professor of Psychiatry

From Division of Neurology, Duke University Medical Center, Durham, North Carolina

Table 1. *Intraoperative BAEPs: Surgical Procedures Monitored*

1. Procedures in the cerebellopontine angle (CPA)
   a. Acoustic neuroma resection
   b. Microvascular decompression of cranial nerves
   c. Retrolabyrinthine vestibular neurectomy
   d. Other CPA tumor resections
2. Other posterior fossa procedures
   a. Basilar artery aneurysm
   b. Posterior fossa AVMs
   c. Intrinsic brain-stem tumors

peripheral auditory structures. More recently, BAEPs have been applied to other posterior fossa procedures including resection of vascular abnormalities or brain-stem tumors. These procedures are less likely to threaten the auditory nerve, and BAEPs are employed primarily to assess brain-stem function.

BRAIN-STEM AUDITORY EVOKED POTENTIALS

Technique of Intraoperative Recording

The use of acoustically shielded headphones in the operating room is precluded by their mass, which intrudes into the operative field. A wide variety of ear insert transducers suitable for operating room use is available. We have successfully used inexpensive microstereo earphones in over 150 posterior fossa surgical cases.[27, 28, 30] They can easily be placed at the opening of the ear canal and covered with water-resistant tape to avoid contamination from surgical fluids. Evoked potential equipment manufacturers offer molded ear inserts connected by several inches of a polyvinyl tube to a transducer. The displacement of the transducer away from the ear physically removes it from the fluids that may accumulate intraoperatively. The length of the tube delays sound arrival at the cochlea and temporally separates the BAEP from the stimulus artifact generated by the transducer. Absolute latencies of all BAEP waveforms are delayed but interpeak latencies are unaffected by this technique.

Intraoperative BAEP stimulation parameters are very similar to those used in the laboratory. Alternating clicks of 100 μsec duration are used to reduce stimulus artifact that can be a problem at high-intensity stimulation with monophasic pulses. However, rarefaction or condensation clicks can be utilized if they offer better resolution of the BAEP response. The usual stimulus intensity is 70 dBHL, but frequently it is increased to 85 or 95 dBHL to maximize the response. The higher stimulus intensity is often required for waveform resolution due to the large amount of ambient noise present intraoperatively. The ear on the side of the surgical approach is the primary site of stimulation. To reduce transcranial stimulation, white noise 40 dB below the click intensity is delivered to the contralateral ear. Our routine stimulation rate is 31/sec. The range we have used intraoperatively is 11 to 51/sec. An exact fraction of 60 should not be used in order to avoid the incorporation of 60 Hz artifact. Many authors avoid the use of the faster rates because of deterioration of the quality of the BAEP response. However, in our experience, the benefit of a quick turnaround time and earlier demonstration of a significant change outweighs the minor deterioration in response quality. With the 31 Hz stimulation rate, a trial of 2000 replications can be completed in slightly over 1 minute (depending on the number of artifact-contaminated sweeps). After averaging approximately 100 to 200 stimuli (5 to 10 sec), the latency of wave V can frequently be determined and communicated to the surgeon if warranted.

The montage and recording parameters for intraoperative BAEPs are essentially identical to those used in the diagnostic laboratory recordings. Two channel derivations using ipsilateral ear Ai to Cz and contralateral ear Ac to Cz are recorded. A ground is placed at Fz. Two surface electrodes are placed at each site in the event of electrode displacement or dysfunction during the operation. Routine filter settings are a low-frequency filter of 150 Hz and a high-frequency filter of 3000 Hz. A typical trial incorporates the average of 1000 to 4000 stimuli depending on the signal-to-noise ratio. We routinely expand our analysis time to 15 msec because wave V may be displaced beyond 10 msec with operative manipulation.

Analysis of BAEP Response

Wave V is the most easily defined and the most robust waveform in the BAEP. It may be the only component recorded in patients with significant conduction or neurosensory hearing impairments. In the hostile operating room environment, the earlier waveforms may not be as easily resolved. Therefore, all authors have resorted to analyzing the latency and amplitude of wave V as the primary criterion of change in the BAEP.[1, 2, 4, 9, 10, 19, 20, 22, 25–31] Attention is focused on the BAEP response obtained on stimulation of the ear ipsilateral to the surgical approach. Change in the wave V latency is best seen with a serial display of responses including the intraoperative baseline as well as the last several trials. This allows determination of the overall latency and amplitude changes, as well as assessment of rapid changes occurring over the most recent averages. Occasional averages are obtained from stimulation of the contralateral ear to evaluate any alteration in brain-stem function.

Wave V latency changes of less than 0.5 msec are commonly seen early in the operative course.[10, 25, 29, 31] This mild shift occurs during opening and is not associated with direct surgical threat to auditory or brain-stem function. These initial changes are not recorded from stimulation of the contralateral ear and as such are not due to the effects of anesthesia or change in core body temperature. More likely, this mild, unilateral delay of wave V is due to the effects of local temperature change or irrigation solutions. In any case, this mild delay has no associated auditory or neurologic morbidity and is not considered clinically significant.

Although such mild shifts (less than 0.5 msec) can be ignored, there is still no consensus as to the degree of wave V delay or amplitude loss that is clinically important. Definitions of a significant latency shift from baseline have included 0.5 msec,[18] 1.0 msec,[30, 31] 1.5 msec,[10] and 0.07 msec per minute.[10] A loss of greater than 50 per cent of wave V amplitude is also described as indicative of a potentially important change.[10, 31] In our own experience, we have used a 1.0 msec shift as representative of a change that warrants communication with the surgeon.[29, 30] An abrupt shift occurring at a rate greater than 0.1 msec per minute is also cause for concern, even if the total shift of 1.0 msec has not been reached. A wave V amplitude loss of greater than 50 per cent is also probably significant but is rarely seen in the absence of an accompanying latency shift. One author has argued that the total loss of an identifiable wave V is the only change worthy of altering the surgical approach.[9] However, analysis of our data reveals that patients with shifts greater than or equal to 1.0 msec have a risk of auditory morbidity that is significantly different from those having a lesser shift.[29, 30] Therefore, we continue to use the relatively conservative value of 1.0 msec.

BAEPs are extremely sensitive to intraoperative manipulation and as a result will demonstrate changes that are frequently not accompanied by postoperative deficits (false-positive result). Ideally, any monitoring technique should consistently identify those patients at risk for neurophysiologic compromise but not cause unnecessary prolongation or alteration of the surgical procedure. In 70 consecutive cases of microvascular decompression (MVD), 43 per cent of the procedures were altered owing to the development of a shift of greater than 1.0 msec.[29, 30] If the complete loss of wave V was the only criterion utilized in the same operations, 20 per cent of the procedures would have been altered. This is in a clinical setting in which a 12 per cent incidence of auditory morbidity had previously been identified.[28] Thus, the ratio of BAEP changes to expected auditory morbidity was 4:1 or 2:1, depending on the criteria used. Although the stricter criterion may result in some needless adjustment or interruption of the surgical procedure, we feel that it offers the best chance to effect a decline in auditory morbidity.

The demonstration of a significant auditory or neurologic deficit in the absence of BAEP change (false-negative result) has fortunately been extremely rare. We have observed the development of an intraoperative midbrain infarct with the maintenance of normal intraoperative BAEPs.[27] Although this may be termed a false negative, such findings should not be unexpected given the anatomic limitations of the BAEP pathway and its presumed generators. It was this experience that led us to use the upper extremity somatosensory evoked potentials (SEPs) in addition to BAEPs to sample larger areas of the brain stem. Similarly, Raudzens has described a patient with normal intraoperative BAEPs that did not awaken from surgery.[31] The patient presumably suffered diffuse hemispheric injury outside the BAEP-monitored pathways, and as such this also does not represent a true false negative. Jannetta and colleagues have reported a "true" false-negative case of a patient who had a major auditory deficit postoperatively in spite of no intrasurgical change of the BAEPs.[14] Ojemann has described two patients who had the maintenance of an identifiable but altered wave V intraoperatively with a marked loss of functional hearing.[26] It is possible that these "false negatives" were due to damage of the auditory fibers that occurred after the monitoring was discontinued; however, the postoperative BAEPs and hearing evaluations were not described adequately in those reports to assess that possibility. Our experience includes

Table 2. *Intraoperative BAEPs: Mechanisms of Alteration*

1. Transsection of eighth nerve
2. Occlusion of internal auditory artery
3. Retraction or stretching of eighth nerve
4. Manipulation and dissection near eighth nerve
5. Brain-stem ischemia or compression
6. Technical factors
   a. Displacement or malfunction of stimulator
   b. Occlusion of external auditory canal (for example, fluids)
   c. Interfering noise (for example, drilling)
   d. Electrical interference (for example, electrocautery)

a single case of a profound auditory deficit with apparently preserved BAEPs. However, the discrepancy was due to technical error caused by a shorted transducer that delivered bilateral stimulation when the technologist attempted to unilaterally stimulate the ear on the side of surgery. Mechanical pressure on the cable connecting the transducers to the stimulator apparently caused the problem midway through surgery. This latter case emphasizes the need for attention to technical detail in order to avoid misleading intraoperative results.

Mechanism of BAEP Changes

Table 2 lists the most common mechanisms that produce an alteration of the BAEP response. Certainly, transsection of the eighth nerve leads to an abrupt and irreversible loss of wave V and resultant ipsilateral postoperative deafness.[10, 31] Interestingly, preservation of wave I and occasionally of wave II is seen in this setting. This reflects the generation of wave I in the cochlea and distal portion of the eighth nerve and the generation of at least a portion of wave II in the proximal eighth nerve.[22]

Usually, an abrupt loss of all BAEP waveforms is seen with the eighth nerve anatomically intact. The persistent loss of waves I–V and the subsequent deafness is frequently assumed to be due to ischemia affecting the cochlea or distal eighth nerve.[15] Support for this theory is found in experimental work in animal models.[3, 34–36] Sekiya and Møller demonstrated hemorrhages in the area cribosa at the fundus of the internal auditory canal as a result of cerebellar retraction.[36] The hemorrhages appeared to be due to the rupture of the branches of the Internal Auditory Artery (IAA). Thus, ischemia to the peripheral auditory structures is the probable cause of the sudden loss of all components of the auditory response. The loss of wave I, which is generated by the cochlea and distal eighth nerve, is anatomically consistent with this model of ischemic injury. Vasospasm has also been proposed as a cause for the loss of cochlear function during CPA operations, but no clinical or experimental support for this assertion is available.

More commonly, the changes seen intraoperatively are gradual and occur over several minutes.[31] Typically, these gradual changes occur during cerebellar retraction or during manipulation near the eighth nerve. The BAEP changes are primarily a prolongation of waves II–V with a maintenance of wave I.[9, 16, 31] When early waveforms are clearly identified, the change is seen in the I–II or I–III interval. When the changes continue to progress, waves II–V are ultimately lost but wave I is maintained. Sekiya and Møller noted no histologic abnormalities of the eighth nerve or disruption of the arterial supply when similar BAEP changes were seen in the Rhesus monkey model.[36]

The exact mechanical cause of this "conduction block" secondary to operative manipulation remains unclear. The intracranial portions of the eighth nerve are known to be fragile and sensitive to stretch and compression. The proximal portions of the eighth nerve are covered only by central myelin that does not include the perineurium (which offers resistance to stretching) or epineurium (which offers resistance to compression).[22, 35, 36] The prolongation of the I–V interval can occur during cerebellar retraction (presumably because of stretching) or during dissection near the nerve (presumably owing to compression). The BAEP changes have been demonstrated to be reversible (both clinically and experimentally) and offer an opportunity to avert irreversible injury to audition.

This discussion has emphasized BAEP changes secondary to compromise of cochlea or eighth-nerve function. Such lateralized changes are commonly seen during operations in the CPA. Compromise of the brainstem auditory pathways can also contribute to BAEP changes. We have observed two cases of a lateralized compressive or ischemic injury to the brain stem that resulted in a unilateral loss of the later BAEP waveforms. Postoperatively, these patients had moderate neurologic deficits and a localized brain-stem injury confirmed on magnetic resonance imaging. Profound bilateral BAEP changes are secondary to diffuse brain-stem ischemia or compression and are associated with severe brain-stem injuries.[11, 31]

Nonpathologic factors also are noted to influence intraoperative BAEPs. The effects of anesthesia or mild hypothermia are usually minimal.[22, 25] When seen, the associated wave V shifts occur symmetrically and are less than 0.5 msec.[9, 10, 19, 29, 31] There are reports of BAEP responses being lost with change in patient position.[10] This has been interpreted as due to interruption of the posterior fossa vascular supply with change in head position, but could have also resulted from technical factors (for example, displacement of transducer or recording electrodes, occlusion of external auditory canal).

Technical factors can also contribute to changes in the BAEP response. Malfunctioning of the stimulator, displacement of the transducer, or accumulation of fluids in the external auditory canal all lead to an attenuation or loss of an effective auditory stimulus. The hostile intraoperative recording environment includes many devices that produce interfering electrical noise. Many electrical devices, particularly the electrocautery, produce electrical interference that degrades the signal. Drilling to remove bone, in addition to producing electrical interference, produces a masking noise that significantly reduces the BAEP amplitude. At times during the operation, the use of electrocautery or the bone drill may need to be interrupted to allow adequate recording of the BAEP.

Predictive Value of BAEP Changes

Even though the exact indication for adjustment of the surgical approach remains poorly defined, the literature does offer significant

Table 3. *Intraoperative BAEPs: Postoperative Hearing*

UNILATERAL BAEP CHANGE (WAVE V)	AUDITORY OUTCOME
< 1.0 msec delay	No loss of hearing
≥ 1.0 msec delay	Low risk for mild-moderate hearing loss
Transient loss	Moderate risk for mild-moderate hearing loss
Persistent loss	High risk (50 %) for severe hearing loss or deafness

information regarding the predictive value of different BAEP alterations with regard to postoperative auditory function (Table 3).

1. No or mild latency alterations (less than 1.0 msec) (Fig. 1). Boston and colleagues[4] have described mild hearing loss in a patient with only a 0.4 msec shift in wave V latency. In addition, Jannetta[14] has referred to hearing loss in a patient with "no deterioration" of BAEPs. Otherwise, extensive experience has demonstrated that no hearing loss is noted in patients who have little or no wave V shift.[19, 22, 25]

2. Significant latency alterations (1.0 msec or greater) (Fig. 2). Raudzens[31] described mild hearing loss in three of seven patients with a latency shift of greater than 1.0 msec. However, Grundy described no deficits in 23 patients with similar shifts[10]; Friedman identified only 3 patients with transient mild hearing losses in 17 patients with similar intraoperative changes.[9] Our own experience has identified only one mild hearing loss in 16 patients with wave V shifts greater than or equal to 1.0 msec.[29, 30] It is clear from this experience that a moderate latency shift (more than 1.0 msec) is associated with a low risk (approximately 10 per cent) of subsequent hearing loss. The hearing loss identified in this setting is usually mild and is frequently noted only transiently. With latency prolongations of wave V, there is a point at which attenuation begins and may rapidly progress to loss of the component ("cliff effect"). We have noted this with as little as a 1.5 msec shift in some patients,

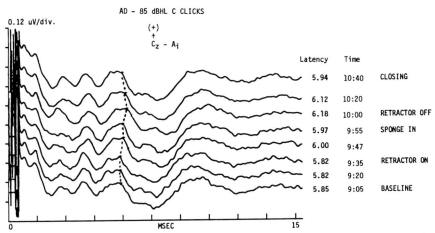

Figure 1. In this and subsequent illustrations, serial BAEPs obtained during microvascular decompression are displayed. The intraoperative baseline is displayed at the bottom with selected non-consecutive responses displayed more superiorly. Latency of wave V, time of day, and associated surgical activity are also listed. The dashed line denotes wave V. (Rate 31 per sec, 2000 trials/average, LFF = 150, HFF = 3000). Note the minimal shift (<0.4 msec) of wave V latency and the maintenance of earlier waveforms. Such minimal changes are seen in the majority of surgeries and do not warrant surgical adjustment.

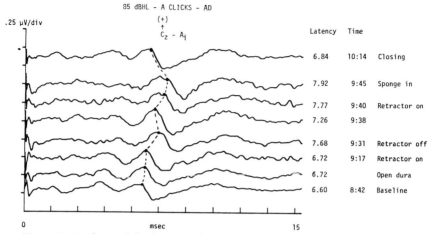

Figure 2. An abrupt shift of wave V latency (1.0 msec) is seen with placement of the retractor at 9:17 and improvement is subsequently demonstrated after removal of the retractor. Replacement of the retractor led to additional wave V shift, but the latency shift improved toward baseline near the conclusion of the procedure. Waves I and III were poorly identified or absent throughout the procedure.

whereas others retain 70 per cent of their original amplitude despite wave V latency shifts of 3.0 msec (9.5 msec absolute).

3. Temporary loss of BAEP waveforms II–V (Fig. 3). The loss of the BAEP response obviously serves as an indication for adjustment of the surgical approach. Although the response frequently returns within minutes, we have seen the persistent absence of wave V for over 45 minutes prior to its return in a patient with normal postoperative hearing. Of 11 patients with the temporary loss of wave

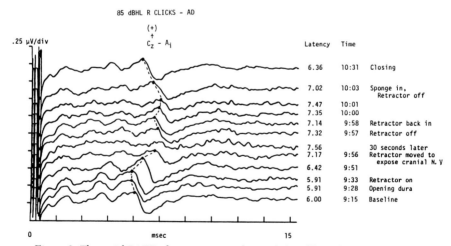

Figure 3. The serial BAEPs demonstrate an abrupt shift and loss of wave V that occurred at 9:56 when the cerebellar retractor was moved to better expose the trigeminal nerve. Return of wave V (although later and decreased in amplitude) is seen 1 minute after removal of retractor. Subsequent replacement of the retractor did not result in significant BAEP changes and the patient had normal postoperative hearing. Waves I and III were lost along with wave V and did not return until last average displayed.

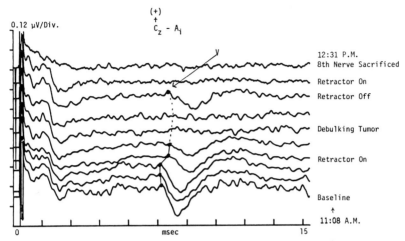

Figure 4. Serial BAEPs obtained ipsilateral to the resection of an acoustic neuroma are displayed. Note the loss of wave V with placement of the retractor and initial debulking of tumor. Wave V is identified after removal of the retractor (arrow) but lost with replacement of the retractor and subsequent sacrifice of eighth nerve in order to achieve adequate resection. Patient was deaf on side of surgery postoperatively.

V during microvascular decompression (MVD), we have noted mild-moderate hearing loss in 3 and normal hearing in 8.[24, 29] Similarly, Friedman[9] reported three patients with the temporary loss of wave V during MVD who had no postoperative deficits. Ojemann,[26] as mentioned above, did note significant hearing loss in two of three patients with the temporary loss of wave V during acoustic neuroma resection. In summary, patients who lose their BAEP response intraoperatively but have it return prior to the conclusion of the procedure almost always have functional hearing postoperatively. However, this population of patients is at risk for a mild to moderate hearing deficit.

4. Persistent loss of BAEP waves II–V or I–V (Fig. 4). In the early series by Raudzens[31] and Grundy,[10] the persistent loss of the later waveforms was strongly associated with postoperative deafness on the operative side. Of the nine patients suffering a persistent loss of waves II–V, seven were noted to be deaf postoperatively and two had severe hearing loss. Subsequently, Ojemann reported that 5 of 13 patients who lost their BAEP responses during acoustic neuroma resection retained functional hearing postoperatively.[26] We have seen three patients with a loss of the later BAEP waveforms during MVD, with two maintaining normal hearing and one with only a mild-moderate deficit.[29, 30] It is of interest that the two patients suffering trigiminal neuralgia who retained normal hearing postoperatively despite persistent loss of BAEP waves II–V had multiple sclerosis. Both had preoperative BAEP abnormality in the form of prolonged interpeak latencies. However, in the majority of reported cases, the intrasurgical loss of waves II–V is associated with significant postoperative hearing loss or deafness.[22]

Wave I may be difficult to resolve in the baseline intraoperative study (particularly in the setting of hearing impairment) or may also disappear intraoperatively without change in wave V. Many authors have begun using recordings of the electrocochleogram (ECochG)[15, 26, 32] or direct eighth-nerve recordings (8NP)[22–24] to better evaluate peripheral auditory structures. When a well-developed wave I or eighth-nerve potential is lost along with the later waveforms, a vascular etiology is suggested.[15] A vascular insult may be more likely to be irreversible, but there are not adequate data in the literature to offer a confident assessment of the predictive value of the loss of waves I–V as compared with the loss of waves II–V alone.

Intraoperative BAEP Interpretation

Despite some variability of different authors' experience with BAEPs, certain recommendations regarding their intraoperative use are still possible.[19, 25] In the absence of any BAEP change, a confident statement can be made to the surgeon that the patient's hearing remains intact and the surgical procedure can continue without immediate concern for compromise of auditory function.

Moderate changes of latency should be reported to the surgeon. The exact magnitude latency change when alteration of the surgical procedure is appropriate remains undetermined. We have used 1.0 msec empirically and the exact number that is most appropriate may vary depending on which surgical procedure is being monitored. In addition, the significance of any latency shift is greater if it occurs rapidly or is associated with cerebellar retraction or dissection near the eighth nerve. Certainly, progressive delays beyond 1.5 msec deserve attention and adjustment of the surgical approach until the response has been stabilized and, we hope, improved.

The disappearance of the BAEP responses must always be reported to the surgeon and if possible a change in the operative procedure should be initiated. Unilateral changes indicate compromise of afferent auditory fibers suggesting that withdrawal or adjustment of the cerebellar retractor is appropriate. Serial trials should then be obtained to assess for the return of the BAEP response. If serial trials do not indicate a return of the waveforms, the surgery can proceed with the probability that postoperative auditory compromise is a likely outcome. It may be appropriate at this point to concentrate further monitoring efforts to the contralateral ear and/ or median SEP (Fig. 5). Bilateral BAEP changes indicate brain-stem compromise and are usually associated with severe neurologic morbidity.

Prevention of Postoperative Complications

Although BAEPs have been demonstrated to be predictive of the postoperative auditory state of the patient, the much larger question is whether BAEPs may actually lessen the operative morbidity. McDaniel and colleagues[20] compared patients undergoing retrolabyrinthine vestibular neurectomy for vertigo both with and without BAEP monitoring. The incidence of significant hearing loss on pure tone audiometry was decreased from 6 to 20 patients to 2 of 20 patients after the institution of BAEP monitoring. Although suggestive, the results were not significant ($P = .18$), owing primarily to the small number of patients studied.

We have carried out a retrospective comparison of the auditory morbidity during retromastoid craniectomy for MVD both before and after the application of intraoperative BAEPs to this procedure.[29, 30] A previous report by Piatt and Wilkins had outlined the results in 152 procedures performed at our institution prior to June 1983. Subsequently, we have

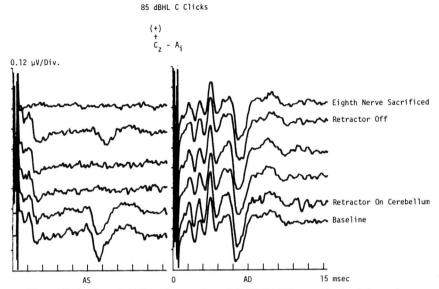

Figure 5. Ipsilateral (AS) and contralateral (AD) BAEPs are obtained from the same patient as in Figure 4. Even with marked ipsilateral BAEP changes, the contralateral BAEP remains stable and indicates that the ipsilateral changes seen are due to eighth nerve injury and not due to brain-stem compromise.

monitored 70 consecutive procedures with BAEPs. All patients had medically intractable trigeminal neuralgia or hemifacial spasm that was treated with MVD of the fifth or seventh cranial nerve via a retromastoid approach. All procedures were performed by a single surgeon using a similar technique. The two groups were similar with respect to age, sex, indication for procedure, and laterality of approach. Postoperative auditory deficits were identified by subjective complaint, clinical bedside testing, and audiometry. Pre- and postsurgical audiometry was performed in approximately 10 per cent of the nonmonitored series and in 61 per cent of the monitored series. All patients were classified as having no deficit (no change in auditory function subjectively or 10 dB or less change on audiometry); mild deficit-mild hearing loss with retention of functional hearing (11 to 30 dBHL loss); profound deficit or loss of functional hearing (greater than 30 dBHL loss or deafness).

The intraoperative BAEP results obtained during this study are demonstrated in Table 4. Forty cases (57 per cent) did not have a latency change in excess of 1.0 msec. Sixteen had a prolongation of wave V latency

Table 4. *Intraoperative BAEP Results: Wave V Prolongation*

MAXIMUM SHIFT	NUMBER OF CASES	AUDITORY DEFICITS
< 1.0 msec	40	none
≥ 1.0 msec	16	1-mild
Transient loss	11	3-mild
Persistent loss	3	1-mild

Table 5. *Audiologic Morbidity after Microvascular Decompression*

MONITORING	TOTAL	NO LOSS	MILD LOSS	PROFOUND LOSS
None	152	134 (88.2%)	8 (5.2%)	10 (6.6%)
BAEP	70	65 (92.9%)	5 (7.1%)	0 (0%)*

*p = 0.02

in excess of 1.0 msec. Fourteen cases demonstrated a loss of an identifiable wave V but with 11 having a return of wave V after adjustment of the surgical approach. Associated auditory morbidity is listed in the right-hand column. The incidence of auditory morbidity of the 40 patients with wave V changes of less than 1.0 msec compared with the 30 patients with the change in excess of 1.0 msec (in whom five auditory deficits occurred) was significant at $P = .01$ (Fischer exact test). In 30 of the cases monitored (43 per cent), a prolongation of wave V latency prompted communication to the surgeon of a potential threat to eighth-nerve function. As a result, the surgical approach was adjusted and in nearly all cases a subsequent improvement in BAEP response was seen. It is this portion of the monitored patients that may have benefited by the use of intraoperative BAEPs to avoid postoperative deficits.

Table 5 compares total audiologic morbidity in these two series. Combining mild and profound deficits, the monitored groups had an incidence of auditory morbidity of 7.1 per cent (5 of 70), compared with the 11.8 per cent incidence (18 of 152) noted in the nonmonitored group. The difference between the monitored and nonmonitored series for all degrees of hearing loss, although suggesting a reduced morbidity, did not reach statistical significance ($P = .21$). The lack of a significant difference was in part due to the inclusion of transient deficits and increased use of audiometry in the monitored series. Both these effects would serve to increase the detection of mild deficits in monitored patients.

Profound auditory deficit or deafness is a much firmer endpoint that is less affected by methods or efforts of detection. No patient in the monitored group had profound hearing loss or deafness as compared with 10 (6.6 per cent) in the nonmonitored group. This decrease in profound loss of auditory function as compared with all other outcomes was significant at the $P = .02$ level (Fischer exact test).

Because of the concern that the incidence of auditory morbidity may be a function of increasing experience of the surgeon, the incidence of auditory compromise in the first half of the nonmonitored series was compared with the second half of that same group. Although other complications did decrease with increasing surgical experience, the incidence of both mild and profound auditory morbidity did not change. Thus, the use of BAEPs resulted in a significant decline and elimination of profound hearing loss as a complication of microvascular decompressive surgery.

OTHER POSTERIOR FOSSA MONITORING TECHNIQUES

Electrocochleogram/Eighth-Nerve Potential

Intraoperative BAEPs can be supplemented by recording of electro-cochleograms (ECochG) and/or direct eighth-nerve potentials (8NP). Complete technical discussions of these techniques are beyond the scope of this article but are readily available in the literature.[15, 22–26, 32] The main focus of both these techniques is to more quickly and confidently identify evidence of peripheral auditory system dysfunction. Wave I is the most difficult component of the BAEP response to identify, and both these techniques shorten the time it takes for confident identification of wave I.

ECochGs are recorded from a needle electrode placed through the inferior portion of the tympanic membrane to rest on the promontory of the medial wall of the middle ear. This active electrode is referenced to the ipsilateral earlobe or mastoid. The ECochG response consists of a polyphasic short-latency deflection (cochlear microphonic [CM]) and a later relatively large deflection (N1). The CM is thought to be generated by the hair cells of the inner ear. Alternating clicks cannot be used to record the CM as it is a phase-dependent response and will cancel. The N1 is the compound action potential generated in the eighth nerve. The average latency of the N1 response is approximately 2.6 msec and is significantly later than the wave I latency seen in BAEP recording. The CM recording allows assessment of cochlear function and sometimes assists in localizing and characterizing the etiology of the intraoperative change; for example, CM is lost in occlusion of IAA, while it is spared in eighth-nerve transsection.[22, 26] The CM and N1 can remain unchanged in the setting of severe hearing loss and as such cannot be used without accompanying BAEPs.[26] The invasive nature of the recording electrode and the technical difficulties of obtaining adequate recordings has limited the use of the ECochG in intraoperative monitoring.[19, 22, 25]

Møller and colleagues[22–24] have developed a technique of directly recording from the eighth nerve near its entry zone into the brain stem. The latency of this eighth-nerve potential (8NP) is 0.5 to 1.0 msec later than the BAEP wave-I latency. The technique involves placement of a fine, multistrand Teflon-coated wire with a cotton tip directly on the proximal eighth nerve. It is referenced to a needle electrode placed in the wound margin. The response is a large positive-negative-positive triphasic potential that is presumably due to the action potential of the afferent auditory fibers passing directly under the recording electrode. The main advantage of the 8NP is its large amplitude, which allows identification of the response after a single or at most a few stimuli. This reduces the time needed to detect any change in the eighth-nerve response. Clinical experience with this technique is more limited than with BAEPs, and the exact character and degree of shift that is clinically significant remains to be clarified. The obvious disadvantage of this technique is that the 8NP cannot be recorded during the initial retraction of the cerebellum, which is frequently accompanied by BAEP changes and possible compromise of eighth-nerve function. The technique also involves the active participation of the surgeon for placement of the eighth-nerve electrode, which intrudes somewhat into the operative field. Technically, the 8NP is more easily recorded than the ECochG and is increasingly being utilized in tandem with intraoperative BAEPs.

Upper-Extremity SEPs in Posterior Fossa Surgery

Although BAEPs appear to be very sensitive to compromise of eighth-nerve or pontine function, they are unable to assess midbrain or medullary function that lies outside the central auditory pathway being monitored. Subsequent to the development of an intraoperative midbrain infarct in a patient with no significant BAEP abnormality, we have added upper-extremity somatosensory evoked potential (SEP) monitoring to surgical procedures in the posterior fossa.[27] The use of SEPs allows assessment not only of medullary and midbrain function but also subcortical and cortical function. Reports of false-negative BAEPs include descriptions of bilateral thalamic or hemispheric injury that may have been detected intraoperatively by the use of SEP technique.[11, 31] Other reports have subsequently appeared that describe the use of upper-extremity SEPs in a series of patients undergoing posterior fossa brain-stem or vascular surgical procedures.[8, 17]

Obtaining intraoperative SEPs is technically very similar to routine diagnostic studies. The median nerve is stimulated at the wrist using short EEG-type needle electrodes placed subdermally near the median nerve. Care must be taken to secure the stimulating electrodes to avoid displacement during the surgical procedure. The stimulation intensity is adjusted (in the range of 20 to 39 mA) with a duration of 100 to 200 msec at a rate of 11 to 31/sec. Low- and high-frequency filters are set at 30 Hz and 3000 Hz, respectively. Recording electrodes are placed at Erb's point (EP), over the fifth cervical vertebra (S5C), at Fpz, and midway between the parasagittal central and parietal electrodes on the contralateral scalp (C_c'). The shoulder opposite the site of stimulation is used as a noncephalic reference (NCR). Four channel recordings are obtained using the following montage: EP_i–EP_c, S5C–Fp_z, C_c'–NCR, and C_c'–Fp_z (i = ipsilateral and c = contralateral to the site of stimulation). The analysis time is 30 msec. Five hundred to 2000 responses are averaged during each trial requiring 1 to 2 minutes for data acquisition. The patient is instrumented for bilateral stimulation, but the upper-extremity contralateral to the surgical approach is used as the primary site of SEP stimulation. Ipsilateral median nerve stimulation is used if SEP changes are seen on contralateral median nerve stimulation. This allows assessment as to whether the changes are symmetric (suggesting effects of anesthesia) or asymmetric (suggesting focal neurologic compromise). It must be emphasized that halogenated inhalation agents in high concentration significantly delay and attenuate the N20 response. A balanced anesthetic including fentanyl, nitrous oxide, and barbituates is an alternative that interferes minimally with SEP recording, although bolus injections of narcotics produce transient SEP latency shifts in some patients.

For interpretation of the intraoperative SEP, attention is focused on the prominent negative component occurring at approximately 20 msec absolute latency (N20) in the C_c'–Fp_z derivation. This waveform is presumed to be generated by the underlying somatosensory cortex and thus demonstrates an intact somatosensory pathway. A broad negativity with a similar latency is seen on the C_c'–NCR derivation. This waveform is labeled N18 and is subcortically generated.[6, 21] The exact site of its generation is unknown, but it is assumed to arise in brain-stem structures such that it may not be sensitive to midbrain or thalamic compromise. The N18 may be minimally affected when the N20 is obliterated by a midbrain lesion. Thus, the N20, although more affected by anesthetic agents, serves as the primary focus of interpretation of the intraoperative SEP.

We empirically have used a 1 msec shift of N20 latency or 50 per cent loss of amplitude as evidence of significant change. Unfortunately, the clinical experience with SEP changes during posterior fossa surgical procedures is very limited. Initial reports during basilar artery aneurysm surgery have been unimpressive with a high incidence of false-negative results.[8, 17] Experience is too limited in posterior fossa tumor procedures to offer an adequate assessment of its clinical utility.

CONCLUSIONS

Extensive clinical experience has demonstrated that intraoperative BAEPs are a reliable method of monitoring auditory nerve and brain-stem function during posterior fossa surgery. With faster rates of stimulation, minute-to-minute assessment of auditory function is possible. Supplementation of the BAEP response with direct eighth-nerve recordings may further improve the rapidity with which eighth-nerve compromise can be identified. BAEPs are sensitive only to auditory nerve and pontine dysfunction; significant midbrain or medullary injury can occur without significant change in BAEPs. The addition of median nerve SEPs to posterior fossa surgical procedures may identify these injuries, although clinical experience with this technique is limited.

Intraoperative BAEPs are extremely sensitive to possible neurophysiologic compromise, and the identification of BAEP changes far exceeds the expected incidence of postoperative complications. However, the loss of the later BAEP waveforms should serve as an indication for adjustment of the surgical approach in an attempt to preserve hearing. Similarly, a moderate latency shift (for example, greater than 1.0 msec) particularly if rapid and associated with cerebellar retraction or dissection near the eighth nerve, should be addressed and corrected. Adjustment of the surgical approach routinely leads to an improvement in the BAEP response and potentially avoids irreversible injury to brain-stem or auditory function. Fortunately, the incidence of false-negative BAEP results has been extremely rare.

With the recent demonstration of a significant decline in postoperative auditory morbidity with the use of intraoperative BAEPs, arguments for its use in many posterior fossa procedures (particularly those focusing on the cerebellopontine angle) have been strengthened. Additional clinical experience and refinements of the technique should further improve its reliability and its effectiveness in decreasing operative complications in a number of clinical settings.

REFERENCES

1. Abramson M, Stein BM, Pedley TA, et al: Intraoperative BAER Monitoring and hearing preservation in the treatment of acoustic neuromas. Laryngoscope 95:1318–1322, 1985
2. Allen A, Starr A, Nudleman K: Assessment of sensory function in the operating room utilizing cerebral evoked potentials: A study of fifty-six surgically anesthetized patients. Clin Neurosurg 28:457–481, 1981

3. Andoh A: An experimental study on the surgical vulnerability of the auditory tract. Neurol Med Chir (Tokyo) 25:787–92, 1985
4. Boston JR, Deneault LG, Kronk L, et al: Automated monitoring of BAEPs in the operating room. J Clin Monit 1:161–167, 1985
5. Bursick DM, Vries JK, Sclabussi RJ, et al: Intraoperative BAEPs as adjunct to posterior fossa surgery in children. In Nadar RM, Barber C (eds): International Evoked Potentials Symposium. 1982, pp 565–571
6. Desmedt JE, Chevon G: Noncephalic reference recording of early somatosensory potentials to finger stimulation in adult or aging man: Differentiation of widespread N18 and contralateral N20 from the pre-rolandic P22 and N30 components. Electroencephalogr Clin Neurophys 52:553–570, 1981
7. Erwin CW, Gulevich SJ: Evaluation of transducers for obtaining intra-operative short-latency auditory evoked potentials. Electroencephalogr Clin Neurophysiol 61:194–196, 1985
8. Friedman WA, Kaplan BL, Day AL, et al: Evoked potential monitoring during aneurysm operation: Observations after fifty cases. Neurosurg 20:678–687, 1987
9. Friedman WA, Kaplan BJ, Gravenstein D, et al: Intraoperative brainstem auditory evoked potentials during posterior fossa microvascular decompression. J Neurosurg 62:552–557, 1985
10. Grundy BL, Janetta PJ, Procopio PT, et al: Intraoperative monitoring of brainstem auditory evoked potentials. J Neurosurg 57:556–575, 1982
11. Hahn JF, Latchan VP: Evoked potentials in the operating room. Clin Neurosurg 31:389–403, 1983
12. Hashimoto I, Ishiyama Y, Totsuka G, et al: Monitoring brainstem function during posterior fossa surgery with brainstem auditory evoked potentials. In Barber C (ed): Evoked Potentials. Lancaster, England, MTP Press, 1980, pp 377–390
13. Jacobson GP, Tew JM: Intra-operative Evoked Potential Monitoring. J Clin Neurophysiol 4(2):146–176, 1987
14. Jannetta PJ, Møller AR, Møller MB: Technique of hearing preservation in small acoustic neuromas. Ann Surg 200:513–523, 1984
15. Levine RA, Montgomery WW, Ojemann RG, et al: Monitoring auditory evoked potentials during acoustic neuroma surgery: Insights into the mechanism of the hearing loss. Ann Otol Rhinol Laryngol 93:116–23, 1984
16. Levine RA, Montgomery WW, Ojemann RG, et al: Evoked potential detection of hearing loss during acoustic neuroma surgery. Neurology 28:339, 1978
17. Little JR, Lesser RP, Luders H: Electrophysiological monitoring during basilar aneurysm operation. Neurosurgery 20:421–427, 1987
18. Little JR, Lesser RP, Luders H, et al: Brainstem auditory evoked potentials in posterior circulation surgery. Neurosurgery 12:496–502, 1983
19. Luders H: Surgical Monitoring with Auditory Evoked Potentials. New York, American Academy of Neurology Evoked Potential Course, 1987
20. McDaniel AB, Silverstein H, Norrell H: Retrolabyrinthine vestibular neurectomy with and without monitoring of eighth nerve potentials. Am J Otol (suppl):23–26, 1985
21. Mauguiere F, Desmedt JE, Courjon J: Neural generators of N18 and P14 far-field somatosensory evoked potentials studied in patients with lesions of the thalamus or thalamo-cortical radiations. Electroencephalogr Clin Neurophysiol 56:283–292, 1983
22. Møller AR: Evoked Potentials in Intraoperative Monitoring. Baltimore, Williams and Wilkens, 1988, pp 27–67
23. Møller AR, Jannetta PJ: Monitoring auditory functions during cranial nerve microvascular decompression operations by direct recording from the eighth nerve. J Neurosurg 59:493–499, 1983
24. Møller AR, Jannetta PJ: Monitoring auditory nerve potentials during operations in the cerebellopontine angle. Otolaryngol Head Neck Surg 92:434–439, 1984
25. Nuwer M: Evoked Potential Monitoring in the Operating Room. New York, Raven Press, 1986, pp 149–171
26. Ojemann RG, Levine RA, Montgomery WM, et al: Use of intraoperative auditory evoked potentials to preserve hearing in unilateral acoustic neuroma removal. J Neurosurg 61:938–948, 1984
27. Piatt JH, Radtke RA, Erwin CW: Limitations of brainstem auditory evoked potentials for intra-operative monitoring of posterior fossa surgery. Neurosurg 16:818–821, 1985

28. Piatt JH, Wilkins RH: Treatment of tic douloureux and hemifacial spasm by posterior fossa exploration: Therapeutic implications of various neurovascular relations. Neurosurg 14:462–471, 1984
29. Radtke RA, Erwin CW, Wilkins, RH: Intraoperative BAEPs: Significant decrease in postoperative auditory deficit. Neurology, in press, 1988
30. Radtke RA, Erwin CW, Wilkins RH, et al: Interoperative brainstem auditory evoked potentials (BAEPs): Significant decrease in post-operative auditory deficit. Neurology 37(suppl 1):219, 1987
31. Raudzens PA, Shetter AG: Intraoperative monitoring of brainstem auditory evoked potentials. J Neurosurg 57:341–348, 1982
32. Sabin HI, Bentivoglio P, Symon L, et al: Intraoperative electrocochleography to monitor cochlear potentials during acoustic neuroma excision. Acta Neurochir 85:110–116, 1987
33. Sanders RA, Duncan PG, McCullough JW: Clinical experience with brainstem audiometry performed under general anesthesia. J Otolaryngol, 8:24–31, 1979
34. Sekiya T, Iwabuchi T, Andoh A, et al: Changes of the auditory system after cerebello-pontine angle manipulations. Neurosurg 12:80–85, 1983
35. Sekiya T, Iwabuchi T, Kamata S, et al: Changes of auditory evoked potentials during cerebello-pontine angle manipulations. J Neurosurg 63:598–607, 1983
36. Sekiya T, Møller AR: Effects of cerebellar retraction on the cochlear nerve: An experimental study on rhesus monkeys. Acta Neurochir 90:45–52, 1988
37. Silverstein H, McDaniel AB, Norrell H: Hearing preservation after acoustic neuroma surgery using intraoperative direct eighth cranial nerve monitoring. Am J Otol (suppl):99–106, 1985
38. Stockard JJ, Rossiter JS, Jones TA, et al: Effects of centrally acting drugs on BAEPs. Electroencephalogr Clin Neurophysiol 43:550–551, 1977

Division of Neurology
Box 2905
Duke University Medical Center
Durham, North Carolina 27710

Use of Peripheral Nerve Action Potentials for Intraoperative Monitoring

Kevin R. Nelson, MD*

Intraoperative evoked potentials have become a standard of practice for many surgical procedures.[43] Most commonly, central sensory pathways are monitored during spinal surgery, allowing the surgeon to quickly detect and correct spinal cord dysfunction that may occur during the procedure.

Neurophysiologic monitoring during cranial and peripheral nerve surgery has been practiced for several years. The trigeminal,[64] facial,[50] and acoustic nerves[38–40, 50, 55] have been monitored with scalp-recorded evoked potentials or nerve action potentials from electrodes directly on the nerves.[11, 71, 73] In addition, electrodes can be inserted in facial muscles to record the neurotonic discharges that indicate mechanical stimulation of the nerve caused by surgical manipulation.[16]

Intraoperative scalp somatosensory recording is of value for detection of nerve root avulsion,[31, 60, 61] brachial plexus lesions,[42] plexus injury from surgical posturing,[35] or sciatic nerve injury from leg manipulation during hip arthroplasty.[59] Motor cerebral cortex has been stimulated and potentials recorded from the brachial plexus in the evaluation of plexus injuries.[29] Stimulation of the surgically exposed ulnar nerve has isolated lesions at the elbow by recording compound motor and sensory action potentials from skin surface electrodes.[6, 37]

This article confines itself to the assessment of peripheral nerve injuries with intraoperative nerve action potentials (INAP) recorded by electrodes placed directly on the nerve. Principles of peripheral nerve injury, as well as the clinical use and recording techniques of INAP, are discussed.

PATHOLOGIC AND PHYSIOLOGIC BASES OF PERIPHERAL NERVE INJURY

A peripheral nerve can be traumatized by compression, laceration, streching, ischemia, or a combination of factors (for example, gunshot

*Assistant Professor of Neurology, and Director, Electromyography Laboratory, University of Kentucky, Lexington, Kentucky

wounds). Most investigations have used the classification proposed by Seddon[53, 54] and modified by Sunderland.[63]

Neuropraxia results from a focal conduction block without structural changes in the axon. This may be metabolic (for example, ischemic) or associated with intussusception of myelin and nodal demyelination.[46] This conduction block is reversible over days to weeks and is usually not accompanied by signs of denervation in distal tissues.

Axonotmesis is characterized by disruption of axons but with preserved endoneurium. Axonal injury produces Wallerian degeneration and denervation. Recovery depends on nerve regeneration with axonal sprouts traveling approximately 1 to 2 mm per day.[5, 69]

Neurotmesis involves injury to both axons and connective tissue elements. Sunderland divides this further by the degree of connective tissue disruption. Third-degree injuries occur when fasicular structure is maintained with damage to endoneurial architecture. In fourth-degree injuries, the overall nerve integrity is maintained, but the perineurium is disturbed; the entire nerve and epineurium is disrupted with fifth-degree injuries.

Several factors are important to neural recovery. With failed reinnervation, a slow loss of axons proximal to the injury may occur[58, 63] and would emphasize the importance of early treatment. In contrast, others have observed conduction for several months in nerve fibers proximal to axonal transection in animals.[9] If the basal lamina is intact, Schwann cells align to form tubes and direct the regeneration of axonal sprouts.[15, 58] Reactive fibrosis imposes an important barrier to regeneration, particularly in stretch injuries where the fibrosis may extend for a considerable distance. Regeneration will obviously be impeded if the transected ends of a nerve are not apposed.

Following axonal injury, conduction velocity proximal to the injury site is reduced to 60 per cent to 70 per cent of normal,[8] whereas the distal response disappears in 4 to 5 days.[13] As the nerve regenerates, the initial axonal sprouts are devoid of myelin and may be similar to demyelinated fibers that do not utilize saltatory conduction.[4] With remyelination, the myelin sheath is thinner and the internodal distance shorter.[51] The conduction velocity in axons distal to the injury remains below normal.[2, 5, 7, 65]

A neuroma incontinuity develops when the epineurium remains intact yet there is intraneuronal fibrosis intermixed with axons that are often misdirected. This neuroma is considered to be a major barrier to axons attempting to course their way to the end organ[52, 58] and is a source of ectopic discharges.[36]

Many issues on the surgical repair of peripheral nerve injuries are not agreed on, yet several management principles are uniform. If the neuroma contains regenerating axons, then an external neurolysis is performed whereby the nerve is longitudinally incised and the scar tissue encasing the nerve dissected away. This is believed to reduce high intraneuronal pressure, improve blood flow, and alleviate the physical barriers of regeneration. Internal neurolysis consists of tracing the fasicles through the injury site and surgically releasing them.

If no functioning axons cross the injury site, the nerve ends are trimmed and sutured, or an intervening graft is placed if the ends cannot be apposed. A primary repair is done only on nerves acutely and "cleanly" transected.

Frequently the clinical evaluation or conventional electromyography/ nerve conduction studies (EMG/NCS) do not detect axons that have regenerated and crossed the injury site for a few millimeters or centimeters without reinnervating distal tissues. For neuromas, visual inspection and palpation at the time of surgery cannot reliably determine the extent of intraneurial connective tissue[53] and whether the neuroma contains axons. Intraneuronal saline injections have been used to separate fasicles and improve examination during surgery. These injections acutely reduce the nerve's response to stimulation[20] and likely cause demyelination[10] in a region that has already sustained injury.

These methods alone usually do not detect regenerating axons crossing an injury before profound changes have occurred in distal denervated tissues. Early in the patient's course, INAP recording determines if an injury contains regenerating axons. If an INAP demonstrates regenerating axons, then a neurolysis is undertaken. An absent INAP indicates that no viable nervous tissue is present, and resection of the neuroma with suture or graft repair is often performed.

CLINICAL ASPECTS OF INTRAOPERATIVE NERVE ACTION POTENTIALS

INAP recording identifies functional neuronal elements within both neuromas and peripheral nerve tumors. Since the initial report on INAP by Kline,[23] several centers have advocated the use INAP in the management of peripheral nerve injuries.[17, 19, 24, 67, 71] A neurolysis was performed on neural elements with an INAP response. Resection with graft or suture was undertaken in those nerves with an absent INAP, or when the INAP was judged inadequate.[71] Recording techniques have varied considerably and there has been disagreement on what INAP parameters qualify a neural element for neurolysis or resection.[28, 70] In several investigations, Kline has used a nonaveraged INAP and feels that an absent response indicates the nerve lacks the number of axons required for clinically significant recovery.[23, 28] With his techniques, amplitudes of fewer than 20 μV are considered unreliable yet would indicate neurolysis.[28]

Van Beek and colleagues[71] studied 14 patients with INAP: 4 with brachial plexus and 10 with various single peripheral nerve injuries. Signal averaging was used. When present, amplitudes of INAP ranged from 5 to 63 μV. Although these authors felt that absolute neurophysiologic criteria were lacking, a neurolysis was performed when the INAP amplitude exceeded 40 μV. Four patients had resection with a recordable INAP whose amplitude was below 40 μV. Clinical results were not given. In another four patients, the INAP amplitude altered surgical treatment. Two patients underwent neurolysis instead of resection (INAP amplitudes of 45 and 63 μV); another two with an absent INAP received grafts rather than neurolysis. Follow-up was limited; in one case primitive sensation returned to the hand of a grafted median nerve. Conduction velocity below 30 m/sec was believed to represent an unfavorable sign because the nerve was felt to contain predominately small nonmotor axons. The method of conduction velocity calculation was not described, nor were values stated.

Kline and Judice[26] have reported the most complete analysis of INAP with detailed clinical evaluation and prolonged follow-up. One hundred seventy-one consecutive patients with brachial plexus lesions were studied over a 12-year period. Each patient received at least 1½ years of follow-up that included muscle strength grading. A total of 438 neural elements were evaluated with INAP. Nearly all patients underwent surgery less than 6 months following their injury. Those injuries sustained by patients consisted of stretch (60), gunshot (46), tumor (23), iatrogenic (18), and lacerations with continuity (8) or without (16). Conventional EMG/NCS was carried out in over 95 per cent of cases, and histologic examination was performed on all tissue resected because of an absent INAP. Data analysis was based on injury type and whether the injury was clinically complete or incomplete. Neurophysiologic data reported were limited to the presence or absence of INAP. If an INAP were recorded, a neurolysis was performed. An absent INAP dictated element resection followed by end-to-end suture or grafting. Recovery was judged adequate if a proximal muscle innervated by that element contracted against gravity and some resistance, and a distal muscle contracted against gravity.

In this study, INAP was the most effective means of detecting axons crossing the injury site that were capable of clinically significant regeneration. This was best evaluated in clinically complete injuries by comparing INAP to EMG/NCS and intraoperative visualization of the motor response to nerve stimulation. Particularly for completely injured elements, the decision between neurolysis or resection is most critical.

Of the 96 clinically complete gunshot wounds (GSW), 37 elements had an INAP. In these 37, 32 elements were treated with neurolysis and 31 recovered. Fifty-five elements underwent resection, and 29 recovered. Eight clinically complete elements had EMG/NCS evidence of an incomplete lesion. Whether these eight had an INAP recorded is not stated. A minimum of 29 elements had a INAP present yet a complete lesion on EMG/NCS; 13 had no visually observable motor response to intraoperative nerve stimulation.

One hundred and fourteen elements with a clinically complete stretch injury were studied. Thirty-one had an INAP recorded of which 26 responded to neurolysis; 27 of 55 with an absent INAP recovered after resection. Only three elements had an EMG/NCS incomplete lesion, and at least 18 patients with an INAP present had a complete injury by both EMG/NCS and observation of motor response to intraoperative stimulation. This again confirms the sensitivity of INAP for detecting axons crossing the injury site.

Clinically complete laceration injuries and those of iatrogenic etiology were combined. Thirty-two of 33 were complete by EMG/NCS, and 30 of 35 by intraoperative observation of motor response after nerve stimulation. In contrast, 11 of 35 had an INAP present. In the total 35 elements, all nine treated with neurolysis recovered as did 12 of 16 with resection.

The value of INAP over conventional EMG/NCS was also shown in a previous study by Kline[22] where eight patients with injury to nerves of the lower extremities had a recordable INAP with a complete lesion by clinical and EMG/NCS examination. All were "improved" with neurolysis. No element had an absent INAP with an incomplete EMG/NCS injury.

The acceptance of INAP superiority for detecting regenerating axons crossing the injury is founded on clinical outcome, and assumes that resection (which was dictated by an absent INAP) does not adversely affect outcome compared with neurolysis. A controlled study is lacking. It is clear that those elements with a recordable INAP are less severely injured. In an earlier investigation that combined injuries to the brachial plexus and large nerves of the arms and legs,[27] Kline reported three patients who underwent nerve resection despite the presence of an INAP. Histologic examination showed that the neuroma contained large numbers of axons in marked contrast to the specimens from the 89 patients who lacked an INAP response. This agrees with a primate study that found that INAP amplitude directly correlated with the number of axons within the neuroma.[25]

The INAP was important in determining the prognosis of clinically complete lesions by injury location. On the basis of the data published, combined lower plexus injuries (roots to lower trunk, medial cord) can be compared with combined upper plexus injuries (roots to upper and middle trunks, lateral and posterior cords). With a present INAP, 24 of 25 upper plexus lesions responded to neurolysis as did 8 of 9 lower plexus injuries. In contradistinction, 17 of 45 upper plexus elements without an INAP recovered following resection, but none of the 12 lower plexus injuries recovered. It is unlikely that resection itself is responsible for this difference. Thus, an absence of lower plexus axons detected by INAP indicates a poor prognosis. In addition, a recordable INAP reflects regenerating axons that are clinically important and with this measure are independent of the distance to target tissues. Whether the degree of recovery is influenced by distance was not addressed by this or any other investigation.

In the evaluation of incompletely injured neural elements, INAP, EMG/NCS, and intraoperative motor observation are similar in the ability to detect axons crossing the injury site.

Of the 38 elements with a clinically incomplete GSW, 35 had an INAP present and all responded to neurolysis. In the 38, one element had a complete lesion on EMG/NCS and three a complete lesion on intraoperative motor observation. The three elements with an absent INAP also had no visible motor response to intraoperative nerve stimulation; and all three achieved recovery following resection and suture repair (two lateral cord to median nerve, one medial cord to median nerve). One of these three elements had EMG/NCS evidence of incomplete injury, and another had a complete EMG/NCS lesion.

Thirty-four elements had incomplete stretch injuries; all had an INAP response. Three patients had complete lesions by EMG/NCS and three by intraoperative motor observation. Thirty-two responded to neurolysis, and the two that did not respond had incomplete lesions by EMG/NCS and intraoperative observation.

No attempt was made to correlate clinical recovery to INAP parameters

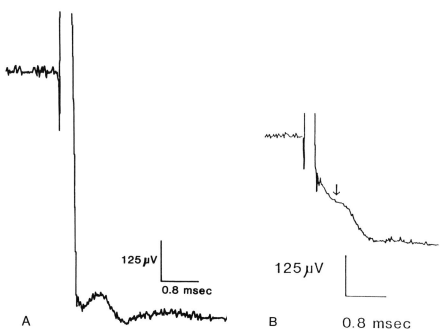

Figure 1. INAP obtained during resection of posterior tibial neurofibroma. *A*, INAP prior to resection. *B*, INAP recorded distal to the neuroma after stimulation of a single fascicle compressed by the tumor. Arrow denotes onset of INAP superimposed on the tail of shock artifact.

(for example, amplitude) in either complete or incomplete injuries. Kline and Judice also believed that the INAP was also of value in the resection of brachial plexus tumors. When INAP identified intact fascicles, efforts were made to preserve that fascicle, especially if the tumor was not malignant (Fig. 1). A fascicle was sacrificed with benign neurofibromas if no INAP was recorded. No consideration was given for compression producing an absent INAP by a neuropraxic injury.

Some surgeons have advocated perineurial rather than epineural repair of nerves. This controversy has been reviewed elsewhere.[48] For perineural suturing, sensory and motor fascicles must be identified for alignment. Single fascicles can be stimulated and recordings obtained directly from fascicles,[73] or surface electrodes placed over sensory branches (for example, superficial radial) or muscle.

TECHNIQUE OF INTRAOPERATIVE NERVE ACTION POTENTIAL RECORDING

For most procedures, neurophysiologic surgical monitoring must provide rapid and reliable data on neural structures at risk. Stimulation and recording sites are usually outside the surgical field to limit the mutual interference between the surgeon and monitoring. In contrast, INAP demands that stimulation and recording involve neural elements within the

STIMULATE   RECORD

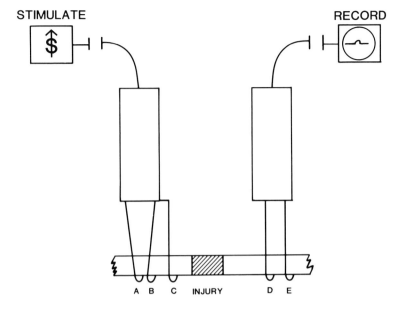

Figure 2. Representation of INAP recording technique
A-Stimulating anode
B-Stimulating cathode
C-Patient ground isolated from stimulus
D-Recording G_1
E-Recording G_2

surgical site and the surgeon take an active neurophysiologic role. The operative procedure is directly altered by efforts to obtain an INAP recording, and the INAP response usually determines if neurolysis or resection is undertaken.

To record an INAP, bipolar stimulating electrodes are placed proximally and the cathode nearest the injury (Fig. 2). A response is obtained by distal recording electrodes, with G_1 oriented toward the stimulating cathode. Because most neural elements contain both motor and sensory fibers, the INAP is neither exclusively orthodromic nor antidromic.

Preparation

The clinical neurophysiologist should be in the operating suite as the patient is positioned. This allows placement of ground electrodes at distant sites as well as surface sensory or motor electrodes. More important, the recording equipment may be located to ensure the clinical neurophysiologist a clear view of the operative field. This view enables the neurophysiologist to make certain that the surgeon has applied the electrodes to the nerve correctly, to troubleshoot in the event of an inadequate response or artifact interference, and to observe a clinical motor response after stimulation of the nerve. As the patient is prepared for surgery, anesthetic monitoring, surgical equipment (for example, a microscope), and scrub nurse all cluster

around the operating table and may prevent proper positioning of neurophysiologic monitoring equipment. Placement of other equipment and
personnel is often less critical.

The limb should be safely immobilized in the event a powerful
contraction ensues, yet the extremity must be visible so a clinical response
can be observed. Specific posture depends on the particular nerve being
studied and the location of injury.

Adequate exposure of the nerve is fundamentally important, and often
this requires a more extensive exposure than when an INAP is not recorded.
A minimum of 5 cm is necessary between stimulating and recording
electrodes, and often greater separation is desirable. It is imperative that
electrodes lift the nerve free from the surrounding tissue and fluid. Blood
(and cerebrospinal fluid if present) is irrigated away from the electrodes,
and the nerve is maintained moist.

Surgeons wish to complete their task with a minimum of interference
and in a timely fashion. Preoperative equipment checks are mandatory.
Kline and colleagues[24] has advocated that the recording electrodes be
initially placed just above the injury so that it can be determined if axons
are reaching the injury site and the recording equipment is functioning
properly. For surgeons or assistants unfamiliar with INAP procedure, a
diagram (similar to Fig. 2) may facilitate proper electrode orientation.

Instrumentation

The differential amplifier for INAP should have high-input impedance
and good common mode rejection[18] as required for recording other low-
amplitude biologic signals. Rapid recovery amplifiers[72] are particularly
helpful in suppressing the frequent problem of shock artifact. Signal storage
is necessary so that a detailed waveform analysis can be undertaken.
Whether signal averaging detects axons capable of regeneration is dis-
puted.[28, 70] Most modern amplifiers have the capacity of signal averaging.
Unlike others,[19, 24, 68, 71] a standard EMG instrument is utilized at the
University of Kentucky: TE-42 unit (TECA Corp., Pleasantville, New
York).

Investigators have used different filter bandpasses. Kline and
colleagues[24, 26] as well as Van Beek and colleagues[71] have utilized the narrow
bandpass of 300 Hz and 3 kHz. More open bandpasses of 20 Hz and 20
kHz were reported by Terzis and Publicover[68] as well as Kaplan and co-
workers,[19] who employed 0.1 Hz and 30 kHz. At the University of Kentucky,
a bandpass of 16 Hz and 16 kHz is used that is similar to routine clinical
motor conduction studies and nerve action potential recordings from animals
under experimental conditions.[9] If shock artifact is unusually troublesome,
the high bandpass filter (low-frequency cutoff) can be raised to avoid higher
capacitance and slower discharge times of the resistance/capacitance filter.

Selection of amplifier gain depends on the amplitude of the response
recorded, and should allow the waveform to be at least 1 cm in height.
Typically, gains of 20 to 1000 μV/cm are utilized. Most investigators have
not given amplitudes recorded from normal neural elements or those
containing neuromas.[26, 73] The element in question may be compared with
another felt to be unaffected.[73] Van Beek and colleagues[71] reported the

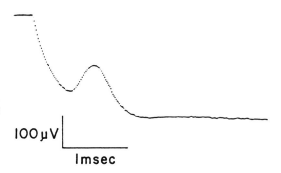

Figure 3. Posterior tibial INAP. The lesion was shrapnel injury with previous neurolysis. Conventional NCS studies revealed an absent response with stimulation above the injury and recording from abductor hallicus.

following INAP amplitudes (microvolts) in 8 neuromas: ulnar-45,60,63; median-20,63; peroneal-5(3). In elements felt to be normal, amplitudes ranged from 0.5 to 2.0 mV. These values are in agreement with those obtained with our techniques that typically do not use signal averaging (Fig. 3). Of interest, Lambert and Dyck[30] have shown that with monopolar in vitro recordings of the sural nerve, amplitudes recording from whole nerve or fascicles are similar. They state that amplitude depends on density of axons. This has obvious implications for neuromas that contain variable degrees of fibrosis so the amplitude of the INAP may not directly reflect the number of axons depolarizing at the recording electrode.

Time base depends on the distance between stimulation and recording electrodes (Fig. 4). A neural element may conduct up to 100 m/sec and would appear 0.5 msec following stimulation if the distance between stimulating and recording electrodes were 5 cm. For most applications, a time base of 0.5 msec per cm (sweep duration of 5 msec) is necessary to separate the INAP response from stimulus artifact and reliably measure the latency of waveform onset. A time base of 1 msec per cm is acceptable with greater separation between stimulating and recording electrodes.

Electrodes

INAP electrodes are not commercially available and must be custom-made. Details on materials and construction are provided in the Appendix. There are several practical considerations in electrode design.

Although some investigators have used stainless steel wire as the stimulating or recording surface,[19, 21, 71] platinum-iridium is recommended. Stimulating electrodes polarize, causing electrolysis and subsequent release of toxic heavy metals into the surrounding tissues.[33] This is particularly true when repetitive stimulation is delivered, and with such metals as silver. For most large nerves (for example, radial, posterior tibial), 18ga wire is of sufficient strength and size. Mounted electroencephalographic needle electrodes (Grass Instrument Co, Quincy, Massachusetts) work well for delicate neural elements (Fig. 5). The wire is hook-shaped so the nerve can be cradled by the electrode. Specific configuration is dictated by the electrode's function. Stimulating anode and cathode are mounted closely together to limit current spread and reduce shock artifact. A hooked ground may be placed just distal to the cathode, situating the ground between stimulation

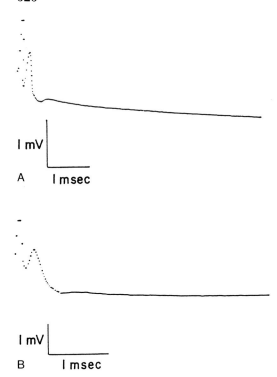

Figure 4. Contusion isolated to the axillary nerve 4 months before INAP recording. Clinical and EMG examination revealed no voluntary activity in the deltoid. INAP is recorded from the axillary nerve after stimulation of the posterior cord of the brachial plexus. Postoperative recovery time was too brief to determine whether the INAP represents regenerating axons or whether the INAP was recorded proximal to the nerve injury. *A*, Time base of 1 msec per cm. Shock artifact obscures INAP. *B*, Time base of 0.5 msec/cm.

and recording electrodes. Occasionally, a stimulation probe cathode is used (G in Fig. 5), with an anode plate or hook as close as possible to the cathode to limit current spread.

Recording electrodes are similar to those used for stimulation. There is greater distance between G_1 (active electrode) and G_2 (reference electrode) than stimulating anode/cathode. This greater separation enhances amplitude in bipolar recordings. Whether recordings are monopolar or bipolar can be difficult to determine. Of the axons that cross the G_1 site, a variable number will reach the more distal G_2. If axons terminate between G_1 and G_2, what appears to be a bipolar recording may in fact be monopolar. This condition is similar to the crush preparations used in experimental animal techniques.[34, 57] Gradually moving the recording electrodes distally until a response is no longer present may give an approximation of where axons terminate.

Electrode handles must allow easy manipulation to facilitate placement and minimize trauma to the nerve. Electrodes can be hand-held, and the mechanical manipulators used by some[73] are not necessary. Handles as well as electrode leads are color-coded. This enables proper alignment and rapid differentiation between stimulating anode/cathode and recording G_1/G_2.

Stimulation

Either constant voltage or constant current stimulation can be used. We utilize the constant voltage stimulator provided with the clinical EMG/NCS instrument. Intraoperative supramaximal stimulation requires much

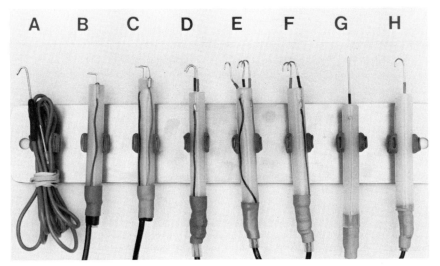

Figure 5. Electrode array used for INAP recording. Holder is sterilized with electrodes in place. Towel clips on each end secure holder near the recording site.
A-Hooked ground. Situated directly on the nerve or in adjacent tissues.
B-Fine recording electrodes for small neural elements.
C-Fine bipolar stimulating electrodes with ground.
D-Bipolar recording electrodes
E-Bipolar stimulating electrodes (bent toward each other) with ground
F-Bipolar stimulating electrodes
G-Monopolar stimulating probe (cathode)
H-Monopolar hook stimulating electrode (anode)

less current density than routine nerve conduction studies. This is attributed to reduced resistance for direct nerve stimulation because intervening tissue and fluid are absent. Supramaximal stimulation is reached at fewer than 75V (usually 25 to 50V), with a stimulus duration of 0.05 msec. Stimulation is usually triggered manually to allow adequate analysis, although rates of 0.5 to 1 Hz are sometimes used for frequent waveform acquisition and monitoring.

Other Technical Considerations

The operating suite is a hostile environment for recording INAPs. There are many potential sources of radiated 60 Hz line frequency artifact. A few of the more common include blood and blanket warmers, anesthetic equipment, microscope, and operating lights. The clinical neurophysiologist must be vigilant for sources of 60 Hz interference. It is best detected when the time base is increased to 10 msec per cm, and may be obscured with the shorter sweep durations used for INAP acquisition. Identification and elimination of the artifact source is the best solution. The use of short recording leads (50 cm or less) with the preamplifier near the recording electrodes is helpful. Driven shielded cables may also reduce interference.[18]

Ground currents may develop within ground loops when recording instruments grounded to the patient are also connected to widely spaced outlet grounds. Such ground current will produce line frequency interference.

Because the surgeon is actively participating in the recording procedure, cautery interference is not a problem as it can be with other types of neurophysiologic monitoring.

After a nerve is stimulated, muscles may contract if axons through the injury are preserved or if the nerve branches between stimulation and lesion. Muscle contraction can also be caused by failure to elevate the stimulating electrodes from surrounding tissues, or stimulus current can spread to other physically close neural elements. A large compound muscle action potential will volume conduct to the recording site and obscure a smaller INAP. Repositioning the stimulating electrodes, reducing stimulus intensity, or neuromuscular blockade will resolve the difficulty.

Shock artifact is a frequent problem. This occurs when stimulus current reaches the recording electrodes either by volume conduction or ground currents. Often the stimulus artifact overloads the amplifier, or the stimulus duration may extend to the recorded response (see Figs. 1 and 4). Several maneuvers will reduce the magnitude of the problem: Using the lowest stimulus intensity that evokes a supramaximal response, short stimulus durations (0.05 msec), stimulus units isolated from patient ground, and proper bandpass. Lifting the nerve from surrounding tissue and irrigation of blood and fluid limits stimulus spread to the recording electrodes. Overlap of stimulating and recording cables should be avoided. A low-resistive patient ground between stimulating and recording sites reduces shock artifact by creating an intervening isopotential field. Lengthening the distance between stimulating and recording electrodes will usually help because there is a steep drop-off in stimulus current with distance. Reorienting the stimulating and recording electrodes can also be of value. G_1 is maintained on the nerve and G_2 is placed in adjacent tissues so that the G_1/G_2 axis is perpendicular to the stimulating cathode/anode axis. This monopolar recording minimizes the difference in stimulus current between G_1 and G_2.

Technical aspects unique to the surgical procedure may obscure an INAP response. Unknowingly to the neurophysiologist, the anesthesiologist may administer neuromuscular blockade drugs that prevent a clinically observable motor response. The surgeon may apply a tourniquet to produce a bloodless field. The nerve will become ischemic with reversible loss of the INAP. Kline[21] recommends tourniquet release for 15 to 20 min before recording. Unlike cortically recorded evoked potentials, anesthetic depression of INAP does not occur.

Once an INAP is obtained, some have suggested that a conduction velocity be calculated,[67, 71, 73] although it is uncertain if this conduction velocity was used to make a surgical decision. We do not routinely calculate conduction velocity because measurement of distance is often cumbersome. Temperature in the elevated nerve is considerably less than the patient's core temperature, and nerve temperature cannot be easily controlled under these conditions.

SUMMARY

Following a physical injury to peripheral nerve, clinical evaluation and the use of conventional EMG/NCS is often unable to determine whether axons are crossing the site of injury before severe changes in distal tissues occur. The INAP recording identifies functional axons within neuromas before other signs of reinnervation have developed. In clinically complete lesions, recording an INAP across the injury indicates the presence of regenerating axons, and neurolysis of the encasing connective tissue is recommended. If an INAP is absent, resection of the dense neuroma is usually undertaken with end-to-end suture or graft. A present INAP indicates clinically significant regenerating axons even with large distances to target tissue. An absent INAP for injuries far from target tissue indicates a poor prognosis. In clinically incomplete lesions, INAP recording is of no value over the clinical examination and EMG/NCS. INAP can aid peripheral nerve tumor resection by identification of intact nerve fascicles.

INAP responses are obtained by placing platinum-iridium bipolar stimulating electrodes proximal to the injury. The INAP is then recorded by distal electrodes. A standard EMG/NCS instrument with an isolated stimulation unit can be used with the appropriate gain and time base settings. Stimulus intensity required for a supramaximal response is usually less than 75 V at 0.05 msec duration. Frequency bandpass is similar to that for conventional EMG/NCS studies. Electrodes must elevate the nerve during the recording. Artifact from 60 Hz line frequency and stimulus are common problems.

APPENDIX: ELECTRODE CONSTRUCTION

PETER BURBANK, CBET*

Materials†

1. Nylon rod, 5/16 in. diameter (McMaster-Carr Co, Chicago, Illinois; part #8538K15).
2. Polyolefin shrink tubing of ½ in. outside diameter, clear double wall preferred (Partsmasters, Inc., Dallas, Texas).
3. Platinum-iridium wire, 0.040 in. diameter (18ga) (supplied by local jeweler).
4. Belden low-noise instrumentation cable #9452 with graphite-cloth runner (supplied by local electronics distributor).

Methods

A 3½ in. length of rod is selected. The cable end of the rod is flattened for ½ in. with a belt sander to one half of the rod's original diameter. Burrs are then removed. A suitable length of cable (for example, 1.5 to 6 ft) is

---

*Biomedical Instrumentation, University of Kentucky, Lexington, Kentucky.
†Materials are supplied in English units of measurement.

stripped of the outer jacket to expose inner wires for 4 in. The inner wires are held along the length of the rod and the unstripped jacket is centered in the flattened area of the rod's cable end. To form a strain relief and anchor, a short ring of polyolefin tubing is shrunk around the cable and rod at the flattened area. The red and black inner wires are stretched along the rod and cut ¼ in. from the rod end. These wires are then soldered to 1½ in. platinum-iridium electrode wire tips. An excellent side-to-side solder joint can be made using Superior flux #30 (water rinse). The wire tips are fixed to the sides of the nylon rod with cyanoacrylate. A 3 in. length of polyolefin is shrunk over the rod and wires. Heat is applied from the electrode to cable end, moving slowly to avoid bubbles and assure melting of the inner tubing. The electrode wire is then bent to the desired shape with round-nose pliers and polished smooth.

Monopolar electrode holders have a hole centered in the rod's end to hold the electrode wire. This hole is met by a perpendicular side hole ⅜ in. from the electrode end. An endodontic barbed broach (#45) is used to round the junction of the end and side holes to facilitate insertion of the electrode wire. This wire is cemented in place and the cable connection soldered at the side of the rod. Polyolefin tubing is placed as previously described.

Electrodes are gas-sterilized.

ACKNOWLEDGMENT

The author expresses his deep appreciation to Lori Pederson for her valuable assistance in the preparation of this manuscript.

REFERENCES

1. Abramson M, Stein BM, Pedley TA, et al: Intraoperative BAER monitoring and hearing preservation in the treatment of acoustic neuromas. Laryngoscope 95:1318–1322, 1985
2. Ballantyne JP, Campbell MJ: Electrophysiological study after surgical repair of sectioned human peripheral nerves. J Neurol Neurosurg Psychiatry 36:797–805, 1973
3. Benecke JE Jr, Calder HB, Chadwick G: Facial nerve monitoring during acoustic neuroma removal. Laryngoscope 97:697–700, 1987
4. Bostock H, Sears TA: The internodal axon membrane: Electrical excitability and continuous conduction in segmental demyelination. J Physiol 280:273–301, 1978
5. Buchthal F, Kuhl V: Nerve conduction, tactile sensibility, and the electromyogram after suture or compression of peripheral nerve: A longitudinal study in man. J Neurol Neurosurg Psychiatry 42:436–451, 1979
6. Campbell WW, Sahni SK, Pridgeon RM, et al: Intraoperative electroneurography: Management of ulnar neuropathy at the elbow. Muscle Nerve 11:75–81, 1988
7. Cragg BG, Thomas PK: The conduction velocity of regenerated peripheral nerve fibres. J Physiol 171:164–175, 1964
8. Cragg BG, Thomas PK: Changes in conduction velocity and fibre size proximal to peripheral nerve lesions. J Physiol 157:315–327, 1961
9. Davis LA, Gordon T, Hoffer JA, et al: Compound action potentials recorded from mammalian peripheral nerves following ligation or resuturing. J Physiol 285:543–559, 1978
10. Dyck PJ, Lais AC, Hansen SM, et al: Technique assessment of demyelination from endoneurial injection. Exp Neurol 77:359–377, 1982
11. Friedman WA, Kaplan BJ, Gravenstein D, et al: Intraoperative brain-stem auditory

evoked potentials during posterior fossa microvascular decompression. J Neurosurg 62:552–557, 1985

12. Gantz BJ: Intraoperative facial nerve monitoring. Am J Otol (suppl):58–61, 1985

13. Gilliatt RW, Hjorth RJ: Nerve conduction during Wallerian degeneration in the baboon. J Neurol Neurosurg Psychiatry 35:335–341, 1972

14. Grundy BL, Jannetta PJ, Lina A, et al: Intraoperative monitoring of brainstem auditory evoked potentials. J Neurosurg 57:674–677, 1981

15. Haftek J, Thomas PK: Electron-microscope observations on the effects of localized crush injuries on the connective tissues of peripheral nerve. J Anat 103:233–243, 1968

16. Harner SG, Daube JR, Ebersold MJ: Electrophysiologic monitoring of facial nerve during temporal bone surgery. Laryngoscope 96:65–69, 1986

17. Hudson AR: Peripheral nerve surgery. In Dyck PJ, Thomas PK, Lambert EH (eds): Peripheral Neuropathy, 2nd ed. Philadelphia, W.B. Saunders, 1984, p 420

18. The International Federation of Societies for Electroencephalography and Clinical Neurophysiology: Recommendations for the Practice of Clinical Neurophysiology. Amsterdam, Elsevier, 1983

19. Kaplan BJ, Gravenstein D, Friedman WA: Intraoperative electrophysiology in treatment of peripheral nerve injuries. J Fla Med Assoc 71:400–403, 1984

20. Kline DG: Evaluation of the neuroma in continuity. In Omar G, Spinner M (eds): Management of Peripheral Nerve Problems. Philadelphia, W.B. Saunders, 1980, p 450

21. Kline DG: Physiological and clinical factors contributing to the timing of nerve repair. In Clinical Neurosurgery. Baltimore, Williams & Wilkins, 1977, p 425

22. Kline DG: Operative management of major nerve lesions of the lower extremity. Surg Clin North Am 52:1247–1265, 1972

23. Kline DG, Dejonge BR: Evoked potentials to evaluate peripheral nerve injury. Surg Gynec Obstet 127:1239–1248, 1968

24. Kline DG, Hackett ER: Management of the neuroma in continuity. In Wilkins RH, Rengachary SS (eds): Neurosurgery. New York, McGraw-Hill, 1985, p 1864

25. Kline DG, Hackett ER, May PR: Evaluation of nerve injuries by evoked potentials and electromyography. J Neurosurg 31:128–136, 1969

26. Kline DG, Judice DJ: Operative management of selected brachial plexus lesions. J Neurosurg 58:631–649, 1983

27. Kline DG, Nulsen FE: The neuroma in continuity. Its preoperative and operative management. Surg Clin North Am 52:1189–1209, 1972

28. Kline DG, Happel L, Hackett E, et al: Clinical use of nerve stimulation. Plast Reconstr Surg 75:764–765, 1985

29. Kondo M, Matsuda H, Miyawaki Y, et al: A new method of electrodiagnosis during operations on the brachial plexus and peripheral nerve injuries. The value of motor nerve action potentials evoked by trans-skull motor area stimulation. Int Orthop 9:115–121, 1985

30. Lambert EH, Dyck PJ: Compound action potentials of sural nerve in vitro in peripheral neuropathy. In Dyck PJ, Thomas PK, Lambert EH, et al (eds): Peripheral Neuropathy, 2nd ed. Philadelphia, W.B. Saunders, 1984, p 1030

31. Landi A, Copeland SA, Wynn Parry CB, et al: The role of somatosensory evoked potentials and nerve conduction studies in the surgical management of brachial plexus injuries. J Bone Joint Surg 62B:492–496, 1980

32. Levine RA, Ojemann RG, Montgomery WW, et al: Monitoring auditory evoked potentials during acoustic neuroma surgery: Insights into the mechanism of the hearing loss. Ann Otol Rhinol Laryngol 93:116–123, 1984

33. Loeb GE, Gans C: Electromyography for Experimentalists. Chicago, University of Chicago Press, 1986

34. Low PA, McLeod JG: Refractory period, conduction of trains of impulses, and effect of temperature on conduction in chronic hypertrophic neuropathy. J Neurol Neurosurg Psychiatry 40:434–447, 1977

35. Mahla ME, Long DM, McKennett J, et al: Detection of brachial plexus dysfunction by somatosensory evoked potential monitoring—A report of two cases. Anesthesiology 60:248–252, 1984

36. Meyer RA, Raja SN, Campbell JN, et al: Neural activity originating from a neuroma in the baboon. Brain Res 325:255–260, 1985

37. Miller RG: The cubital tunnel syndrome: Diagnosis and precise localization. Ann Neurol 6:56–59, 1979
38. Moller, AR, Janetta PJ: Microvascular decompression in hemifacial spasm: Intraoperative electrophysiological observations. Neurosurgery 16:612–618, 1985
39. Moller AR, Jannetta PJ: Monitoring auditory nerve potentials during operations in the cerebellopontine angle. Otolaryngol Head Neck Surg 92:434–439, 1984
40. Moller AR, Jannetta PJ: Monitoring auditory functions during cranial nerve microvascular decompression operations by direct recording from the eighth nerve. J Neurosurg 59:493–499, 1983
41. Nagano A, Tsuyama N, Hara T, et al: Brachial plexus injuries. Prognosis of postganglionic lesions. Arch Orthop Trauma Surg 102:172–178, 1984
42. Nashold BS, Ovelmen-Levitt J, Sharpe R, et al: Intraoperative evoked potentials recorded in man directly from dorsal roots and spinal cord. J Neurosurg 62:680–693, 1985
43. Nuwer, MR: Evoked potential monitoring in the operating room. New York, Raven Press, 1986
44. Piatt JH Jr, Radtke RA, Erwin CW: Limitations of brain stem auditory evoked potentials for intraoperative monitoring during a posterior fossa operation: Case report and technical note. Neurosurgery 16:818–821, 1985
45. Publicover NG, Terzis JK: Physiologic assessment of nerve injuries. In Terzis JK (ed): Microreconstruction of Nerve Injuries. Philadelphia, W.B. Saunders, 1987, p 83
46. Ochoa J, Fowler TJ, Gilliatt RW: Anatomical changes in peripheral nerves compressed by a pneumatic torniquet. J Anat 113:433–455, 1972
47. Ojemann RG, Levine RA, Montgomery WM, et al: Use of intraoperative auditory evoked potentials to preserve hearing in unilateral acoustic neuroma removal. J Neurosurg 61:938–948, 1984
48. Orgel MG: Epineurial versus perineurial repair of peripheral nerves. Clin Plastic Surg 11:101–104, 1984
49. Prass RL, Luders H: Acoustic (loudspeaker) facial electromyographic monitoring: Part 1. Evoked electromyographic activity during acoustic neuroma resection. Neurosurgery 19:392–400, 1986
50. Richmond IL, Mahla M: Use of antidromic recording to monitor facial nerve function intraoperatively. Neurosurgery 16:458–462, 1985
51. Saida K, Sumner AJ, Saida T, et al: Antiserum-mediated demyelination: Relationship between remyelination and functional recovery. Ann Neurol 8:12, 1980
52. Schaumburg HH, Spencer PS, Thomas PK: Disorders of Peripheral Nerves. Philadelphia, F.A. Davis Company, 1983, p 188
53. Seddon H: Surgical Disorders of the Peripheral Nerves, 2nd ed. Edinburgh, Churchill Livingston, 1975
54. Seddon HJ: Three types of nerve injury. Brain 66:237, 1943
55. Silverstein H, McDaniel AB, Norrell H: Hearing preservation after acoustic neuroma surgery using intraoperative direct eighth cranial nerve monitoring. Am J Otol (suppl):99–106, 1985
56. Silverstein H, McDaniel A, Wazen J, et al: Retrolabyrinthine vestibular neurectomy with simultaneous monitoring of eighth nerve and brain stem auditory evoked potentials. Otolaryngol Head Neck Surg 93:736–742, 1985
57. Smith KJ, Hall SM: Nerve conduction during peripheral demyelination and remyelination. J Neurol Sci 48:201–219, 1980
58. Spencer PS: The traumatic neuroma and proximal stump. Bull Hosp Joint Dis 35:85–102, 1974
59. Stone RG, Weeks LE, Hajdu M, et al: Evaluation of sciatic nerve compromise during total hip arthroplasty. Clin Orthop 201:26–31, 1985
60. Sugioka H: Evoked potentials in the investigation of traumatic lesions of the peripheral nerve and the brachial plexus. Clin Orthop 184:85–92, 1984
61. Sugioka H, Tsuyama N, Hara T, et al: Investigation of brachial plexus injuries by intraoperative cortical somatosensory evoked potentials. Arch Orthop Trauma Surg 99:143–151, 1982
62. Sugita K, Kobayashi S, Matsuga N, et al: Microsurgery for acoustic neurinoma—lateral position and preservation of facial and cochlear nerves. Neurol Med Chir (Tokyo) 19:637–641, 1979
63. Sunderland, S: Nerves and nerve injuries, 2nd ed. Edinburgh, Livingston, 1978

64. Takayasu M, Shibuya M, Suzuki Y, et al: Trigeminal sensory evoked potentials in patients with trigeminal neurinoma: Report of two cases. Neurosurgery 20:453–456, 1987
65. Tallis R, Staniforth P, Fisher TR: Neurophysiological studies of autogenous sural nerve grafts. J Neurol Neurosurg Psychiatry 41:677–683, 1978
66. Terzis JK: Sensory mapping. Clin Plastic Surg 3:59–64, 1976
67. Terzis JK, Dykes RW, Hakstian RW: Electrophysiological recordings in peripheral nerve surgery: A review. J Hand Surg 1:52–66, 1976
68. Terzis JK, Publicover NG: Clinical application of electrophysiologic recordings. *In* Terzis JK (ed): Microreconstruction of Nerve Injuries. Philadelphia, W.B. Saunders, 1987, p 203
69. Trojaborg W: Rate of recovery in motor and sensory fibres of the radial nerve: Clinical and electrophysiological aspects. J Neurol Neurosurg Psychiatry 33:625–638, 1970
70. Van Beek AL: Reply. Plast Reconstr Surg 75:765, 1985
71. Van Beek A, Hubble B, Kinkead L, et al: Clinical use of nerve stimulation and recording techniques. Plast Reconstr Surg 71:225–240, 1983
72. Walker DD, Kimura J: A fast-recovery electrode amplifier for electrophysiology. Electroencephalogr Clin Neurophysiol 45:789–792, 1978
73. Williams HB, Terzis JK: Single fascicular recordings: An intraoperative diagnostic tool for the management of peripheral nerve lesions. Plast Reconstr Surg 57:562–569, 1976

Electromyography Laboratory
University of Kentucky
Lexington, Kentucky 40536-0084

Cumulative Index 1988

Volume 6

February Endocrinology of Neuropsychiatric Disorders, pages 1–239

May Neurologic Complications of Transplants, pages 241–427

August Muscle Disease, pages 429–648

November Evoked Potentials, pages 649–951

Note: Page numbers of issue and article titles are in **boldface** type.

Abscess, of brain. See *Brain, abscess of.*

Acetazolamide, for treatment of hyperkalemic periodic paralysis, 491
  for treatment of hypokalemic periodic paralysis, 487–488
  for treatment of paramyotonia, 492–493

Acetylcholine receptor antibody, in graft-versus-host disease, 394–398

Acl-Coa dehydrogenase deficiencies, 567–568

Acromegaly-increased growth hormone, 583–584

ACTH, and dexamethasone suppression test, 24–25

Action potentials, versus synaptic potentials, in BAEP generation, 696

Adenovirus infection, of CNS, in bone marrow transplantation, 379

Adrenal insufficiency, clinical pattern of, 577–578
  metabolic impact of, 578
  muscle disorders associated with, 575–578

Adrenal tissue transplantation, to brain, 405–407, 410, 413–415

Adrenocortex. See *Hypothalamic-pituitary-adrenocortex axis.*

AEPs. See *Auditory evoked potentials (AEPs).*

Affective disorders, dexamethasone suppression test sensitivity in, 26–28
  in children and adolescents, **41–54**
    alternate techniques of measurement of, 48

biologic markers in, 44
dexamathasone suppression test in, 45–48
growth hormone in, 48–50
hypothalamic-pituitary-adrenocortex axis in, 44
melatonin in, 50–51
thyrotropin-releasing hormone effects in, 50
thyroid function in, **55–82**
  and tricyclic antidepressants, 66–67
  antidepressant effects on hypothalamic-pituitary–adrenocortex axis, 67–68
  antithyroid antibodies, 66
  thyrotropin-releasing hormone test, 57–66, 68–70
    and dexamethasone suppression test, 62–63
    and monoamine metabolites, 63–64
    and REM latence, 63
    blunting, 58–59
    in depression, 64
    multiple pituitary faults, 64
    prediction of treatment outcome, 62
    side effects and confounding variables, 58
    state-trait considerations, 59
    technique, 57–58
    test-retest reliability, 59
    thyrotropin blunting, 64–66
    variance sources, 59–62
Age, effects on SEPs, 844–849
Aging, brain tissue transplantation and, 408

Agoraphobia, 135–138
AIDS virus (human immunodeficiency virus)
    infection, of CNS, in transplantation,
    313
Alcoholic myopathy syndromes, 598
Alcoholism, thyroid function in, 70–71
    thyrotropin-releasing hormone in, 71–73
Allograft, infection transmitted with, 243
    rejection of, in cytomegalovirus infection,
        313
    survival of, antiepileptic drugs and, 289
Alzheimer's disease, **149–157**
    brain tissue transplantation and, 407
    cortisol in, 150–151
    growth hormone in, 152–154
    somatostatin in, 154–155
    thyrotropin in, 155
Amiodarone neuromyopathy, 605
Ammonia, in hepatic encephalopathy, 338–
    339
Amphiphilic drug myopathy, 601–606
    effects on lysosomes producing vacuolar
        myopathy, 603–605
    effects on surface membrane and associ-
        ated myofiber necrosis, 602–603
    general aspects of amphiphilic drug reac-
        tions on, 606
Amplifiers, differential, 650–651
    of evoked response system, 649–651
Analog-to-digital (A/D) converter, 651–652
Aneurysms, SEPs for monitoring following,
    892–893
Anorexia nervosa, **195–212**
    arginine vasopressin in, 203
    growth hormone in, 199–201
    hypothalamic-pituitary-adrenocortex axis
        in, 195–197
    hypothalamic-pituitary-ovarian axis in,
        195–197
    neurotransmitters in, 205
    thyroid function in, 201–203
Antibodies, antithyroid, 66
Anticoagulants, in stroke, in renal transplan-
    tation, 321–322
Antidepressants, and thyroid hormones, 66–
    67
    tricyclic, and hypothalamic-pituitary-adre-
        nal axis, 67–68, 229–230
Antiepileptic drugs, in transplantation, 291–
    292
    allograft survival and, 289
    of liver, 343
Antimicrotubule myopathy, 607–609
Antithymocyte globulin therapy, side effects
    of, 273
Anxiety disorders, **131–148**
    and primary endocrine diseases, 141–142
    endocrine changes in, 132–141
        generalized anxiety disorder, 139
        obsessive-compulsive disorder, 139–140

panic disorder with and without agora-
    phobia, 135–138
post-traumatic stress disorder, 140–141
simple phobia, 133–135
social phobia, 135
state of anxiety in, 131–132
Aorta, crossclamping of, in spinal surgery,
    SEPs for monitoring following, 888–889
Aphasia, in cyclosporine therapy, 267
Apomorphine, in affectively ill children and
    adolescents, 49–50
Aspergillus infection, of CNS, in transplan-
    tation, 251–252
    of bone marrow, 378
    of heart, 352–353
    of kidney, 311–312
Aspirin, in stroke prevention, in renal trans-
    plantation, 321–322
Ataxia, heredodegenerative, brain tissue
    transplantation and, 410
Attention deficit hyperactivity disorder,
    111–129
    etiology of, 112–115
    growth hormone studies in, 117–125
    neuroanatomic hypothesis in, 116–117
    regulatory neurotransmitters, 115–116
Audiometry, frequency-specific, 797–800
    types of, 791–792
Auditory brain-stem response (ABR), in
    evaluation of hearing, 792
Auditory brain-stem response (ABR) testing,
    for identification of hearing impairment
    in infants, 794–797
Auditory evoked potentials (AEPs), classifi-
    cation of, 792–793
    in assessment of hearing, **791–808**
Azathioprine, for treatment of inflammatory
    myopathies, 556
Azathioprine therapy, complications of, 273
    in liver transplantation, 341–342
    in renal transplantation, 317–318

Bacteremia, in transplantation, from *Liste-
    ria*, 248
    from *Strongyloides*, 254–255
BAEPs. See *Brain-stem auditory evoked po-
    tentials*.
Becker's muscular dystrophy, and Du-
    chenne's muscular dystrophy, genetics
    of, 439–445. See also *Duchenne's mus-
    cular dystrophy*.
    clinical features of, 436–438
    laboratory studies in, 438
    recent advances in, **436–453**
Benzodiazepines, 230–231
Biologic markers, and thyrotropin-releasing
    hormone test, 62–64

dexamethasone suppression test and, 31–35

in affectively ill children and adolescents, 44

Bipolar disorder, rapid cycling, 56–57

BK virus infection, of CNS, in transplantation, 256

Blood-brain barrier disruption, in brain tissue transplantation, 412

Body myositis, inclusion, 550

Body surface area, and thyrotropin blunting, 61

Bone marrow transplantation. See also *Graft-versus-host disease.*

complications of, **377–387**

cerebellar syndromes, 382–383

CNS infections, 377–380

encephalopathy, 380–381

graft-versus-host disease, 384

malignancies, 382

peripheral neuropathy, 383–384

seizures, 281–284, 292

spinal cord syndromes, 382–383

vascular, 380

Brachial plexopathy, in heart transplantation, 350–351

Brain, abscess of, in transplantation, 244–247, 249, 252

of heart, 351–357

of kidney, 312

adrenal tissue transplantation to, 405–407, 410, 413–415

ischemia of, in heart transplantation, 349–350

transplantation of tissue in, **405–420**

blood-brain barrier disruption in, 412

cell culture in, 416–417

fetal tissue in, 415–416

graft composition for, 411

graft growth limitations in, 411

immunologic considerations in, 412–413

in aging, 408

in Alzheimer's disease, 407

in genetic defects, 409–410

in heredodegenerative ataxia, 410

in hormonal disorders, 409

in Huntington's disease, 407–408

in pain modification, 410

in parkinsonism, 405–407, 413–415

in trauma, 408

site for, 411

suspensions versus fragments in, 412

trophic factors in, 410–411, 417

Brain tissue measures, in major depression, 8–10

serotonin, and suicide, 91

Brain-stem and cerebrum maturation, effects on SEPs, 843–844

Brain-stem auditory evoked potentials (BAEPs), abnormalities of, 780–787

in brain-stem ischemia, 786

in disorders of myelin, 784–785

in head trauma, 786

in posterior fossa tumors, 785

in toxic/metabolic encephalopathies, 785–786

anatomic and physiologic bases of, **681–704**

for diagnosis of multiple sclerosis, 867–871

future directions in, 699–700

generators of, 682–684, 696–698

anatomic sources of, 684–696

wave I, 684–686, 688

wave II, 687–690

wave III, 690–692

wave IIN, 690

wave IN, 686–687, 688

wave IV, 692–693

wave V, 693–694

wave VI, 694–695

wave VII, 695–696

at scalp, reflection of, 773–775

in evaluation of CNS, **771–789**

in infants, 786–787

intraoperative monitoring of, **899–915**

and prevention of postoperative complications, 908–910

interpretation of, 908

response of, alterations in, predictive value of, 904–908

analysis of, 901–903

mechanism of alteration in, 903–904

technique of, 900–901

recording techniques of, 682, 771–773

slow negativity in, 696

upper extremity, in posterior fossa surgery, 911–913

waveform identification and interpretation of, 776–780

bifid waves, 776–777

effects of click polarity on, 779–780

Mega-I waves, 776–779

wave V, 779

wave VI-on-V, 779

Brain-stem ischemia, in abnormalities of BAEPs, 786

Brain-stem/auditory function, intraoperative monitoring of, **899–915**

Bromide, in seizures, in transplantation, 292

Bulimia nervosa, 203–205

Busulfan therapy, complications of, 283, 290

Calcium metabolism, disorders of, in primary and secondary hyperparathyroidism and metabolic bone disease, 585–587

Candida infection, of CNS, in transplantation, 252–253
  of bone marrow, 378
  of heart, 356
Candidemia, in transplantation, 253
"Capillary lead" syndrome, in cyclosporine therapy, 288
Carbamazepine, 68
  in transplantation, 291–292
  allograft survival and, 289
Carbohydrate metabolism, premenstrual changes and, 179
Carcinoma, of CNS, in renal transplantation, 314
Carnitine deficiency, 566–567
Carnitine palmityl transferase deficiency, 565–566
Carotid endarterectomy, in renal transplantation, 322
  SEPs for monitoring following, 892–893
Carpal tunnel syndrome, from uremia, 316
Catecholamines, and suicidal behavior, 94–95
Cavernous sinus thrombosis, in renal transplantation, 312
Cell culture, in brain tissue transplantation, 416–417
Central auditory dysfunction, AEPs in diagnosis of, 803–804
Central conduction time (CCT), of motor tracts, 763–767
Central core disease, 501–503
Central motor pathways, assessment of function of, TCS for, 751–770
Central nervous system, disorders of, myalgia and, 630
  evaluation of, BAEPs in, 771–789
  SEPs in, 809–823
  infection of. See under *Infection*.
  intraoperative monitoring of, SEPs for, 881–898
  involvement in Duchenne's muscular dystrophy, 435
  primary lymphoma of, in transplantation, 297–303
Central pontine myelinolysis, in renal transplantation, 318
Centronuclear/myotubular myopathy, 509–512
Cerebellar dysfunction, in bone marrow transplantation, 382–383
  in cytarabine therapy, 272–273
Cerebral hemispheres, monitoring of, 892–893
Cerebral hemorrhage, in transplantation, of bone marrow, 380
  of heart, 350
  of kidney, 320
  of liver, 333–334
Cerebral ischemia, SEPs for monitoring of, 892

Cerebrospinal fluid, 5-hydroxyindoleacetic acid levels, and suicidal behavior, 88–90
  in major depression, 8–10
Cerebrovascular accident. See *Stroke*.
Cerebrovascular disorders, in heart transplantation, 349–350, 362
Children, SEPs in, **839–859**
Children and adolescents, affective disorders in, **41–54**
  alternate techniques of measurement, 48
  biologic markers, 44
  dexamethasone suppression test, 45–48
  growth hormone, 48–50
  hypothalamic-pituitary-adrenal axis, 44
  melatonin, 50–51
  thyrotropin-releasing hormone, 50
  attention deficit hyperactivity disorder in, **111–129**
Children's depression inventory, 48
Chloride conductance, abnormalities of, myotonia as cause of, 477–479
Chloroquine neuromyopathy, 604–605
Cholesterol levels, in cyclosporine therapy, in liver transplantation, 288–289
Clofibrate, as cause of necrotizing myopathy, 594–595
Clonidine, growth hormone response to, in attention deficit hyperactivity disorder, 117–125
  in schizophrenia, 105
  in affectively ill children and adolescents, 49–50
CNS. See *Central nervous system*.
Coccidioides infection, of CNS, in heart transplantation, 357–358
Colchicine myoneuropathy, 607–609
Coma, in liver transplantation, 330, 332, 338–340
  in transplantation, 246
  SEPs for assessment of, in infants and children, 851–852
Confusion, in CNS infection, in transplantation, 246
Congenital fiber-type disproportion myopathy, 512–513
Congenital muscular dystrophies, **519–528**
  classification of, 520
  clinical syndromes of, 521–526
  definition of, 519
  Fukuyama-type, 523–524
  historical perspective, 519–520
  hypotonic-sclerotic, 523
  mild, 521–522
  severe, 522–523
  with autosomal dominant inheritance, 526
  with cerebral involvement, 523–526
  with cerebro-ocular anomalies, 525–526
  with hypomyelination, 524–525
  without cerebral involvement, 521–523

Congenital myopathies, 499–518
Consciousness, altered, in CNS infection, in transplantation, 245
Corticosteroid therapy, complications of, in transplantation, 267–269
  of heart, 361
  of kidney, 307, 317
  of liver, 341
Corticosteroids, and suicide, 85–86
Corticotropin-releasing factor, in Alzheimer's disease, 150
  stimulation test, in major depression, 13–15
Cortisol, and premenstrual changes, 180–181
  and thyrotropin blunting, 60
  assay method, in dexamethasone suppression test, 23
  hypersecretion of, and suicide behavior, 87–88
  in affectively ill children and adolescents, 44
  in Alzheimer's disease, 150–151
  in schizophrenia, 106–107
  suppression index of, 47–48
Cranial nerve palsy, in renal transplantation, 318
  in transplantation, 246
Creatine kinase, determination of, role in genetics of Duchenne's muscular dystrophy and Becker's muscular dystrophy, 443
  elevations in, in Duchenne's muscular dystrophy, 435
Cryptococcus infection, of CNS, in transplantation, 250–251
  of heart, 357
  of kidney, 311–312
Cyclophosphamide therapy, seizures in, 290
Cyclosporin, for treatment of inflammatory myopathies, 556
Cyclosporine therapy, complications of, 261–267, 283–284
  in transplantation, of bone marrow, 382–383
  of heart, 286–287, 361
  of kidney, 285, 317–318
  of liver, 288–289, 340–341, 343
  of pancreas, 373
  seizures in, 286–290
  in heart transplantation, 286–287
  in liver transplantation, 288–289
Cytarabine therapy, complications of, 272–273
Cytomegaloviral infection, of CNS, in transplantation, 244, 255
  of bone marrow, 379
  of heart, 358–359
  of kidney, 312–313

Depression, dexamethasone suppression test in, 21–39
  factors influencing results of, 22–26
  test status of, 26–31
  hypothalamic-pituitary-adrenocorticol axis in, 1–19
  basal versus challenge paradigms, cerebrospinal fluid and brain tissue measures, 8–10
  plasma measures, 4–6
  saliva measures, 8
  urine measures, 6–8
  basal versus challenge paradigms in, 4–10
  challenge paradigms, 10–16
  ACTH stimulation testing, 10–11
  corticotropin-releasing hormone stimulation test, 13–15
  glucocorticoid receptors, 11–13
  metyrapone, 10
  physostigmine stimulation, 16
  RU486, 13
  vasopressin, 15–16
  physiology of, 1–4
  thyroid hormone levels, 55–56
  thyrotropin-releasing hormone effects of, 64, 69
Dermatomyositis, associated with connective tissue disorders, 549
  associated with malignancy, 548–549
  clinical features of, 546–547
  drug-induced, 549
  juvenile, clinical features of, 547–548
Descending inhibitory pathways, role of, in BAEP generation, 697
Desmethylimipramine, 49
Dexamethasone suppression test, and depression, 21–39
  biologic marker analysis of, 31–35
  factors influencing results of, 22–26
  ACTH levels, 24–25
  cortisol assay method, 23
  other glucocorticoids, 23–24
  plasma dexamethasone in psychiatric patients, 25–26
  test conditions and criteria, 22–23
  test status, 26–31
  clinical outcome and dexamethasone response, 30–31
  sensitivity in major depression, 26–28
  specificity for major depression, 28–29
  treatment response and suppressor status, 29–30
  and suicide, 86–87
  and thyrotropin-releasing hormone test, 62–63
  in affectively ill children and adolescents, 45–48
  in schizophrenia, 106–107

Dexamethasone therapy, complications of, 267–269
Diabetes insipidus, brain tissue transplantation and, 409
Dialysis disequilibrium syndrome, 317
Dialysis encephalopathy, 284, 317
20,25-Diazacholesterol, as cause of myotonic syndrome, 479–480
Digital filtering, for analyzing evoked potentials, 655
Dopamine, and thyrotropin blunting, 60–61
D-Penicillamine, role of, in polymyositis and dermatomyositis, 549
Duchenne's muscular dystrophy, and Becker's muscular dystrophy, genetics of, 439–445
  carrier detection and prenatal diagnosis of, 442
  creatine kinase determination in, 443
  DNA analysis in, 443–445
  manifesting carriers of, 439–440
  molecular investigations, 440–442
  pedigree analysis in, 442–443
  variations and outliers of, 438
cardiac involvement, 433–434
central nervous system involvement, 435
clinical features of, 430–433
creatine kinase elevations in, 435
electromyography in, 435
gastrointestinal involvement, 434–435
laboratory studies in, 435
muscle biopsy in, 436
nonskeletal muscle involvement, 433
recent advances in, **429–453**
treatment of, 445–447

Electrocochleogram/eighth-nerve potential, recording of, for intraoperative monitoring, 910–911
Electrode construction, 929–930
Electrolyte imbalance, in liver transplantation, 343–344
Electromyography, in Duchenne's muscular dystrophy, 435
  in evaluation of inflammatory myopathies, 551
Electroretinography, anatomic and physiologic bases of, **657–667**
  flash, 660–663
  pattern, 663–666
Encephalitis, in transplantation, 244–247
  of heart, 358–359
  of kidney, 312–313
Encephalomyopathy(ies), mitochondrial, **529–543**
Encephalopathy, dialysis, 284, 317
  in cyclosporine therapy, 264, 266
  in cytarabine therapy, 272–273

in transplantation, of bone marrow, 380–381, 398
  of heart, 349–350, 362
  of kidney, 285–286
  of liver, 330, 332, 338–340
  of pancreas, 369–371
  metabolic, in graft-versus-host disease, 398
    in heart transplantation, 362
    in pancreas transplantation, 371
  rejection, in renal transplantation, 285–286
  uremic, 316–317
Endarterectomy, carotid, SEPs for monitoring following, 892–893
Endocarditis, marantic, in bone marrow transplantation, 380
Endocrine disorders, associated with myalgia, 627
Endocrine myopathies, **575–592**
Endocrine ophthalmopathy, 581–582
Epilepsy, myoclonic, with ragged red fibers (MERRF), 532
Epsilon-aminocaproic acid, as cause of necrotizing myopathy, 595
Epstein-Barr virus, transplantation and, in CNS infection, 255
  primary CNS lymphoma and, 299–300
Equilibrium disturbances, from renal dialysis, 317
Etretinate, as cause of necrotizing myopathy, 595
Evoked potentials, analysis of, methods for, 655–656
  auditory, in assessment of hearing, **791–808**. See also *Auditory evoked potentials.*
  brain-stem auditory, anatomic and physiologic bases of, **681–704**. See also *Brain-stem auditory evoked potentials.*
    in evaluation of CNS, **771–789**. See also *Brain-stem auditory evoked potentials.*
  brain-stem auditory (BAEPs), **899–915**. See also *Brain-stem auditory evoked potentials.*
  definition of, 649
  for diagnosis of multiple sclerosis, **861–880**. See also *Multiple sclerosis, diagnosis of.*
  issue on, **649–933**
  somatosensory, for evaluation of peripheral nervous system, **825–838**. See also *Somatosensory evoked potentials.*
    in evaluation of CNS, **809–823**. See also *Somatosensory evoked potentials.*
  median nerve, anatomic and physiologic bases of, **705–733**. See also *Somatosensory evoked potentials, of median nerve.*

visual, anatomic and physiologic bases of, 667–679
Evoked response system, components of, 649–655
Extrapyramidal disorders, 159–172
in Huntington's disease, 161–165
in Parkinson's disease, 160–161
in tardive dyskinesia, 165–168
Eye, evaluation of, using VEPs and electroretinograms, 657–679. See also Visual system.

Fabry's disease, thromboembolic events and, in renal transplant patient, 308–309
Far-field SEPs, physioanatomic substrates of, 708–715
scalp-recorded, 708–710
and cervical-recorded short-latency potentials, 710–715
physioanatomic mechanism of, 722–725
Fatty acid oxidation, abnormalities of, evaluation of patients with, 569–571
treatment for patients with, 571
in skeletal muscle, 563–564
Femoral nerve compression, in renal transplantation, 316
Fetal tissue transplantation, 415–416
Fever, in CNS infection, in transplantation, 245–246
Fiber tract geometry, effects of, in BAEP generation, 696
Fibrinolysis, decreased, in renal transplantation, 308
Fingerprint body myopathy, 506–507
"Floppy infant" syndrome, 499–518
Fourier transformation, for analyzing evoked potentials, 655
Fungal infection, of CNS, in transplantation, 250–254, 352–353, 356–357, 378

Genetic disorders, brain tissue transplantation and, 409–410
Globulin, antithymocyte, side effects of, 273
Glucocorticoid excess, clinical pattern of, 575–576
laboratory results in, 576
Glucocorticoid therapy. See Corticosteroid therapy.
Glucocorticoids, cellular actions of, 576–577
in dexamethasone suppression test, 23–24
receptors in major depression, 11–13
Goldman-Hodgkin-Katz equation, 474
Gonadal hormones, premenstrual changes, 181–183
Gonadotropin-releasing hormone deficiency, brain tissue transplantation and, 409

Graft-versus-host disease, chronic, 389–390
complications of, 384, 389–403
CNS effects, 398
myasthenia gravis, 394–398
myositis, 390–394
peripheral neuropathy, 398
Granulomatosis, Wegener's, thromboembolic events and, in renal transplant patient, 308–309
Gray matter structures, as generators of SEPs, 736
Growth hormone, in affectively ill children and adolescents, 48–50
in Alzheimer's disease, 152–154
in anorexia nervosa, 199–201
in attention deficit hyperactivity disorder, 117–125
in Huntington's disease, 164–165
in Parkinson's disease, 161
in schizophrenia, 103–106
in tardive dyskinesia, 168
Guillain-Barré syndrome, in cytarabine therapy, 273
in renal transplantation, 313

Hallucinations, in cyclosporine therapy, 266
in pancreas transplantation, 373
Head, trauma to, in abnormalities of BAEPs, 786
Headache, in CNS infection, in transplantation, 245–247
Hearing, assessment of, AEPs in, 791–808. See also Auditory evoked potentials.
Hearing aid, amplification of, monitoring of, 804–805
Hearing impairment, in infants, identification of, ABR testing for, 794–797
AEPs for, 793–797
behavioral testing for, 794
frequency-specific audiometry for, 797–800
Hearing loss, cochlear, AEPs in diagnosis of, 801–802
conductive, AEPs in diagnosis of, 800–801
etiology of, differential diagnosis of, AEPs in, 800–804
management of, 804–805
nonorganic, AEPs in diagnosis of, 804
retrocochlear, AEPs in diagnosis of, 802–803
Heart transplantation, complications of, 349–365
cerebrovascular disorders, 362
immunosuppressive therapy and, 361
infection, 351–359
lymphoma, 359–361
metabolic encephalopathy, 362
perioperative, 349–351
psychosis, 361–362
seizures, 286–287

Height, effects on SEPs, 844–849
Hemiparesis, in CNS infection, in transplantation, 246
Hemorrhage, cerebral, in transplantation, of bone marrow, 380
of heart, 350
of kidney, 309
of liver, 333–334
Heparin, in stroke, in renal transplantation, 322
Hepatitis, post-transplant, 244
Herpesvirus infection. See also *Varicella-zoster virus infection.*
of CNS, in transplantation, 244, 255–256
of bone marrow, 379
of heart, 358–359
Hiccough, in corticosteroid therapy, 269
Homeostasis, premenstrual changes, 185–186
Hormonal disorders, brain tissue transplantation and, 409
Human immunodeficiency virus infection, of CNS, in renal transplantation, 313
Huntington's disease, 161–165
brain tissue transplantation and, 407–408
5Hydroxytryptophan, in affective ill children and adolescents, 49–50
Hypercoagulability, in renal transplantation, 307–308
Hyperglycemia, nonketotic, in liver transplantation, seizures in, 287–288
Hyperlipidemia, in renal transplantation, strokes and, 306–307
Hyperparathyroidism, primary, 585
secondary, and renal failure, 586
Hypertension, in renal transplantation, 309, 318
Hypokalemic myopathy, 597
Hypomagnesemia, in cyclosporine therapy, 266–267
seizures in, 288
Hypoparathyroidism, chronic myopathy in, 589
muscle disorders associated with, 587–589
Hypopituitarism, 584
Hypoplasia, type II, 513–514
Hypothalamic-pituitary-adrenocortical axis, and psychotropic medications, **225–234**
antidepressants, 229–230
benzodiazepines, 230–231
lithium, 226–227
neuroleptics/antipsychotics, 228–229
withdrawal effects, 231
in affectively ill children and adolescents, 44
in anorexia nervosa, 197–199
in major depression, **1–19**
basal versus challenge paradigms, 4–10
cerebrospinal fluid and brain tissue measures, 8–10

plasma measures, 4–6
saliva measures, 8
urine measures, 6–8
challenge paradigms, 10–16
ACTH stimulation test, 10–11
corticotropin-releasing hormone stimulation test, 13–15
glucocorticoid receptors, 11–13
metyrapone, 10
physostigmine stimulation, 16
RU486, 13
vasopressin, 15–16
physiology of, 1–4
in suicide, 85–88, 92–95
Hypothalamic-pituitary-ovarian axis, and suicidal behavior, 88
premenstrual changes, 179–180
Hypothyroidism, 582–583
Hypotonia, benign congenital, 514–515

Ibotenic acid, in Huntington's disease, 407–408
Immunology, brain tissue transplantation and, 412–413
Immunosuppressive therapy. See also specific drug.
complications of, **261–278**
from antithymocyte globulin, 274
from azathioprine, 274
from corticosteroids, 267–269
from cyclosporine, 261–267
from cytarabine, 273–274
from methotrexate, 269–271
from OKT3 monoclonal antibody, 271–273
in transplantation, of bone marrow, 382–383
of heart, 361
of kidney, 317–318
of pancreas, 373
infection risk and, 241–242
period of greatest vulnerability during, 244
lymphoma in, in transplantation, 298–300, 359–361
neoplasms and, in renal transplantation, 313–315
"steroid sparing", 242
Infants, (BAEPs) in, 786–787
SEPs in, **839–859**
with hearing impairment, identification of, 793–797
Infarction, cerebral, in liver transplantation, 287
Infection, CNS, in transplantation, **241–260**
acid fast bacteria in, 249–250
Aspergillus in, 251–252, 311–312, 352–353, 378
brain abscess. See *Brain, abscess of.*

Candida in, 252–253, 356, 378
causes of, 247–250
Cryptococcus in, 250–251, 311–312, 357
diagnosis of, 256–257
during early period (first month), 243
during intermediate period (months 2 to 6), 244
during late period (after 6 months), 244
fungal organisms in, 250–254, 352–353, 356–357, 378
herpesviruses in. See *Herpesvirus infection; Varicella–zoster virus infection.*
imaging techniques in, 352, 354, 356
immunosuppression in, 241–242
Listeria in, 247–248, 311–312, 357–358
meningoencephalitis, 351–357
Mucoraceae in, 253–254, 356
Nocardia in, 356
nosocomial, 243
of bone marrow, 377–380
of heart, 351–359
of kidney, 309–313, 320
of liver, 332, 337
of pancreas, absence of, 373
parasites in, 254–255, 353–356, 379
phycomycetes in, 356–357
signs and symptoms of, 244–247
Strongyloides in, 254–255
timetable of, 242–244
Toxoplasma in, 353–356
viral. See *Viral infection.*
Inflammatory myopathies, **545–561**
classification of, 546
clinical features of, 546–550
diagnosis of, 546
diagnostic studies of, 550–554
epidemiology of, 545
pathogenesis of, 554–555
treatment of, 556–557
Input system, of evoked response system, 649–651
Insulin, in affectively ill children and adolescents, 49
in Huntington's disease, 165
in Parkinson's disease, 161
Intracranial lesions, transplant patients with, management of, role of stereotactic biopsy in, **637–642**
Ion channels, membrane, in myotonia, 475–476
Ipecac myopathy, 598–599
Ischemia, brain-stem, in abnormalities of BAEPs, 786
cerebral, in heart transplantation, 349–350
in pancreas transplantation, 369–370
SEPs for monitoring of, 892

spinal cord, as complication of spinal surgery, in animal models, SEPs for monitoring following, 889–890
systemic, SEPs for monitoring of, 892

JC virus infection, of CNS, in transplantation, 256

Kainic acid, in Huntington's disease, 407–408
Kearns-Sayre syndrome, 530–531
Kidney, failure of, complications of, 316–317
seizures in, 284
transplantation of, antiepileptic drug effects on, 289
complications of, **305–325**
central pontine myelinolysis, 318
CNS infections, 245, 247
from immunosuppressive therapy, 317–318
from renal failure, 316–317
gradual onset dysfunction, 320–321
infection risk after, 243–244
infectious, 309–313
malignant hypertension, 318
neoplastic, 313–315
rapid onset dysfunction, 320
seizures, 284–286
stroke, 305–309
surgical, 315–316
transient dysfunction, 318–320
treatment of, 321–322

L-Dopa, growth hormone response to, in attention deficit hyperactivity disorder, 117–125
in affectively ill children and adolescents, 49–50
Leg aches, idiopathic, in children, 623–624
Lesions, compressive, SEPs for assessment of, 855
peripheral, SEPs for assessment of, 856
structural, SEPs for assessment of, 855
Leukemia, in bone marrow transplantation, 382
Leukoencephalopathy, in methotrexate therapy, 271
in transplantation, of bone marrow, 380–381
of kidney, 312
of liver, 288–289, 341–342
progressive multifocal, in transplantation, 256, 312, 341–342
Lipid metabolism, disorders of, myopathies caused by, **563–574**

Lipid storage myopathy, 569

Lipomatosis, epidural, in corticosteroid therapy, 269

Listeria infection, of CNS, in transplantation, 247–248
   of heart, 357–358
   of kidney, 311–312

Lithium, and hypothalamic-pituitary-adrenocortical axis, 67–68, 226–227

Liver transplantation, complications of, **327–348**
   coma, 330, 332, 338–340
   electrolyte abnormalities, 343–344
   encephalopathy, 330, 332, 338–340
   seizures, 287–289, 292, 330–331, 333, 342–343

Lovastin, as cause of necrotizing myopathy, 594

Lung-heart transplantation, seizures in, 286–287

Luteinizing hormone-releasing hormone, in schizophrenia, 106

Lymphoma, in transplantation, **297–303**
   of heart, 359–361
   of kidney, 314

Magnetic resonance imaging, and evoked potentials, for diagnosis of multiple sclerosis, 875

Malignancy, in bone marrow transplantation, 382
   in renal transplantation, 314, 320–321

Mania, thyrotropin-releasing hormone effects, 69

Marantic endocarditis, in bone marrow transplantation, 380

Maturation, in infants and children, effects on SEPs, 841–849

Mazindol, for treatment of Duchenne's muscular dystrophy, 447

Measles encephalitis, in renal transplantation, 312

Median nerve SEPs. See *Somatosensory evoked potentials, of median nerve.*

Mega-I waves, in generation of BAEPs, 776–779

Melanocyte-stimulating hormone, 180–181

MELAS, 531–532

Melatonin, and premenstrual changes, 180–181
   in affectively ill children and adolescents, 50–51
   in Parkinson's disease, 161

Meningismus, in CNS infection, in transplantation, 246

Meningitis, in transplantation, 244–247
   cryptococcal, 250–251
   from *Listeria*, 248

   in methotrexate therapy, 270
   in OKT3 monoclonal antibody therapy, 271–272
   of heart, 357–358
   of kidney, 312
   of pancreas, 371

Meningoencephalitis, in heart transplantation, 352–357

Mental disturbance, in corticosteroid therapy, 268–269

Metabolic abnormalities, in transplantation, of bone marrow, 380–381
   of heart, 362
   of kidney, 319–321
   of liver, 332
   of pancreas, 371

Metabolic encephalopathy, in graft-versus-host disease, 398

Metastasis, to CNS, in renal transplantation, 314

Methotrexate, for treatment of inflammatory myopathies, 556

Methotrexate therapy, complications of, 269–271, 380–381

Methylprednisolone therapy, complications of, 267–269, 283–284
   seizures in, 290–291

Metyrapone, in major depression, 10

Mineral and electrolyte disorders, associated with myalgia, 627

Mineralocorticoids, premenstrual changes, 178–179

Mitochondrial encephalomyopathies, **529–543**
   biochemical aspects, 534–537
   evaluation of patients with, 538–539
   genetics of, 538
   historical aspects, 533–534
   treatment of, 539–540
   with lactic acidosis and stroke-like episodes (MELAS), 531–532

Mitral valve prolapse, in patients with myotonic dystrophy, 459–460

Mixed nerve stimulation, in evaluation of radiolopathies, 831

MN-SEPs. See *Somatosensory evoked potentials, median nerve.*

Monitoring, intraoperative, BAEPs for, **899–915**
   peripheral nerve action potentials for, **917–933**

Monoamine metabolites, and thyrotropin-releasing hormone test, 63–64

Monoamine oxidase inhibitors, 68

Monoclonal antibody OKT3 therapy, complications of, in transplantation, 271–272
   of liver, 341
   of pancreas, 373

Motor cortex localization, SEPs for detection of, 893–894

Motor evoked potentials, for diagnosis of
multiple sclerosis, 874–875
Motor neuron disorders, myalgia and, 629–
630
Motor tracts, central conduction time of,
763–767
Motor-evoked potentials, anatomic and
physiologic bases of, **751–770**
methods of, 751–763
TCS for obtaining, 751–770
MRI. See *Magnetic resonance imaging.*
Mucoraceae infection, of CNS, in heart
transplantation, 356
in transplantation, 253–254
Multicore disease, 507
Multiple sclerosis, diagnosis of, BAEPs for,
867–871
combined evoked potential studies for,
873–874
evoked potentials for, **861–880**
motor evoked potentials for, 874–875
MRI and evoked potentials for, 875
PSVEPs for, 862–867
short-latency SEPs for, 871–873
evaluation of patients with, SEPs for,
812–815
Multisystem triglyceride storage disorder,
578–569
Muscle development, role of somatomedins
in, 584–585
Muscle disorders, asociated with pituitary
dysfunction, 583–585
associated with adrenal malfunction, 575–
578
associated with hypoparathyroidism and
pseudohypoparathyroidism, 587–589
associated with thyroid disease, 578–583
issue on, **429–642**
Muscle fatty acid metabolism, clinical abnormalities of, 565–569
Muscle(s), skeletal, normal fatty acid oxidation in, 563–564
use and overuse of, 622–623
Muscular dystrophy. See specific types, for
example, *Duchenne's muscular dystrophy, Becker's muscular dystrophy.*
Myalgia, **621–636**
classification of, 622
drugs and toxins associated with, 628
evaluation of, 630–632
inflammatory and immune disorders associated with, 624–625
metabolic defects associated with, 625–
628
muscle use and overuse as cause of, 622–
623
neurologic disorders associated with, 628–
630
pathophysiology of, 621–622
treatment of, 632–633

Myasthenia gravis, in graft-versus-host dis-
ease, 394–398
Mycobacterium tuberculosis, in CNS infec-
tion, in transplantation, 249–250
Myelin, disorders of, resulting in abnormalities of BAEPs, 784–785
Myelinolysis, central pontine, in renal transplantation, 318
Myelitis, transverse, in renal transplantation, 313
Myelopathy, in cytarabine therapy, 272
in renal transplantation, 320
transverse, in methotrexate therapy, 270
Myoglobinuria, toxic, 595–596
Myopathy, in corticosteroid therapy, 269
Myopathy syndromes, unproved, 612–613
Myopathy(ies). See also under specific
types, e.g., *Nemaline myopathy.*
caused by disorders of lipid metabolism,
563–574
congenital, **499–518**
drug-induced, risk factors in, 613–614
endocrine, **575–592**
inflammatory, **545–561**. See also *Inflammatory myopathies.*
lysis of myofibrils in type I fibers, 509
myalgia and, 628–639
toxic, **593–619**
with cardiomyopathy, 612
with disturbed maturation, 509–515
with neuropathy, 612
with peripheral crescent, 509
with tubular aggregates, 506
Myositis, in graft-versus-host disease, 390–
394
Myotonia, **473–484**
electrical excitability in muscle, 474–477
in myotonic dystrophy, 458
physiologic basis of, 477–481
treatment of, 481–482
types of, 473–474
Myotonic dystrophy, **455–472**
clinical features of, 455–463
muscular manifestations, 455–458
myotonia in, 458
nonmuscular manifestations, 458–463
congenital, 462–463
etiology and pathogenesis of, 463–466
incidence and epidemiology of, 463
laboratory studies in, 466–468
treatment of, 468–470
Myotonic syndromes, 473–474
with abnormal sodium channels, 480–481
with multiple membrane abnormalities,
479–480

Necrotizing myopathy, 593–595
focal, 600–601
focal fibrosing, 600–601

Nemaline myopathy, 503–506
Neoplasms, in bone marrow transplantation, 382
  in renal transplantation, 313–315, 320–321
Nerve injury(ies), SEPs for evaluation of, 826–827
Neural grafts. See Brain, transplantation in.
Neurodegenerative disorders, SEPs for assessment of, 852–855
Neuroleptic drugs, and hypothalamic-pituitary–adrenocortical axis, 228–229
  and prolactin, 213–223
Neurologic disorders, associated with myalgia, 628–630
Neuropathy, compressive, in pancreas transplantation, 371, 373
  in renal transplantation, 316
  in cyclosporine therapy, 266
  myalgia and, 629
  peripheral. See Peripheral neuropathy.
Neuropsychiatric disorders, and premenstrual changes, 173–194
  and schizophrenias, 103–109
  and suicide, 83–102
  in affectively ill children and adolescents, 41–54
  in Alzheimer's disease, 149–157
  in anorexia nervosa and bulimia nervosa, 195–212
  in attention deficit hyperactivity disorder, 111–129
  in depression, dexamethasone suppression test for, 21–39
    hypothalamic-pituitary-adrenocortical axis, 1–19
  in extrapyramidal system disorders, 159–172
  prolactin and, and neuroleptic drugs, 213–223
  psychotropic medications and hypothalamic-pituitary–adrenal regulation in, 225–234
  thyroid function in affective disorders and alcoholism, 55–82
Neurotransmitters, in anorexia nervosa, 2–5
Newborns, high-risk, SEPs for assessment of, 852
Nifedipine, for treatment of myotonia, 482
Nocardia infection, of CNS, in transplantation, 249
Nocturnal cramps, 623
Nosocomial infection, in organ transplantation, 243

Obsessive-compulsive disorder, 139–140
OKT3 (Orthoclone) monoclonal antibody therapy, complications of, in transplantation, 271–272

  of liver, 341
  of pancreas, 373
Opiates, endogenous, 176–177
Opportunistic infection, post-transplant, 244. See also specific organism.
Organophosphate(s), and "agonist-induced" myopathy, 599–600
Osteomalacia, 586

Pain modification, brain tissue transplantation and, 410
Pancreas transplantation, complications of, 367–376
Panic disorders, 135–138
Papovavirus infection, of CNS, in transplantation, 256, 312
Paramyotonia, 491–493
  treatment of, 492–493
Paramyotonia congenita, with abnormal sodium channels, 480
Parasite infections, of CNS, in transplantation, 254–255, 353–356, 379–380
Parkinsonism, adrenal tissue transplantation and, 405–407, 413–415
  in cytarabine therapy, 273
Parkinson's disease, 160–161
Patient compliance, prolactin levels and, 218
Pattern recognition, and signal extraction, for analyzing evoked potentials, 655–656
Pattern-shift visual evoked potentials (PSVEPs), for diagnosis of multiple sclerosis, 862–867
Periodic paralyses, 485–498
  classification of, 485–493
  evaluation of, 493–494
  hyperkalemic, 490–491
    treatment of, 491
  hypokalemic, 486–488
    treatment of, 487–488
  normokalemic, 491
  thyrotoxic, 488–489
    clinical presentation of, 580
    treatment of, 489, 580
Peripheral nerve action potentials, for intraoperative monitoring, 917–933
  clinical aspects of, 919–922
  recording of, technique of, 922–928
    environmental factors affecting, 927–928
    instrumentation, 924–926
    preparation, 923–924
    role of electrodes in, 926
    stimulation, 926–927
Peripheral nerve disease, evaluation of SEPs in, 826–828
  assessment of specific nerves, 826
Peripheral nerve injury, pathologic and physiologic bases of, 917–919

Peripheral nerve lesions, SEPs for assessment of, 856
Peripheral nerve maturation, effects on SEPs, 842
Peripheral nervous system, evaluation of, **825–838**
Peripheral neuropathies, SEPs for evaluation of, 827
Peripheral neuropathy, in cyclosporine therapy, 272
  in graft-versus-host disease, 398
  in transplantation, of bone marrow, 383–384
    of heart, 350–351
    of kidney, 321
    of pancreas, 371
Peroneal neuropathy, in heart transplantation, 351
Phencyclidine intoxication, 596–597
Phenobarbital, allograft survival and, 289
  in transplantation, 291–292
Phenytoin, allograft survival and, 289
  in transplantation, 291–292
Phobias, simple, 133–135
  social, 135
Photoreceptors, types and functions of, 658
Phrenic nerve injury, in heart transplantation, 351
Phycomycetes infection, of CNS, in heart transplantation, 356
Physostigmine stimulation, in major depression, 16
Pituitary. See *Hypothalamic-pituitary-adrenocortical axis.*
Pituitary dysfunction, muscle disorders associated with, 583–585
Pituitary gland, transplantation of, 409
Platelet seotonin levels, and suicidal behavior, 90–91
Plexopathy(ies), evaluation of, electrophysiology in, 834–836
Polyarteritis nodosa, thromboembolic events and, in renal transplant patient, 308–309
Polycystic kidney disease, cerebral hemorrhage with, in renal transplantation, 309
Polymyositis, associated with connective tissue disorders, 549
  associated with malignancy, 548–549
  clinical features of, 546–547
  drug-induced, 549
  juvenile, clinical features of, 547–548
  versus toxic myopathies, 611–612
  with acquired immunodeficiency syndrome, 549–550
Posterior fossa monitoring techniques, 910–913
Posterior fossa tumors, in abnormalities of BAEPs, 785

Potassium, for treatment of hypokalemic periodic paralysis, 487
  for treatment of thyrotoxic periodic paralysis, 489
Prednisolone, for treatment of inflammatory myopathies, 556
Prednisone, for treatment of Duchenne's muscular dystrophy, 447
  for treatment of inflammatory myopathies, 556
Prednisone therapy, allograft survival and, 289
  complications of, 267–269, 361
Premenstrual changes, **173–194**
  description and definition of, 173–175
  future studies of, 187
  homeostasis impairment in, 185–186
  multiple cyclic changes in, 183–185
  transitory-change hypotheses in, 175–183
    carbohydrate metabolism, 179
    gonadal hormones, 181–183
    hypothalamic-pituitary-thyroid axis, 179–180
    melanocyte-stimulating hormone, melatonin, testosterone, and cortisol, 180–181
    mineralocorticoids and vasopressin, 178–179
    opiates, endogenous, 176–177
    prolactin, 175–176
    prostaglandins, 177–178
Procainamide, as cause of necrotizing myopathy, 595
  for treatment of myotonia, 481
Progressive encephalopathies, SEPs for assessment of, in infants and children, 851–852
Progressive multifocal leukoencephalopathy, in transplantation, 256
  of kidney, 312
  of liver, 341–342
Progressive systemic sclerosis, thromboembolic events and, in renal transplant patient, 308–309
Prolactin, and neuroleptic drugs, **213–223**
  chronic effects of, 217–218
  clinical response to, 216–217
  in Parkinson's disease, 160–161
  in schizophrenia, apomorphine effect, 105
  in tardive dyskinesia, 168
  patient compliance, 218
  premenstrual changes, 175–176
  research studies of, 220–221
  side effects of, 219
  symptomatic relapse, and withdrawal, 219–220
  in Huntington's disease, 164
Propranolol, for treatment of thyrotoxic periodic paralysis, 489, 580

Prostaglandins, premenstrual changes, 177–178
Pseudallescheria boydii infection, of CNS, in heart transplantation, 357–358
Pseudohypoparathyroidism, muscle disorders associated with, 587–589
Pseudotumor cerebri, in corticosteroid therapy, 269
PSVEPs. See *Pattern-shift visual evoked potentials.*
Psychiatric disorders, in corticosteroid disorders, 268–269
Psychiatric patients, dexamethasone plasma levels in, 25–26
Psychosis, in heart transplantation, 350, 361–362
Psychotropic medications, and hypothalamic-pituitary–adrenal regulation, **225–234**
    antidepressants, 229–230
    benzodiazepines, 230–231
    lithium, 226–227
    neuroleptics/antipsychotics, 228–229
    withdrawal effects of, 231
PTH, systemic actions of, 586–587
PTN-SEPs. See *Somatosensory evoked potentials, posterior tibial nerve.*
Purkinje cells, transplantation of, 410

Quinine, for treatment of myotonia, 481
Quinolinic acid, in Huntington's disease, 407–408

Radiculopathy, in renal transplantation, 320
Radioculopathy(ies), evaluation of, electrophysiology in, 828–834
Receiver operating characteristic (ROC), 31–35
Receptors, serotonin, and suicide, 91–92
Recurrent laryngeal nerve injury, in heart transplantation, 351
Reducing body myopathy, 508
Rejection encephalopathy, in renal transplantation, 285–286
REM latency, and thyrotropin-releasing hormone test, 63
Respiratory insufficiency, in patients with myotonic dystrophy, 460–461
Resting cramps, 623
Retina, anatomy and physiology of, 657–660
Rhinocerebral mucormycosis, in transplantation, 253–254
Rhizopus infection, of CNS, in heart transplantation, 356
Risk factors, in suicidal behavior, 83–84
RU486, 13
Ruvalcaba-Myhre-Smith syndrome, 569

Schizophrenia, **103–109**
    dexamethasone suppression test and, 106–107
    growth hormone response to, 103–105
Sclerosis, multiple. See *Multiple sclerosis.*
    progressive systemic, thromboembolic events and, in renal transplant patient, 308–309
Scoliosis, as complication of spinal surgery, SEPs for monitoring following, 887
Segmental cutaneous nerve stimulation, in evaluation of radiolopathies, 831–834
Seizures, in transplantation, 245–246, **279–296**
    antiepileptic drug therapy versus allograft survival in, 289
    diagnosis of, 279–281
    etiology of, 279–280
    in cyclosporine therapy, 262–264, 290, 340
    in immunosuppressive therapy, 290
    of bone marrow, 281–284
    of heart and heart-lung, 286–287
    of kidney, 284–286, 319
    of liver, 287–289, 330–331, 333, 340, 342–343
    of pancreas, 370
    therapy for, 291–292
SEPs. See *Somatosensory evoked potentials.*
Septal cells, transplantation of, 409
Serotonin, and suicidal behavior, 88–94
    5-hydroxyindoleacetic acid in cerebrospinal fluid, 88–90
Shiverer mouse, brain tissue transplantation and, 409–410
Signal analysis, methods for, 655–656
    principles of, **649–656**
Signal averaging, principles of, **652–656**
Skin lesions, cryptococcal, in transplantation, 250–251
Sleep, and growth hormone, 49
    in infants and children, effects on SEPs, 850–851
Slow negativity, as source of BAEPs, 696
Sodium abnormalities, in liver transplantation, 344
Somatomedins, role of, in muscle development, 584–585
Somatosensory evoked potentials (SEPs), far-field, physiological substrates of, 708–715. See also *Far–field SEPs.*
    for detection of motor cortex localization, 893–894
    for evaluation of peripheral nervous system, **825–838**
    for evaluation of plexopathies, 834–836
    for evaluation of radioculopathies, 828–834
    for intraoperative monitoring of cerebral and spinal cord function, **881–898**

for monitoring of cerebral hemispheres, 892–893

in evaluation of CNS, **809–823**
  as a guide to prognosis, 817–818
  clinical applications, 812–821
    for detection of lesions in central so-matosensory pathways, 812–817
    in defining extent of neuropathological involvement, 820
    in determining whether sensory symp-toms have organic basis, 820–821
    to prevent or minimize neurological problems, 819–821
  in peripheral nerve disease, 826–828. See also *Peripheral nerve disease, evalua-tion of SEPs in.*

median nerve, multiple wavelets over ris-ing and descending phases of negative peak in, 725–729

median nerve (MN-SEP), in infants and children, **839–859**
  clinical applications of, 851–856
  effects of maturation on, 841–849
  effects of sleep on, 850–851
  generators of, 840
  methodologies in, 839–841

of median nerve, anatomic and physio-logic bases of, **705–733**
  late peaks in, 719–722
  recording of, four-channel short-latency, 715
  recording technique of, 705–707
  technical problems with recording of, 707–708

posterior tibial nerve, anatomic and physi-ologic bases of, **735–749**
  generators of, 735–747
    cortical components, 741–747
    spinal components, 736–740
    subcortical scalp-recorded compo-nents, 740–741
  in infants and children, **839–859**
    generators of, 840
  of white matter, 735–736

scalp-recorded, early, topographic charac-teristics of, 715–719
  physioanatomical substrates of, 715–722

short-latency, for diagnosis of multiple sclerosis, 871–873

Somatostatin, and thyrotropin blunting, 61
  in Alzheimer's disease, 154–155

Spinal cord, infarction/ischemia of, in pan-creas transplantation, 370
  in renal transplantation, 315–316

Spinal cord ischemia, as complication of spinal surgery, in animal models, SEPs for monitoring following, 889–890

Spinal cord maturation, effects on SEPs, 842–843

Spinal cord syndromes, in bone marrow transplantation, 382–383

Spinal surgery, SEPs for monitoring follow-ing, 882–891
  changes in, 890–891
  in animal models, 889–890
  in clinical settings, 887–889
  patient-related factors, 886–887
  recording techniques, 882–886

Spironolactone, for treatment of hypoka-lemic periodic paralysis, 488
  for treatment of thyrotoxic periodic paral-ysis, 489

Stationary field potentials, physioanatomic mechanism of, 722–725

Status epilepticus, nonconvulsive, in renal transplantation, 319

Stereotactic biopsy, accuracy and complica-tions of, 640
  role of, in management of transplant pa-tients with intracranial lesions, **637–642**

Steroid myopathy, treatment of, 577

Stress disorder, post-traumatic, 140–141

Stroke, in transplantation, of bone marrow, 380
  of kidney, 305–309, 320–322
  of pancreas, 370

Stroke-like syndrome, in methotrexate ther-apy, 270–271

Strongyloides infection, of CNS, in trans-plantation, 254–255

Suicide, **83–102**
  and catecholamines, 94–95
  and dexamethasone suppression test, 47
  and growth hormone in affectively ill chil-dren and adolescents, 50
  biologic risk markers of, 83–84
  future research of, 95–96
  hypothalamic-pituitary-adrenal axis in, 85–88
  hypothalamic-pituitary-thyroid axis, 88
  serotonin studies of, 88–94
    and hypothalamic-pituitary-adrenal functioning, 92–95
    5-hydroxyindoleaacetic acid in cerebro-spinal fluid, 88–90
    in brain, 91
    in platelets, 90–91
    limitations of, 92
    postmortem studies of, 91
    receptor binding in, 91–92
  testosterone and, 88

Synaptic potentials, versus action potentials, in BAEP generation, 696

Systemic ischemia, SEPs for monitoring of, 892

Systemic lupus erythematosus, thromboem-bolic events and, in renal transplant pa-tient, 308

Tardive dyskinesia, 165–168
TCS. See *Transcranial stimulation.*
Testosterone, and suicidal behavior, 88
  premenstrual changes, 180–181
Tetany, 587–589
Thiazides, for treatment of hyperkalemic periodic paralysis, 491
Thrombocytopenia, in bone marrow transplantation, 283
Thromboembolic events, in renal transplantation, 305–309
Thyroid disease, muscle disorders associated with, 578–583
Thyroid function, in affective disorders, **55–82**
  and tricyclic antidepressants, 66–67
  antidepressant drugs and hypothalamic-pituitary-adrenal axis, 67–68
  antithyroid antibodies, 66
  serum thyroid hormone levels, 55–57
  thyrotropin-releasing hormone effects, 68–70
  thyrotropin-releasing hormone test, 57–66
  in alcoholism, 70–71
  in anorexia nervosa, 70–71
Thyroid-stimulating hormone, in affectively ill children and adolescents, 50
  in Parkinson's disease, 161
Thyrotoxic myopathy, 578–580
Thyrotoxicosis, metabolic changes caused by, 579
  physiologic changes associated with, 579
Thyrotropin, blunting, 64–66
  in Alzheimer's disease, 155
Thyrotropin-releasing hormone. See also *Thyroid function.*
  in alcoholism, 71–73
  in schizophrenia, 105–106
Tocainamide, for treatment of paramyotonia, 492
Toxic myopathies, **593–619**
  differential diagnosis of, 609–614
  recognition of, 609–612
  versus polymyositis, 611–612
Toxic/metabolic encephalopathies, in abnormalities of BAEPs, 785–786
Toxoplasma infection, of CNS, in transplantation, 254
  of bone marrow, 379–380
  of heart, 353–356
Traimterene, for treatment of hypokalemic periodic paralysis, 488
Transcranial stimulation (TCS), magnetic, method of, 752–756
  of brain, methods of, 751
Transient ischemic attack, in renal transplantation, 318–319
Transplant patients with intracranial lesions,

management of, role of steretactic biopsy in, **637–642**
Transplantation, antiepileptic drug use in, **279–296**
  bone marrow, complications of, **377–387**
    seizures in, 281–284, 292
  brain tissue, **405–420**
  cardiac, complications of, **349–365**
    seizures in, 286–287
  CNS infection in. See *Infection, CNS.*
  graft-versus-host disease in, complications of, **389–403**
  immunosuppressive agents in. See *Immunosuppressive therapy.*
  liver, complications of, **327–348**
    seizures in, 287–289, 292
  lung-heart, seizures in, 286–287
  lymphoma in, **297–303**, 314, 359–361
  pancreas, complications of, **367–376**
  pituitary gland, 409
  renal, antiepileptic drug effects on, 289
    CNS infections in, 245, 247
    complications of, **305–325**
    infection risk after, 243–244
    seizures in, 284–286
  seizures and, **279–296**
Transverse myelitis, in renal transplantation, 313
Transverse myelopathy, in methotrexate therapy, 270
Trauma, brain tissue transplantation and, 408
  to head, in abnormalities of BAEPs, 786
Tremor, in cyclosporine therapy, 262–263, 266, 340
Triamcinalone therapy, complications of, 269
Trilaminar myopathy, 507–508
Tuberculosis, of CNS, in transplantation, 249–250
Tumors, in central somatosensory pathways, direction of, using SEPs, 812–817
  of spine, as complication of spinal surgery, SEPs for monitoring following, 887–888
  posterior fossa, in abnormalities of BAEPs, 785

Uremia, complications of, in renal transplantation, 307–308, 316–317

Valproic acid, allograft survival and, 289
  in transplantation, 291–292
Varicella-zoster virus infection, of CNS, in transplantation, 255–256
  of bone marrow, 379
  of heart, 359
  of kidney, 312

of peripheral nerves, in pancreas transplantation, 371
Vasopressin, and premenstrual changes, 178–179
in anorexia nervosa, 203
in major depression, 15–16
VEPs. See *Evoked potentials, visual.*
Verapamil, for treatment of myalgia, 632
Viral infection, immunosuppressive effects of, 242
of CNS, in transplantation, 244, 255–256
of bone marrow, 379
of heart, 358–359
of kidney, 312–313
Visual system, central, anatomy and physiology of, 667–669
function of, VEPs and electroretinograms for studying, **657–670**
Vitamin D metabolism, disorders of, in primary and secondary hyperparathyroidism and metabolic bone disease, 585–587

Warfarin, in stroke, in renal transplantation, 322

Wave I, as source of BAEPs, 684–686, 688
Wave II, as source of BAEPs, 687–690
Wave III, as source of BAEPs, 690–692
Wave IIN, as source of BAEPs, 690
Wave IN, as source of BAEPs, 686–687, 688
Wave IV, as source of BAEPs, 692–693
Wave V, as source of BAEPs, 693–694
in generation of BAEPs, 779
intraoperative monitoring of, 901–903
Wave VI, as source of BAEPs, 694–695
Wave VII, as source of BAEPs, 695–696
Wave VI-on-V, in generation of BAEPs, 779
Wave(s), bifid, in generation of BAEPs, 776–777
Weakness, in corticosteroid therapy, 269
Wegener's granulomatosis, thromboembolic events and, in renal transplant patient, 308–309
White matter fiber tracts, as generators of SEPs, 735–736

Zebra body myopathy, 508
Zidovudine, as cause of necrotizing myopathy, 595

U.S. Postal Service

STATEMENT OF OWNERSHIP, MANAGEMENT AND CIRCULATION
Required by 39 U.S.C. 3685

1A. TITLE OF PUBLICATION	1B. PUBLICATION NO.	2. DATE OF FILING
NEUROLOGIC CLINICS OF NORTH AMERICA	0 7 3 3 8 6 1 9	7-31-88

3. FREQUENCY OF ISSUE	3A. NO. OF ISSUES PUBLISHED ANNUALLY	3B. ANNUAL SUBSCRIPTION PRICE
FOUR ISSUES PER YEAR (FEB, MAY, AUG, NOV.)	FOUR	66.00

4. COMPLETE MAILING ADDRESS OF KNOWN OFFICE OF PUBLICATION *(Street, City, County, State and ZIP+4 Code) (Not printers)*

CURTIS CENTER INDEPENDENCE SQUARE WEST, PHILA. PA. 19106-3399

5. COMPLETE MAILING ADDRESS OF THE HEADQUARTERS OF GENERAL BUSINESS OFFICES OF THE PUBLISHER *(Not printer)*

CURTIS CENTER INDEPENDENCE SQUARE WEST, PHILA. PA. 19106-3399

6. FULL NAMES AND COMPLETE MAILING ADDRESS OF PUBLISHER, EDITOR, AND MANAGING EDITOR *(This item MUST NOT be blank)*

PUBLISHER *(Name and Complete Mailing Address)*

JOAN BLUMBERG,
W.B. SAUNDERS COMPANY, CURTIS CENTER INDEPENDENCE SQUARE WEST, PHILA. PA 19106-3399

EDITOR *(Name and Complete Mailing Address)*

BRENDA FRANK,
W.B. SAUNDERS COMPANY, CURTIS CENTER INDEPENDENCE SQUARE WEST, PHILA. PA. 19106-3399

MANAGING EDITOR *(Name and Complete Mailing Address)*

BARBARA COHEN-KLIGERMAN,
W.B. SAUNDERS COMPANY, CURTIS CENTER INDEPENDENCE SQUARE WEST, PHILA. PA. 19106-3399

7. OWNER *(If owned by a corporation, its name and address must be stated and also immediately thereunder the names and addresses of stockholders owning or holding 1 percent or more of total amount of stock. If not owned by a corporation, the names and addresses of the individual owners must be given. If owned by a partnership or other unincorporated firm, its name and address, as well as that of each individual must be given. If the publication is published by a nonprofit organization, its name and address must be stated.) (Item must be completed.)*

FULL NAME	COMPLETE MAILING ADDRESS
W.B. SAUNDERS INC. STOCK IS	
100% OWNED BY HARCOURT BRACE	
JOVANOVICH, INC.	

8. KNOWN BONDHOLDERS, MORTGAGEES, AND OTHER SECURITY HOLDERS OWNING OR HOLDING 1 PERCENT OR MORE OF TOTAL AMOUNT OF BONDS, MORTGAGES OR OTHER SECURITIES *(If there are none, so state)*

FULL NAME	COMPLETE MAILING ADDRESS
NONE	

9. FOR COMPLETION BY NONPROFIT ORGANIZATIONS AUTHORIZED TO MAIL AT SPECIAL RATES *(Section 423.12 DMM only)*
The purpose, function, and nonprofit status of this organization and the exempt status for Federal income tax purposes *(Check one)*

(1) ☐ HAS NOT CHANGED DURING PRECEDING 12 MONTHS	(2) ☐ HAS CHANGED DURING PRECEDING 12 MONTHS	*(If changed, publisher must submit explanation of change with this statement.)*

10. EXTENT AND NATURE OF CIRCULATION *(See instructions on reverse side)*	AVERAGE NO. COPIES EACH ISSUE DURING PRECEDING 12 MONTHS	ACTUAL NO. COPIES OF SINGLE ISSUE PUBLISHED NEAREST TO FILING DATE
A. TOTAL NO. COPIES *(Net Press Run)*	6,875	7,000
B. PAID AND/OR REQUESTED CIRCULATION 1. Sales through dealers and carriers, street vendors and counter sales		
2. Mail Subscription *(Paid and/or requested)*	3,795	3,809
C. TOTAL PAID AND/OR REQUESTED CIRCULATION *(Sum of 10B1 and 10B2)*	3,795	3,809
D. FREE DISTRIBUTION BY MAIL, CARRIER OR OTHER MEANS SAMPLES, COMPLIMENTARY, AND OTHER FREE COPIES	76	76
E. TOTAL DISTRIBUTION *(Sum of C and D)*	3,871	3,885
F. COPIES NOT DISTRIBUTED 1. Office use, left over, unaccounted, spoiled after printing	3,004	3,115
2. Return from News Agents		
G. TOTAL *(Sum of E, F1 and 2—should equal net press run shown in A)*	6,875	7,000

11. I certify that the statements made by me above are correct and complete

SIGNATURE AND TITLE OF EDITOR, PUBLISHER, BUSINESS MANAGER, OR OWNER

Lisa Kennedy, Business Manager

PS Form **3526**, Dec. 1985 *(See instruction on reverse)*

Changing Your Address?

Make sure your subscription changes too! When you notify us of your new address, you can help make our job easier by including an exact copy of your Clinics label number with your old address (see illustration below.) This number identifies you to our computer system and will speed the processing of your address change. Please be sure this label number accompanies your old address and your corrected address—you can send an old Clinics label with your number on it or just copy it exactly and send it to the address listed below.

We appreciate your help in our attempt to give you continuous coverage. Thank you.

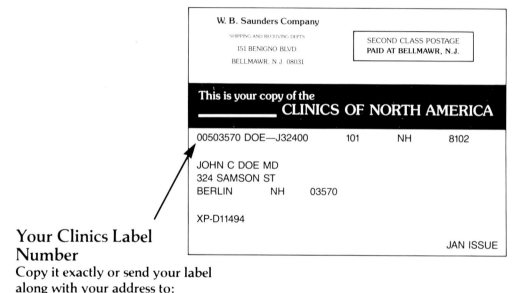

W. B. Saunders Company

SHIPPING AND RECEIVING DEPTS

151 BENIGNO BLVD

BELLMAWR, N.J. 08031

SECOND CLASS POSTAGE
PAID AT BELLMAWR, N.J.

This is your copy of the
_____ CLINICS OF NORTH AMERICA

00503570 DOE—J32400   101   NH   8102

JOHN C DOE MD
324 SAMSON ST
BERLIN   NH   03570

XP-D11494

JAN ISSUE

Your Clinics Label Number
Copy it exactly or send your label
along with your address to:
W. B. Saunders Company, Fulfillment Services
The Curtis Center
Independence Square West, Philadelphia, PA 19106-3399.

Please allow four to six weeks for delivery of new subscriptions and for processing address changes.